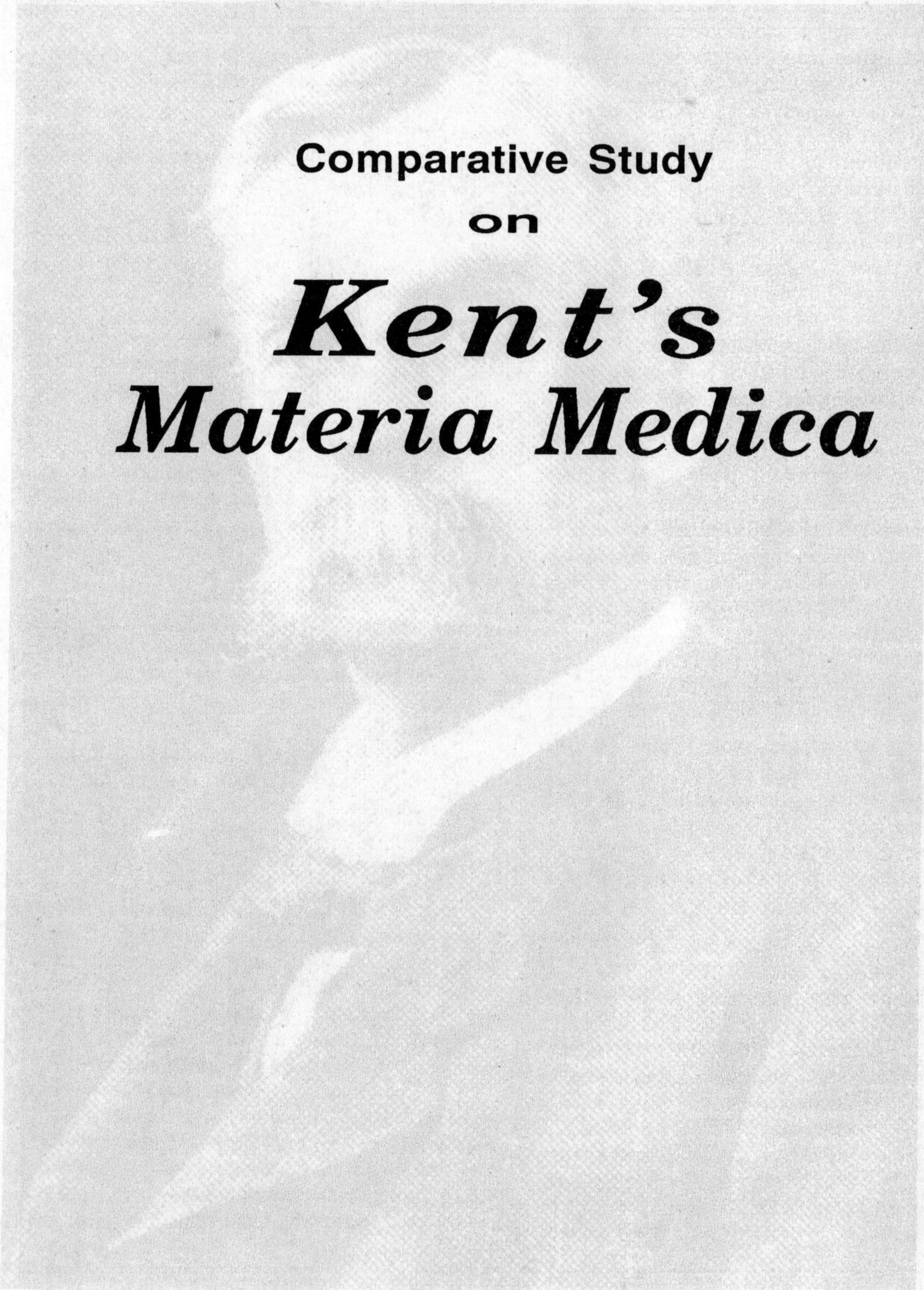

Comparative Study on

Kent's Materia Medica

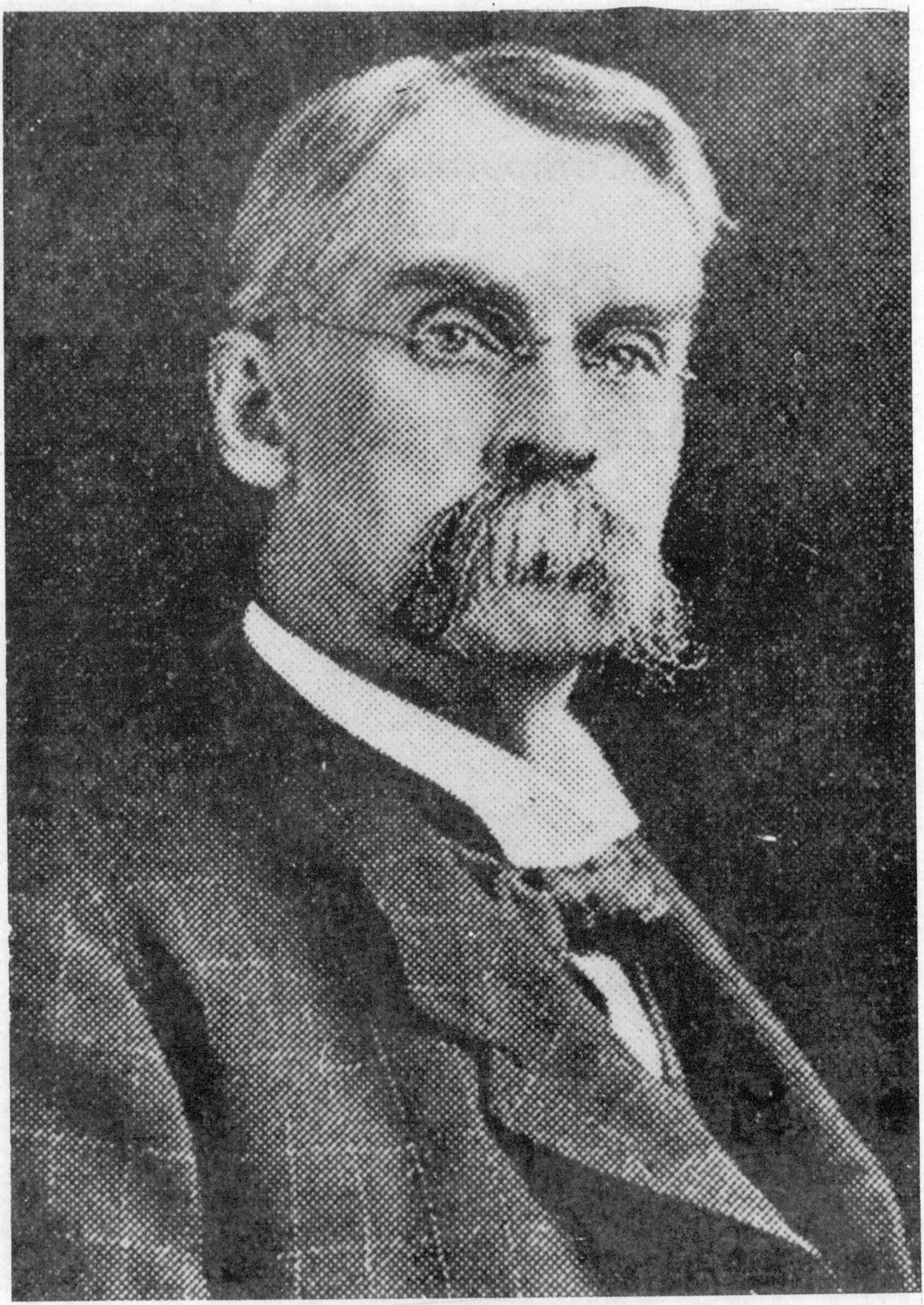

Comparative Study

on

Kent's Materia Medica

A. Gaskin (U.K.)

B. JAIN PUBLISHERS PVT. LTD.

First edition 1994
Reprint Edition 1995

Published by
B. Jain Publishers (P) Ltd.
1921, St. No. 10th, Chuna Mandi
Paharganj, New Delhi - 110 055 INDIA

Printed in India by :
J.J. Offset Printers

Price : **Rs. 100.00**

ISBN-81-7021-732-6

BOOK CODE : *B-3957*

Compiler's Note

I would like to thank some people, without whom none of this would have happened;

David Mundy, who drew my attention to the greatness of Kent's work,

Lorraine Walton, who inspired me to actually do the task of compilation,

Chris Date, who was the software wizard who made it feasible,

Alison Hargreaves, without whom it would never have seen the light of day.

And finally my mum and dad.

Work hard, play hard, read Kent!

INDEX / CONTENTS

ABIES NIGRA

NUX VOM - Sensation of a lump in the stomach (BRY). In chronic cases SEP is more apt to be indicated, and follows NUX well, but quarrels with BRY; associate this with the pressure on the vertex and you have the typical NUX condition. Sensation comes on an hour after eating, showing that there has been an attempt at digestion, but in ABIES NIGRA it comes at once.......... *808*

ABROTANUM

IOD - He is relieved while eating and he is relieved while in motion. In spite of the hunger and much eating HE STILL EMACIATES. "Living well and yet growing thin" was one of Hering's keynotes of IODINE. As in NAT MUR and ABROT he emaciates while he has at the same time an enormous appetite. The nutrition is so disturbed that there is no making of flesh, and hence the emaciation. *601*

CIMIC - Mental states following the disappearance of rheumatism is a strong feature. The rheumatism gets better but the mental state gets worse. Sometimes the rheumatism disappears in short order and the mind is not disturbed, but then it is because a diarrhoea has come on, with great soreness and aching in the bowels, or because a flow from the uterus has given relief. There must be some relief or a disturbance will take place, like ABROT. *32*

KALMIA - "Wandering rheumatic pains in the region of the heart". "When articular rheumatism has been treated externally and cardiac symptoms ensue". Rheumatism that goes from the lower to the upper limbs. Not uncommonly you will meet such things. These "rubbers" that go around the streets with a strong liniment and considerable magnetism frequently cause a rheumatism to leave the knee joint and, when it does that, the heart is likely to be the organ that suffers. Then KALMIA, AURUM, BRYONIA, RHUS-TOX, LEDUM, CALC, ABROTANUM and sometimes CACTUS are remedies that prove suitable for such cardiac affections. *670*

In acute endocarditis the principal remedies are SPONG, ABROT, SEP and KALM. NAJA in valvular diseases................. *941*

ACETIC ACID

RUMEX is one of the most valuable palliatives in advanced phthisis; it will often carry a case through another winter. With RUMEX, PULSATILLA, SENEGA, ARS and NUX VOM you can patch up the last years of a phthisical patient. You will see ACETIC ACID recommended for the diarrhoea in phthisis. You had better let such conditions alone, unless they are very marked. If the diarrhoea is very exhausting use some simple medicine like this one (RUMEX) to slack it up. But the phthisical patient is better off with a little diarrhoea, a loose morning stool. It is the same with the night sweats; if he does not have them he will have something more violent. The allopath stops the diarrhoea and night sweats and then has to feed morphine to his patient because of the consequent sufferings. The more you undertake to relieve the outward conditions, these vents, the more harm you will do the patient, and if you go on you will have to abandon your homoeopathy and give morphine, which is really a crime. *888*

ACONITE

Get the pace, the periodicity of remedies. Some remedies have a continued fever, some a remittent, others an intermittent fever. In ACON, BELL and BRY we have 3 different paces, 3 different motions, 3 different forms of velocity; so in SULPH, GRAPH, NAT-M, CARBO-V - a different form, a different development. Some would not hesitate in a continued fever to give BELL but its complaints come on in great haste, with great violence and have nothing in their nature like a continued fever. This is not like typhoid. BELL and ACON have no manifestations of typhoid, even if the symptoms are present. Be sure that the remedy has not only the group of symptoms, but also the nature of the case. The typhoid case has a likeness in BRY or RHUS, but not in BELL. We owe no obedience to man, not even to our parents, after we are old enough to think for ourselves. We owe obedience to truth. *769*

Complaints of ACONITE and PULSATILLA come on from getting the feet wet, and these complaints rise upwards, come on through the feet and go upwards and affect the head. BELL complaints come on from exposure of the head and go downwards; sometimes affect the head, sometimes the chest, sometimes the stomach, sometimes centre in the abdomen, sometimes centre in the uterus and ovaries. RHUS has complaints from getting wet, but the complaints are in the parts that are wet. If he gets the legs wet he will have rheumatism in the legs. There is a vast distinction, and this distinction has to be made in almost every prescription you will make. Homoeopathy is a matter of individualisation as to how complaints spread. *241*

If you will observe the weather conditions in sharp climates, such as Minnesota, Massachusetts, or Canada, you will find that the cold spells are very intense and that people, when exposed, come down with complaints very rapidly and violently. That is the way the BELL and ACON cases come on, but GELS complaints do not come from such causes nor appear that way. Its complaints are more insidious and come on with a degree of slowness. A GELS develops its symptoms several days after the exposure, while the ACON cold comes on a few hours after exposure. The ACON child exposed during the day in dry cold weather will have croup before midnight. But in the South diseases are very slow. Like the people themselves, their organs are very slow, and their reaction is slow. Their colds are not taken from the violent cold, but from getting overheated. Hence they take colds, fevers of a low, malarial type; they have congestive headaches and congestive complaints that do not come on suddenly. When we think of the climate and consider the people, and the pace of remedies we see that GELS is a remedy for warm climate, while ACON is a remedy for cold climates. Certain acute complaints in the North will be like ACON while similar complaints will have symptoms in the warmer climate like GELS. The colds and fevers of the mild winters will be more likely to run to GELS, whereas the colds and fevers of a violent winter will be more likely to run to BELL and ACON. It is true that ACON has complaints in hot weather, fevers and dysentery of hot weather, but they are different from the complaints of winter. *543*

ARG-NIT - There is fear of death, the overanxious state, that death is near, and often at times like ACON he predicts the moment he is going to die. *136*

HELL - The woman gets a fixed idea that she is going to die on a certain day - and nothing can get it out of her head. This is not like ACONITE because there is no fear of death. ACONITE has fear of death and fixes the time of death. *567*

CIC - Full of fear; fright will bring on convulsions, like OP, IGN and ACON. *434*

ALL-C - "Hoarse, harsh, ringing, spasmodic cough, excited by a constant tickling in the larynx; cough produces a raw splitting pain in the larynx, so acute and so severe as to compel the patient to crouch from suffering, and to make every effort to suppress the cough". "Severe laryngeal cough which compels the patient to grasp the larynx; feels as if cough would tear it." The child will reach up to the larynx and clutch it. This is wholly different from the ACON condition when the child, after exposure to a dry cold wind, wakes before midnight with a hoarse, barking cough and clutches the larynx. So ACON cannot be substituted for ALL-C... .... *57*

CACTUS - When this constriction comes in the heart and about the chest it makes the patient think he is about to die, and he is at once struck with fear, and it is depicted on the face. He fears death and it seems he is going to die, his pain is so intense. But with this intense pain he has nothing of the anxiety we find in ACON, which has a similar constriction of chest and constriction in the neck. The violent choking in ACON makes him fear he is going to choke to death, and the anxiety is awful. It is not so intense in CACT. *300*

When the uterus is continually oozing, but every little while the flow increases to a gush and with every little gush of bright red blood the woman thinks she is going to faint, or if there is gasping, and the quantity of the flow is not sufficient to account for such prostration, nausea, syncope, pallor, IPECAC is the remedy. When with the gushing of bright red blood there is an overwhelming fear of death, ACONITE. *607*

In many instances we go to a haemorrhage and the pelvic symptoms are prominent and all other symptoms are clouded; there is a gushing flow, the blood is hot, etc. and there are only a few symptoms; but the next time you see the woman she is quiet enough to give other symptoms, and in the course of a few days more symptoms come out, as the haemorrhagic state is the outcome of the chronic condition. This is unlike measles. You do not have to look into the chronic state until the measles or scarlet fever or smallpox is finished; these are acute miasms. But the haemorrhage is part of her constitutional state; it is not a miasm; and hence when it is violent, calling for a remedy, probably the best adapted will be the short acting remedies, such as BELL or even ACON; but then look into the constitutional state for it is likely some remedy will have to follow the ACON or BELL, and commonly it is SULPH, the acute remedy being suitable to the violent action and then followed by its complementary medicine. 971

Then we have SEPTICAEMIC CONDITIONS, with purulent lochia or suppression of the lochia. You may go to a case in which, on the third day, there has been a chill, the lochia has been suppressed, the woman has a high temperature and is covered from head to foot in sweat. As you put your hand under the covers you feel steam come up from the body so that you want to take your hand away; it is so hot. She is dazed and is sensitive over the whole abdomen. You know now the meaning of suppression of the lochia; you have a PUERPERAL FEVER on hand. STUDY CLOSELY FOR SULPHUR instead of hunting around ACON, BRY, BELL, OP etc. With these you will make a total failure in most instances, but SULPH fits into just such a state and has cured many cases of puerperal fever. If it is but a milk fever or mammary indisposition and the chill is only acute then your short acting remedies will do very well and even ACON has been useful, but when it is a case of septicaemia SULPH goes to the very root of it...... *972*

MERC, IPECAC and ACON are frequently indicated in epidemic dysentery that comes in HOT weather, and IPECAC, DULC and MERC are frequently indicated in the dysentery of COLD weather. You should go to the bedside of a case of dysentery with your repertory or go home and send medicine. Your first prescription should cure in epidemic dysentery, and if you work cautiously you will cure every case. It is a very simple condition to cure, but a very bad thing to get mixed up.. *738*

MEASLES when they come out with that purplish colour very often require SULPH. SULPH is a great remedy in measles. A routinist can do pretty well in this disease with PULS and SULPH, occasionally requiring ACON and EUPH........................ *960*

ARN follows well after ACON and is complementary to ACON, IPECAC, and VERATRUM... *148*

AESCULUS

SPONG - Wakens at night in great fear, and it is some time before he can rationalise his surroundings (AESC, LYC, SAMB, LACH, PHOS, CARBO VEG)......................... *938*

He wakes up confused and wonders where he is. You will see that in children especially -they wake up in the morning in a bewildered state, such as you will find in ALUM, AESC, LYC. *69*

CIS - Cold feeling or burning in the nose. This is difficult to distinguish. In acute coryza the nose fills up with thick, yellow mucus, and when this is blown out it leaves the nasal cavity empty, and there is irritation; one will say it is a rawness, and another will describe it as a burning. There is relief when the nose fills up again with mucus. In ARS the mucus in the nose is so acrid that it burns, but in ANT-C, AESC and in CIS when the nose is empty there is a burning or rawness. The sensation of coldness, rawness, or burning is caused by the inhalation of air. *444*

ALOE, much like AESC, has a peculiar engorgement of the veins, causing stiffness and fullness throughout the body, but the greatest disturbance is in the veins of the portal system, with great fullness in the region of the liver, and abdominal, rectal and intestinal fullness. *57*

PULS - Most troublesome constipation with haemorrhoids; violent pains in the haemorrhoids, worse lying down, ameliorated from gentle motion, worse from the warmth of the bed, better moving about in the open air. She becomes so nervous in a room while at rest that the pains seem intensified and she must move about. "Haemorrhoids; painful, protruding, blind, with itching and stitches in anus." The aggravation from lying down in extremely painful haemorrhoids is contrasted with AMM-C which has violently painful haemorrhoids relieved by lying flat on the back. In violently painful haemorrhoids with intense burning, think of ARS and KALI CARB. In those with sticking, tearing pains, study AESC. 867

CARD MAR - Pain in the back under the right scapula (much like CHEL and AESC). 397

BERB - Finally the gouty deposits become prominent in the fingers and after the gout has determined itself then we have sore fingers; but these correspond more closely to LEDUM, SULPH, AESC and LYC where the disease has become marked and located in the joints. 261

AETHUSA

SIL has an aggravation from milk. Many times the infant is unable to take any kind of milk and hence the physician is driven to prescribe all the foods in the market if he does not know the right remedy. NAT-C and SIL are both useful when the mother's milk causes diarrhoea and vomiting. The routinist is likely to give such medicines as AETHUSA, entirely forgetting SIL. The latter, as well as NAT-C, has sour vomiting and curds in the stool. "Aversion to the mother's milk and vomiting" "Diarrhoea from milk". Put these two together. 931

PODO - Vomiting, greenish, profuse, watery, vomits everything; vomiting of milk (CALC, AETH - the latter sometimes retains water); 850

AGARICUS

NIT-AC - Shocks on going to sleep (AGAR, ARG-M, ARS, NAT-M.) 801

SIL - In the male, impotence, weakness of the genitals after coition, easily exhausted, lacks power; exhausted if he has coition with anything like normal frequency; it takes him a week or 10 days to rest up, (AGAR). 933

You will see one suffering from the AESC backache, on attempting to rise from sitting, make many painful efforts before he finally succeeds. This is found in SULPH, PETR and is also cured by AGAR. 39

ARG-M has an itching and burning like AGAR, in the toes, in the ears, and he scratches the part and scratching does not relieve it until the skin is off, until it oozes, but no relief from scratching. 131

PETR cures the itching and burning in frozen parts, but not as prominently as AGAR. AGAR leads all other remedies, especially when the condition affects parts where the tissues are thin over the bones, as over the back of the toes. 819

ALLIUM CEPA

In DULC the coryza is more fluent in the house, in the warmth, and less fluent in the cold air, in a cold room. With the DULC coryza, if the patient should go into a cold room pain will commence in the nasal bones and he will begin to sneeze, and water will be discharged from the nose. That very state would relieve a NUX-V patient. ALL-C is made worse in a warm room; like NUX-V, is better in cold, open air. Commences to sneeze as soon as he gets into a warm room. So that we see the meaning of such things, the necessity of going into particulars and examining every case. 508

PULS - When the hay fever comes on, all the other symptoms are better, she feels nothing except the hay fever, however all the symptoms interweave with each other. The NAT MUR symptoms will be worse in the morning and until toward noon, while in PULS they are worse in the evening, the nose filling up with thick, yellowish-green, ropy mucus, and when the nose has been cleared a dry, burning, smarting feeling remains; if the room is warm at night she cannot sleep. NAT MUR is a little like that in the smarting and inability to sleep at night in a warm room. In NAT MUR too the discharge may continue day and night. We have an acute class in which PULS is sometimes indicated - copious watery discharge which ends in sneezing. In the beginning we will think of CARBO-VEG, ARS, ALL-C, EUPH. With CARBO-VEG there is a watery discharge and the irritation extends into the chest, with hoarseness and rawness. In ALL-C we have one group of symptoms that points to this remedy. Excoriating discharge from the nose and bland discharge from the eyes; in the larynx, sensation as if hooks were there, and sometimes this extends below the larynx; this always means ALL-C; it is also worse in a warm room like PULS. The EUPH looks like ALL-C, only the discharge from the eyes is copious, watery and burning - the lachrymation burns the eyes and excoriates the cheeks; discharge from nose is bland like PULS. *863*

When the (nasal) discharge burns a red streak over the upper lip and about the wings of the nose, with sneezing and profuse watery nasal discharge ARS. Copious acrid lachrymation, and copious bland flow from the nose with sneezing: EUPHRASIA. Copious watery discharge from the eyes and copious acrid watery discharge from the nose: ALLIUM CEPA. But these are not the constitutional remedies; they do not cure, but only palliate during the severe attacks. These symptoms are the outcome of the psoric constitution, and this constitution must be treated by anti-psorics. Sometimes the hay fever is so severe that it seems to be the only manifestation of psora in the patient, but if it is restrained or stopped up by bad treatment he is not well during the whole year. Many a time the hay fever goes through the whole winter and only by constitutional upbuilding can it be mitigated. But with constitutional treatment each yearly attack is lighter, and at the end of treatment he is able to live in his own climate unaffected. He must not go to the mountains to mitigate it. If to any place he should go where the affection would be worse, so that all its manifestations would be apparent. The hay fever will only be cured if the patient is curable, but if not, if his condition is so broken down that he is incurable his hay fever will not be cured. *894*

ALOE

PODO - There body is offensive; offensive sweat; compare SEP, MERC, ALOE, SULPH, MUREX, NUX-V. *851*

KALI-BICH; diarrhoea after beer, like ALOE, CHINA, GAMBOGIA, LYC, MUR-AC and SULPH. *621*

ALOE has diarrhoea from leaving off beer, NUX has diarrhoea from leaving off alcoholic drinks. *808*

PODO - There is much flatus and spluttering, but not so marked as in ALOE. .. *848*

ALOE has involuntary dropping of little hard balls especially in children. Even when old enough to understand about such things, they will pass little balls unnoticed. ... *402*

ALUMINA

MED - Everything seems unreal (ALUM). *728*

CANN SAT - When he speaks it seems as though someone else were speaking (ALUM). *360*

PLUMB - Apoplexy. Stupor, when OP is sufficiently similar to remove the cerebral congestion which always surrounds the apoplectic clot, PLUMB may follow. PLUMB, PHOS and ALUM are three sheet anchors. They conform to the symptoms often when the first state has been like OP. *847*

CALC-P - Every cold settles in the tonsils (BARYTA CARB, ALUMINA). *336*

BELL - This constriction that comes in the sore throat occurs just in the act of swallowing fluids or solids, and that action will force the food and fluids up into the nose, and sometimes out of the nose. Some remedies have it as a paralytic condition, because the muscles of deglutition are paralysed and they do not favour the natural contracting actions to force the food down the oesophagus, and in that way the food is forced up into the nose and causes strangling. In BELL, in its acute states, its inflammatory conditions and its spasms would distinguish it from LACH, where it occurs as a paralytic action after diphtheria, and from ALUMINA, which has a spasm of the oesophagus. These are slow in coming, BELL is early. *245*

ARG-NIT - "Felt as if he had a stick in the throat when swallowing". At once you will see its close relation to HEPAR. In inflammatory conditions of the throat with ulceration. In ARG-NIT he wants to be in a cold room, wants cold air and to swallow cold things. In HEPAR he wants warm things to drink, a warm room, and cannot even put his hand out of bed or his throat will begin paining him. Things, you see, just exactly opposite, but they both have "sticks" in the throat. In dry chronic catarrh ALUM and NAT-MUR have "sticks" in the throat; but in red throat with tumefaction and pain these two remedies give no relief, the former two are better. "Sticks" in the throat like fish-bones. NIT-AC, HEPAR and ARG-NIT are the most striking remedies for the fish-bone sensation. *139*

Potatoes disagree with the COLOC patient, like ALUM, ... *466*

Great straining at stool belongs to many remedies but especially to ALUMINA, ALUMEN, CHINA, NAT MUR, NUX VOM, NUX MOSCH, and SIL. *932*

SELENIUM - Its constipation is much like ALUMEN and ALUMINA. It should be carefully compared with these remedies... .... *912*

SQUILLA has a loose morning cough and a dry evening cough (ALUM, CARBO-VEG, PHOS-AC, SEP, STRAM, PULS). *941*

PSOR - Old gleet, painless discharge; the "last drop"; relaxed and cold genitals; a drop of white or yellow pus after a well selected remedy (SEP, SULPH, ALUM). PSOR is indicated above all others if there is an unusually offensive state of the genitals. THUJ if the odor is of a nauseating, sweet character; warts exposed by rolling back the foreskin; sweet odor in spite of washing. *856*

Now it is a natural feature of gonorrhoea for the discharge to be yellow, or yellowish-green in the early stages, for it then to become lighter and lighter until it is whitish thick or thin, growing lighter in character until it becomes white and gleety. ARG-M is the remedy when the discharge remains yellow. The pain has all ceased, and generally when the pain ceases the discharge soon begins to be lighter, but in the ARG-M cases the pain ceases, it becomes a passive discharge, the urethra loses its sensitivity to pain and the mucus membrane loses its sensation to a great extent, but the thick greenish or yellowish discharge remains. Now, in these thick passive discharges that are long-standing, old cases, we are very much troubled to find remedies. These old stubborn cases that still remain yellow and still remain thick. They will not yield to ordinary remedies and they come under a peculiar class of remedies, ARG-M, ALUM, ALUMN, SULPH. Ones not usually thought of in the early period, but the general constitutional state of the patient forms his symptoms. *133*

ALUMINA SILICATA

The relationship between TUB and CALC is very close. They are interchangeable; that is, the one may be indicated for a while, and then the other. They are both deep acting remedies - also SIL is related to TUB, on the same plane of action, going deep into the life in a similar way; CALC, TUB, SIL and the SILICATES. *1003*

ALUMEN

ALUM comes in very nicely after ALUMEN which has much Alumina in its nature and depends largely upon Alumina, which is its base, for its way of working. It occurs to me to throw out a little hint. When you have a good substantial proving of an oxide or a carbonate and the mental symptoms are well brought out, you can use these, in a measure, in a presumptive way, in prescribing another salt with the same base, which has a few mental symptoms in its proving. For instance, you have a group of symptoms decidedly relating to ALUMEN. The mental symptoms of ALUMEN however, have not been brought out to any extent, but still you have the mental symptoms of the base of ALUMEN, which is the oxide, so that if the patient has the mental symptoms of ALUMINA and the physical symptoms of ALUMEN, you can rationally presume that ALUMEN will cure because of the aluminium in each. *66*

ARG NIT - Here is a striking feature. "Patient cannot lie on the RIGHT side because it brings on so much palpitation." We have plenty of remedies with palpitation worse from lying on the left side, but remedies with palpitation worse lying on the right side are rare (ALUMN, BAD, KALM, KALI NIT, LIL TIG, PLAT, SPONG). This is uncommon, strange, rare and peculiar. *138*

A patient suffered from a pressure in the top of the head, such as I recently described to you under ALUMEN. She would suffer for weeks from that pressure on top of the head, and the only relief she could get was from hard pressure; she tired herself out with hard pressure and would contrive all kinds of weights to put upon the head. That would go away in the night and she would wake up the next morning with constant urging to urinate. The irritable bladder alternated with pain on top of the head. ALUMEN cured. In many of these anti-psoric remedies we have an alternation of states. This illustrates the necessity for getting the symptoms of all the states that present themselves for cure, otherwise you will many times prescribe in a chronic case of psoric character and temporarily relieve it, when back comes another aspect of it. You have only hastened the disease a little faster than it would go if let alone. But that is not homoeopathic prescribing. Be sure, when a remedy presents one state, that it is as clearly indicated in the other state, otherwise that remedy is not the simillimum. You must hunt until you find the remedy that has both states, or you will be disappointed. We sometimes do not discover this alternation of states until we have brought it back two or three times by incorrect prescribing. Some people are so reticent and so difficult to get symptoms from that we do not always get these symptoms. But you examine your record and you find where you have made a foolish prescription, that you drove a new condition away and back came the first trouble and you kept on with this see-saw business. Now remember in doing this your patient is not improving, and that you must re-study the whole case, taking the alternating states into account. ***155***

SELENIUM - Its constipation is much like ALUMEN and ALUMINA. It should be carefully compared with these remedies... .... ***912***

Great straining at stool belongs to many remedies but especially to ALUMINA, ALUMEN, CHINA, NAT MUR, NUX VOM, NUX MOSCH and SIL. ***932***

ALUM - Induration here and there so that it favours lupus and epithelioma in one who is subject to these swellings and eruptions. ALUMINA and ALUMEN, like ARS, LACH, SULPH and CON are medicines that relate to these troubles. Some of these have made brilliant cures where there is infiltration. ***71***

Now it is a natural feature of gonorrhoea for the discharge to be yellow, or yellowish-green in the early stages, for it then to become lighter and lighter until it is whitish thick or thin, growing lighter in character until it becomes white and gleety. ARG-M is the remedy when the discharge remains yellow. The pain has all ceased, and generally when the pain ceases the discharge soon begins to be lighter, but in the ARG-M cases the pain ceases, it becomes a passive discharge, the urethra loses its sensitivity to pain and the mucous membrane loses its sensation to a great extent, but the thick greenish or yellowish discharge remains. Now, in these thick passive discharges that are long-standing, old cases, we are very much troubled to find remedies. These old stubborn cases that still remain yellow and still remain thick. They will not yield to ordinary remedies and they come under a peculiar class of remedies, ARG-M, ALUM, ALUMN, SULPH. Ones not usually thought of in the early period, but the general constitutional state of the patient forms his symptoms. ***133***

AMBRA GRISEA

ASAF - Attacks of dyspnoea after coition, like AMBR. ***186***

AMMONIUM CARBONICUM

LAUR should be compared with CAMPH, AMM-C and SECALE. *694*

PULS - Most troublesome constipation with haemorrhoids; violent pains in the haemorrhoids, worse lying down, ameliorated from gentle motion, worse from the warmth of the bed, better moving about in the open air. She becomes so nervous in a room while at rest that the pains seem intensified and she must move about. "Haemorrhoids; painful, protruding, blind, with itching and stitches in anus." The aggravation from lying down in extremely painful haemorrhoids is contrasted with AMM-C which has violently painful haemorrhoids relieved by lying flat on the back. In violently painful haemorrhoids with intense burning, think of ARS and KALI CARB. In those with sticking, tearing pains, study AESC. Looking over a number of years I have been forced to use in these cases a remedy not yet fully proven. In painful haemorrhoids in a broken down constitution, where the whole disease seems to culminate in the haemorrhoids; bleeding, protruding; a mere touch almost causes a convulsion; it causes her to scream out at the top of her voice; it is so painful that she feels that death would be a relief; she lies in bed holding the nates far apart with her hands; after every stool she has 3 or 4 hours of intense suffering. In these cases look up the PAEONY. The haemorrhoids it cures look like the flowers of the plant, they are so inflamed, so red and bleeding; oozing; tender to touch; patient is so worn out with the pain. It has many times relieved the pain and cured these enormous haemorrhoidal tumours. I have cured them after they have been operated on, and all sorts of violence done to them, without relief. Do not go to this drug if you can find a remedy that covers ALL THE PATIENT. Many patients will not confess to any other symptoms, and some of these will suffer so much from the haemorrhoids that you will really need this remedy. *867*

BAR-C - There are a few remedies that have, in such high degree, this coarse rattling in the chest of old people, that it is well to emphasise it. BAR-C is one of them. SENEGA, AMMONIUM and BARYTA MURIATICA should be compared. When there is coarse rattling in the chest all the time in an old person, an octogenarian, who is pretty comfortable in summer, but miserable all winter from the coarse rattling in the chest, and there are no other symptoms, AMMONIACUM will keep him comfortable. *226*

CAMPH - Old withered up people take cold at every exposure to weather and become cold and chilly. ANT-CRUD, AMM-CARB and CAMPH are wonderful remedies in octogenarians. Every cold seems threatening. Old people don't come down with cold the same as young people; they are prostrated, sinking, have rattling in the chest, and the family think it is the death rattle and that it is grandpa's last spell. These three remedies fit the case, they are like the advanced stage of pneumonia. ANT-T, ANT-C, AMM-C and CAMPH cover these cases in which the hot stage is omitted. *358*

ANACARDIUM

THUJ - Pain localised in small spots. A nail driven in the head, side of the head and forehead like IGN and ANAC. *999*

Another feature to be considered in CROTON TIG is its relation to RHUS. It is an antidote to RHUS. CROTON TIG is closely related in its vesicular symptoms to the RHUS family (particularly RHUS-TOX), ANAC, SEPIA and ANAGALLIS. *481*

CLEM is rather singular about the eruptions. One would not think that from so harmless a little shrub so much trouble would come; but there are persons who are just as sensitive to this vine as to RHUS, and it resembles RHUS to a great extent in its manifestations. It produces just as poisonous a condition as RHUS. Here I might speak of several remedies which relate to the RHUS poison. There are many vesicular remedies that look like RHUS and all of them you will have to use more or less in their antidotal relations to each other, but it is well to be sure in a given case which one of them produced the poison. CROTON TIG, RHUS, RANUNCULUS, ANAC and CLEM at times look so alike that I am unable to tell them apart by their eruptions. They are all similar enough to each other to become universal antidotes. The others are all deeper acting than RHUS. The RANUNCULUS, the little buttercup, has cured epithelioma of the lids. It has cured cancerous affections, so we say it goes deep into the tissues. *446*

ANAGALLIS

Another feature to be considered in CROTON TIG is its relation to RHUS. It is an antidote to RHUS. CROTON TIG is closely related in its vesicular symptoms to the RHUS family (particularly RHUS), ANAC, SEPIA and ANAGALLIS. *481*

ANTIMONIUM CRUDUM

To a great extent ANT TART builds upon the ANT CRUD basis. It forms its chest symptoms to a great extent on that basis. Many of the symptoms are like ANT-C; many symptoms are worse when warmed up, and from too much clothing. You will see this patient sitting up in bed with no clothing around the shoulders or neck and the night gown wide open in order to breathe. Suffocates if the room is too warm. It gets that from the ANT-C. The mucous membranes are covered in thick white mucus like ANT-C. Also he does not want to be meddled with or bothered. Everything is a burden. The child, when sick, does not want to be touched or talked to or looked at. Wants to be let alone. *111*

There are many headaches laid down under ANT-T but ANT-C is more likely to work for ANT headaches, while ANT-T is more likely to work for ANT chest troubles. Both of these remedies have very decided gastric symptoms. Constant nausea, vomiting and indigestion. ANT-T with its difficult breathing is sick at the stomach, loathes everything, loathes food, vomits even water. He has also a docile state and if allowed to be quiet, in spite of all the sufferings, he will fall into a deep sleep, or go into a state of inability to feel. He will cough and sleep and snore through the dyspnoea, so that it is in many ways like ANT-C, but ANT-C has nothing like the copious flow of mucus from the mucous membranes that are inflamed. It has nothing like the passive state of the whole economy. It is not so desperate in its provings, and not so dreadful to look upon. *112*

LYC - While the abdomen is distended he is so nervous that he cannot endure any noise. The noise of the crackling of paper, ringing of bells or slamming of doors goes right through him and causes fainting, like ANT-CRUD, BORAX and NAT-MUR. *704*

CIS - Cold feeling or burning in the nose. This is difficult to distinguish. In acute coryza the nose fills up with thick, yellow mucus, and when this is blown out it leaves the nasal cavity empty, and there is irritation; one will say it is a rawness, and another will describe it as a burning. There is relief when the nose fills up again with mucus. In ARS the mucus in the nose is so acrid that it burns, but in ANT-C, AESC and in CIS when the nose is empty there is a burning or rawness. The sensation of coldness, rawness, or burning is caused by the inhalation of air. *444*

When we have a diarrhoea from acids we sometimes find symptoms running to PHOS-AC. In the diarrhoea from sour wine, such as claret, from acids, vinegar, lemons, be sure to study ANT-C. *822*

SIL - Corns (ANT-CRUD, GRAPH). Rheumatism of the soles of the feet. Cannot walk (ANT-CRUD, MED, RUTA). *934*

The gout goes to different parts and in this instance it goes to the stomach and then BENZ-AC, ANT-C or SANGUINARIA is likely to be useful. When it goes to the throat or is followed by swelling of the tongue MERC and BENZOIC ACID should be thought of. *258*

CAMPH — Old withered up people take cold at every exposure to weather and become cold and chilly. ANT-CRUD, AMM-CARB and CAMPH are wonderful remedies in octogenarians. Every cold seems threatening. Old people don't come down with cold the same as young people; they are prostrated, sinking, have rattling in the chest, and the family think it is the death rattle and that it is grandpa's last spell. These three remedies fit the case, they are like the advanced stage of pneumonia. ANT-T, ANT-C, AMM-C and CAMPH cover these cases in which the hot stage is omitted. *358*

Like ANT-C, ANT-T has been useful in old drunkards. Old drunkards sometimes take on a debilitated form and take frequent colds. After getting over a big debauch, having been many days on one of their times, they become relaxed and cold, and the chest fills up with discharge of mucus and great rattling in the chest. Sometimes there is an irresistable desire for cold things in the stomach, but it is the exception. "Desire for acids or acid fruits" and they make him sick. Troubles brought on in the stomach from vinegar, from sour things, from sour wine, from sour fruits as in ANT-C. *114*

ANTIMONIUM TARTARICUM

The CADMIUM SULPH nausea is distressing. Nauseated all the way down to the abdomen, like IPECAC, ANT-T and ARS. *305*

LYC - In deep seated chest troubles, bronchitis or pneumonia, where the chest is filled up with mucus, it will be seen that the face and forehead are wrinkled from pain, and that the WINGS OF THE NOSE FLAP WITH THE EFFORT TO BREATHE. This occurs with all forms of dyspnoea. We see something like it in ANT TART, the sooty nostrils being wide open and flapping. In ANT TART the rattling of the mucus is heard across the room and the patient is seen to be in distress, but if you see the patient lying in bed with the nose flapping and the forehead wrinkled, with rattling in the chest or a dry hacking cough and no expectoration you will often find the particulars of the examination confirm your mind that it is a case for LYC. *709*

SENEGA - The rattling in the chest is as marked as in ANT-T, the tenacious mucus is as copious, as gluey and as stringy as in KALI BICH, so much is this the case that he can get it only part way up and with a spasmodic effort he swallows it, like SPONG and CAUST. *914*

In old, chronic catarrh of the chest, for the earlier stages of which BRY was the most similar remedy, with this thick, tough, ropy mucus, SENEGA is most suitable, and even when the patient is in the last stages of consumption. The symptoms become most troublesome, the gagging and coughing and effort to expectorate because of the thick, ropy mucus are very distressing. He breaks out in a cold sweat, especially on the upper parts of the body. The chest is full of coarse rales from the tough mucus, which he cannot expectorate. We think in such a case of remedies like ANT TART, PYR, KALI BICH etc. but SENEGA is just as suitable especially when there is a great amount of dryness in the throat and larynx, dryness in the throat during sleep and observed on waking, and inability to expectorate the thick, ropy mucus. *915*

APOC has all the rattling that is found in TARTAR EMETIC, and TARTAR EMETIC has a similar way of filling up the chest, cannot lie down. *128*

AMM-C is a good palliative in the last stages of consumption. A dose of AMM-C when there is great coldness, prostration and weakness in the chest. It is not unlike that sensation of weakness in the chest which is like STANNUM. He can hardly cough out loud, and because of the weakness he cannot expel the mucus, like ANT-T. *100*

CAMPH - Old withered up people take cold at every exposure to weather and become cold and chilly. ANT-CRUD, AMM-CARB and CAMPH are wonderful remedies in octogenarians. Every cold seems threatening. Old people don't come down with cold the same as young people; they are prostrated, sinking, have rattling in the chest, and the family think it is the death rattle and that it is grandpa's last spell. These three remedies fit the case, they are like the advanced stage of pneumonia. ANT-T, ANT-C, AMM-C and CAMPH cover these cases in which the hot stage is omitted. *358*

ANTHRACINUM

Carbuncles that come open upon the neck and upon the back begin with a pustule, and then several come, and they are surrounded by little pustules and papules and there is pitting upon pressure. For these carbuncles you will need to study particularly ARS, ANTHR, LACH, SEC and CROT-H. They are the medicines that have in their nature malignancy and manifestation. *477*

PYR - Violent burning in an abscess (ARS, ANTHR, TARENT-C). *872*

APIS

APOC comes in as a good one to contrast with APIS. You will find it analogous in its symptoms and much like the complaints cured by APIS. You will be astonished in going over the dropsical condition, the rheumatic condition, the tumefaction of the cellular tissues, the dropsy of the sacs, the scanty urine resulting in dropsy; the inflammatory swellings with oedema, at the great resemblances; and if you were to start in with two cases and work them out from their particulars, and if one feature were left out, the aggravation and amelioration, the cold and the heat, in many instances you would not be able to distinguish between APIS and APOC, so near alike are their swellings, their bleedings, their distensions and their disturbances. Both are remedies for dropsy; routinists will try first APIS and then they try APOC and then they will try something else that is good for dropsy. But all the way through APOC is aggravated from cold. His complaints are worse from cold applications. In his distended dropsical state he is chilly, sensitive to air. He has a pain in the stomach, and even vomits from cold drinks. Uneasiness here and there in the body when cold things are in the stomach, you see at once how different that is from APIS. ***123***

APOC has a water constitution, one that takes in water and lets out none. He passes little water, and he perspires scantily or not at all; his skin is dry, sometimes hot, but he is chilly. APIS suffers dreadfully from dry skin, from scanty urine; yet APIS is aggravated everywhere from heat and ameliorated from cold. That is the grand distinguishing feature in the dropsies and rheumatisms and many internal complaints. "Dropsy of serous membranes". Dropsy of the brain, pleura, pericardium, peritoneum, all of these are distended with serum. And there is great suffering, great uneasiness. The inflammatory rheumatism is again like APIS in that it takes on dropsy with it. Inflammation of the joints, of the ankle joints, of the toes, of the fingers, of the joints all over the body. The swelling about the joints pits upon pressure, like APIS. But with the scanty urine, want of sweat, with the febrile condition he is all the time chilly and wants the parts well wrapped where APIS wants them uncovered. One might say "Why, that is only one symptom". All who do not perceive the difference between symptoms predicated of the patient and symptoms predicated of the parts will see that as only one symptom with the rest of them. When he takes up a case and works it out in the Repertory he will use it as one symptom. Yet that one feature will sometimes rule out all the rest because it is predicated of the patient and not predicated alone of his parts. We have many remedies where the patient himself is ameliorated from heat. He wants to be in the heat, he wants to be warm, and yet he wants cold applied to the part. But that which is general is the ruling feature, and if you do not know and distinguish the things that are general from the things that are particular we get our Materia Medica mixed up. We must distinguish the things that belong to the patient himself from the things that belong to his parts........... ***123***

LEDUM is antidotal to LACH, to the poison of insects, to the poison of APIS and to animal poisons. ***695***

BELL - The temperature I described among the generals as being so marked, so intense that you will carry it with you for hours after you have touched a BELL case. It differs wholly from the APIS case, which has a rough rash. BELL smooth and shining. APIS wants to be cool, wants to be uncovered, BELL wants to be warm, wants a warm room; APIS has no thirst to speak of; in BELL it is the exception to have no thirst, generally thirsty for water, a little and often. The intense dryness of the mucous membranes and skin. Coldness of the extremities with hot head.. ***254***

ARS has all the dropsical conditions of APIS and APOC. ***125***

The LIL TIG patient suffocates in a crowded room, in the theatre, in church, like APIS, IOD, KALI IOD, LYC and PULS. *701*

Sometimes the delirium and congestive fulness of the head affecting the mind will increase if the room becomes very warm, or from the heat of the stove, from becoming heated, or from warm covers. In children this will be noticed, whereas if the window is thrown up to relieve the stuffiness of the room the child will sleep quietly. Such remedies as BRY, APIS, PULS and many others come in here. *280*

CON - Mental symptoms, nervous symptoms, trembling in widows and widowers who have suddenly been deprived of their sexual relations. When in a state of considerable vigour, if suddenly deprived, the woman or the man takes on a state of trembling weakness, inability to stand any mental effort, and inability to put the attention upon things said by others. Not so common or so marked in the woman as in the man. When this state comes on in a woman who is of unusual sexual vigour there may be severe congestion of the uterus and ovaries, APIS is more likely to fit her symptoms than CON. But with hysteria and excitability CON is the remedy. *468*

AGAR - Clumsy motion of the fingers and hands. In handling things she drops them. Fingers fly open spasmodically while holding things. You will sometimes cure Bridget in the kitchen with AGAR or APIS when the trouble is that she is continually breaking dishes by letting them fall. These two remedies are opposites. AGAR must stay by the fire, while APIS wants to get out of the kitchen. The awkwardness, clumsiness etc. are both mental and bodily. *43*

A feature of infancy is the following: Child may not have diarrhoea, may even be constipated, but it lies in bed and rolls the head in sleep. BELL and APIS roll head. APIS lies on back with the head on its side. Chewing motion of the jaws; sometimes a sucking; a grinding in the teeth of those who are old and have teeth; rolling the head from side to side; if you lift the eyelids you will find a strabismus. Provers felt as if the eyes were drawn inward. PODO has cured such a strabismus in congestion of the brain following a suddenly suppressed diarrhoea. *851*

MERC - Ears inflamed, with cramp-like pains. MERC has STINGING PAINS LIKE APIS. All routinists will give APIS for stinging pains, and yet it often is MERC that the patient needs. *736*

NIT-AC - Inflammation of throat, tonsils, uvula and soft palate. Uvula and tonsils oedematous (APIS, RHUS-T). Great swelling of the throat and tonsils. Ulceration of tonsils. *798*

PODO - Great soreness of the abdomen before and during the menstrual period (APIS, CIMIC, VESPA, LACH, but these are not so likely to have diarrhoea and, if so, it is not so copious). *849*

STAPH - Crawling etc. in the female external genitals, COFF, PLAT, PETROL, APIS, TARENT HISP, the latter has: While outer parts feel as if insects were biting and crawling, better heat and cold. **947**

SULPH is not so suitable in the cases that come on with rapidity and great violence, with vesicles and enormous blebs, but it suits those cases in which there is first an appearance of a mottled dusky red spot on the face, and a little distance from it another spot and then another, and these, as it were, all run together, and after a week or so it develops into a sluggish erysipelatous state, and the veins seem to be distended, and he is passing into a state towards unconsciousness. You will be astonished to see what SULPH will do in such a case, which comes slowly as if there were a lack of vitality to develop it, a slow, sluggish erysipelatous inflammation. Whereas if it be ARS, APIS or RHUS-TOX it spreads with rapidity. ARS and APIS burn like fire, and RHUS has blisters upon the erysipelatous patches. **967**

In an ABORTION you may have selected BELL, which was suitable while the woman was aborting, and it may have overcome the present state, or you may have selected APIS or SABINA, which was suitable for the early state, and it either postpones or checks the haemorrhage for the time or hurries the expulsion of the foetus; but the haemorrhage starts in again and with its return we have prolonged tribulation. In many of these cases we can do nothing until we put the patient on SULPH. If the symptoms are masked, SULPH stands very high. **971**

MERC is a wonderful remedy to ward off ACUTE HYDROCEPHALUS after measles and scarlatina; the child rolls the head and moans, and the head sweats. It is closely related to APIS, which is also a great remedy after scarlet fever to ward off or cure hydrocephalus. **735**

APOC - A low form of disease, like typhoid fever, has kept him in bed for four or five weeks, and he is emaciated and prostrated, and now he does not again gain flesh, he has no appetite, but he drinks copiously; he seems to want nothing but water. His skin commences to distend, fills up and becomes dropsical. That is like APIS, and APIS would be indicated provided he was always hot and wanted to be uncovered, and wanted cold things. **124**

ARGENTUM METALLICUM

MANG is similar to ARG MET, PHOS, GRAPH and SULPH in its underlying tendency to tuberculosis. **723**

NIT-AC - Shocks on going to sleep (AGAR, ARG-M, ARS, NAT-M.) **801**

SELENIUM is said to be incompatible with CHINA. It is much like SULPH in general action, and PHOS-AC in its action upon the nervous system and genitals. The chest spymptoms and expectoration are like ARG-MET, STANNUM. Its constipation is much like ALUMEN and ALUMINA. It should be carefully compared with these remedies. **912**

ALUM - There is expectoration in some of the coughs, but the cough is usually a constant dry hacking cough, one of those troublesome lingering coughs that has existed for years. It competes with ARG MET in its character of the dry hacking cough, especially associated with weakness, but ARG MET has the cough in the daytime, which is not so in ALUM. The ALUM cough is in the morning. **75**

MANG has a day cough - no cough at night because he is lying. ARG MET has a day cough. Like MANG it refers to the larynx and is ameliorated by lying down. **726**

We would think of ALUM when singers break down in the voice from paralysis or from overwork of the voice. The voice lets down and becomes feeble and when taking cold there starts up a peculiar kind of tickling. ALUM is very useful in these cases. ARG MET was the remedy used by earlier homoeopaths for singers and talkers with much trembling and letting down of the voice before the value of ALUM was known in such conditions. Let me tell you something here about RHUS as I may not think of it again. Many old singers, after taking cold, have a weakness left in the voice, which they notice on beginning to sing. On beginning to sing the voice is weak and husky, but after using it a little while it improves. Give RHUS to all these patients, prima donnas, lawyers, preachers etc. They must warm up the voice and then they are alright, but they say "If I go back into the green-room for a little while, when I commence to sing again I am worse than ever." The voice is better if they stay in a very hot room and keep it in use. This fits into the general state of RHUS. There is a kind of hoarseness that you may discover to be a little different from the paralytic hoarseness of ALUM and ARG MET. This hoarseness of which I speak belongs to this same class of people; on first beginning to use the voice it seems that they must get rid of some mucus by clearing the throat until the voice can get to work. The vocal cords, on beginning to work, are covered with mucus, and on getting rid of it they can do very good work, so long as they keep at it. That is PHOS. In such cases the use of the voice becomes painful. The vocal cords are painful after motion and the larynx is painful to touch. Sometimes this is so marked that it is like stabbing with a knife on trying to use the voice. So we must individualise hoarseness very carefully. Homoeopathy is a matter of discrimination. **76**

MANG - Hoarseness and loss of voice in a chronic state. It is suitable in recurrent cases coming with every spell of damp weather until finally tuberculosis starts. Every cold starts up additional trouble in the larynx, causing a laryngitis. It is a wonderful remedy in speakers and singers, as useful as ARG MET. Constant accumulation of mucus, more forms as soon as he clears it. Hemming all the time and annoying everybody. ARG MET, SIL, SULPH, PHOS and MANG all do that. Each hem brings up a mouthful of mucus.................................. **726**

ARGENTUM NITRICUM

RUTA is sometimes overlooked and RHUS-T or ARG NIT given, or other remedies not fully related to the case are given because RUTA is not well known. ***889***

NUX-V - Driven by impulses to commit acts that verge upon insanity - the destruction of others. NAT-SUL has a strong impulse to destroy himself. ARG NIT also, particularly by jumping from a height, but he avoids placing himself in such a position. 804

ARG-M - He thinks, now he is away from all the troubles of the day and can rest, and the instant sleep comes over him he is roused from head to foot by a shock, and another one, and another one, sometimes the whole night he jerks from head to foot. His limbs jerk up, his lower limbs twitch and jerk, then he gets out of bed and walks - tries to walk it off. This comes out in the proving of ARG NIT, but it belongs as much to ARG MET and ARG MET has long cured it. 130

RUTA - Pain in the eye, above and through the eye when he attempts to use the vision, that is, aggravation from overexertion of the vision. From looking at fine print, fine sewing. This overexertion of vision brings about redness, pain and inability to concentrate the vision on one point. Headache follows. Here ARG NIT resembles RUTA. ARG NIT and NAT MUR are the two most frequently used, but ONOSMODIUM is a very frequently indicated remedy for headaches from eyestrain. But they can easily be differentiated. RUTA is aggravated from cold, wants everything warm, ARG NIT is aggravated from heat, wants to be in a cool place. The patient must be considered. ***890***

When the case is of sycotic origin, small or large gelatinous polypi form in the larynx and they are sore, causing loss of voice, or cracked voice. When they cause choking or uneasiness, HEPAR is one of the remedies. HEPAR, CALC, ARG NIT and NIT AC and sometimes THUJA are the remedies related to such a condition. ***575***

AGAR - In one case, after straining had been given up as unsuccessful, would pass a stool involuntarily. This symptom was known only in ARG NIT (stool and urine). ***45***

BORAX - Quantities of fluid like boiled starch are emitted from the anus; BORAX has that as well as ARG NIT. ***268***

HEPAR is useful in old cases of gleet; also when there is a sensation of a splinter in the urethra. In strictures and constrictions of an inflammatory character, during the inflammation there is a tendency to ulcerate and with this the sensation of a stick is felt. ARG NIT, NIT AC and HEPAR run very close together for this kind of inflammation and will cure the inflammatory stricture before it becomes a complete and permanent fibrinous structure. ***576***

NIT-AC - Prolonged inflammation of the urethra with infiltration, making the urethra feel hard and nodular like a whip-cord (ARG NIT). ***800***

MERC - Paralysis of the lower limbs, and twitching, jerking and quivering of the paralysed parts. ARG NIT, PHOS, SEC, STRAM and MERC have twitching of the muscles of the paralysed parts. ***741***

TUB - When phthisical patients find no comfort except riding in the cold wind - which is a rare symptom but has been noticed. This was a symptom specially marked in the late lamented Gregg of Buffalo. He would ride out in the cold winds by the lake for hours. ARG NIT many times relieved that, but it is a strong symptom of TUB. He finally died of tuberculosis. **1005**

ARNICA

After ACON follow well ARN and BELL. Sometimes it is true it will appear to you that ACON is capable of coping with all there is in the disease. But there seems to be a lingering something that holds on and such medicines as ARN and BELL, and IP and BRY do have to come in to finish up the attack - or sometimes SULPH. Very commonly SIL. So we have to study the relations of medicines. ***30***

In ARS the head symptoms alternate with physical symptoms. We find in PODO the peculiar feature that the headaches alternate with diarrhoea, and one or the other will be present. In ARN the mental symptoms alternate with uterine symptoms. The uterine symptoms, when observed, look like ARN, but these go away in the night and mental symptoms come on, the mind being heavy, gloomy and cloudy. When we have remedies that have these manifestations it requires a greater depth of vision to see the alternation of states, because these things are not always brought out in the provings, for the reason that one prover had one group of symptoms, and another another. Yet a remedy that is capable of bringing out the two groups of symptoms is sufficient to cure this alternation of states. ***156***

PYR - The sore bruised condition is as marked as in ARN and BAPT; the aching in the bones like EUPATORIUM, the restlessness, ameliorated by motion and heat like RHUS. *871*

MANG - Everywhere there is soreness to touch and soreness from jarring. The bones are sore from walking. ARN relieves only a day or two; but in MANG it is deep-seated and prolonged, and we would not think of ARN or BAPT, which would only give relief for a day or so. *722*

PETR - Sore, bruised feeling all over the body, especially in the joints. Rheumatic pain in the joints on motion; sore to touch; sensation as if bruised. It is analogous to ARN in relation to bruises. *817*

CARD MAR - Dragging pain in right hypochondrium when lying on left side; like ARN, MAG-M, NAT-S and PTEL. *397*

DULC is a medicine wonderfully useful in diarrhoea, at the close of summer, hot days and cold nights, with changeable stool; diarrhoea of infants. There seems to be no digestion; yellow, slimy stool; yellow-green stool, with undigested stool; frequent stool, blood in the stool and quite a mass of slime, showing a marked catarrhal state. This gets better and worse; this gets better under ordinary remedies; it will often get better from PULS, because PULS symptoms seem to predominate, and sometimes it is relieved by ARN; but every time the child takes cold it comes back again, and soon the physician will realise that he has not struck the remedy belonging to all the symptoms. It is very often an annoying condition, because the symptoms are not recognised until two or three attacks have come. It is not easy to discover that the attacks come on from cold. *504*

Hot flatus, burning the anus; smells of spoiled eggs, ARN and STAPH. *855*

NUX-V - Pressure and sense of weakness in the left inguinal ring - hence cures hernia in babies (LYC, right side). ARN relieves soreness etc. CON also - it competes with NUX in sense of goneness in the groin.... .... *809*

NUX-V - Labour pains with soreness like ARN - urging etc. *809*

SPONG - at times, after great dyspnoea, white tough mucus forms in the air passages, difficult to expectorate; it comes up and often has to be swallowed (ARN, CAUST, LACH, KALI-C, KALI-S, NUX-MOSCH, SEP, STAPH). *939*

All know about ARNICA but be sure to keep it in its place. The first stage of the injury, where much bruising has been done, and there are none of these pains that I have described, for the first few hours of bruised conditions and concussions and shocks ARNICA is a routine, because it produces states in the human body like it had been bruised. But you will find ARNICA only fits into that one place. ARNICA should never be used for wounds the way lay people use it, because if it is used in full strength it may bring on erysipelas. *589*

HYPERICUM belongs to lacerated wounds and when there is laceration of parts that are full of small nerves, sentient nerves, give it at once. Do not waste time with ARNICA because there is soreness, for the soreness is of much less importance than the danger from nerves in lacerated wounds. In punctured wounds give LEDUM at once. Whatever sequences come on of course have to be met in accordance with the state and symptoms of the case. *590*

When tetanus comes on from punctured wounds in the palms or soles or in other parts, think of HYPERICUM, or when you have a punctured wound to treat, give LEDUM at once and you will prevent tetanus. When the fingernails have been torn, or the nerves in sentient parts like the ends of the fingers have been torn and lacerated, HYPERICUM becomes the remedy. For the bruising of various parts, and when the patient feels as if bruised all over, no matter how extensively he is bruised, ARNICA is generally the remedy. It may be said, for punctured wounds study LEDUM; for lacerated wounds of sentient nerves study HYPERICUM; for bruises study ARNICA; for open lacerations and cuts study CALENDULA. The conditions that come from the external ought to be remedied to a great extent by external means.......... ***696***

HYPERICUM is related also to injuries of the spine higher up. It is not an uncommon thing for a man, while going down stairs, to fall backward, his feet slip from under him, and he strikes his back upon one of the steps and undergoes a sharp injury. Some will at once give RHUS TOX; I have known others to give ARN. HYPERICUM is to be given at once to prevent the kind of inflammation that may come from such an injury. .. ***591***

RUTA - "Pain and lameness in the ankles after a sprain or dislocation." "Lameness after sprains, especially of the wrists and ankles." Immediately after a sprain for the inflammatory state you will most likely need to give ARN; and RHUS will probably follow. But when nodules form in the tendons as a result of the strain RUTA is called for. RUTA is a great remedy for a mere sprain; it has all the soreness and weakness of tendons. ARN, RHUS and CALC are often necessary in a routine way when there is absence of all symptoms except the strain alone. ***891***

BRY is often indicated in injuries to joints where ARN would be a failure........... ***277***

CACT - At the beginning of conplaints, at the beginning of the pneumonia; congestive chill with hot head and cold body (like ARN). ***298***

RUMEX is one of the most valuable palliatives in advanced phthisis; it will often carry a case through another winter. With RUMEX, PULSATILLA, SENEGA, ARS and NUX VOM you can patch up the last years of a phthisical patient. You will see ACETIC ACID recommended for the diarrhoea in phthisis. You had better let such conditions alone, unless they are very marked. If the diarrhoea is very exhausting use some simple medicine like this one (RUMEX) to slack it up. But the phthisical patient is better off with a little diarrhoea, a loose morning stool. It is the same with the night sweats; if he does not have them he will have something more violent.The allopath stops the diarrhoea and night sweats and then has to feed morphine to his patient because of the consequent sufferings.The more you undertake to relieve these outward conditions, these vents, the more harm you will do the patient, and if you go on you will have to abandon your homoeopathy and give morphine, which is really a crime. You will remove the sore bruised aching all over the body of a consumptive by ARN, and it will suit the cough and gagging and retching and make him sleep. Later PYR may be needed for the aching in the bones and distressing cough. You patch him up year after year. Sometimes ARS is the remedy and it has to be more frequently repeated; sometimes it is LYC, PULS, PYR or ARN. These medicines help him along, and they have often to be changed, but finally the breakdown occurs, and these medicines are no longer suitable. An awful dyspnoea gradually creeps on the patient; there is craving for air; the breathing space is becoming diminished. Dropsy comes on in the extremities. The heart gives out; there is emaciation; the hippocratic countenance is seen; there is cold sweat, blue face, sinking. Even now we can palliate with TARENT-C. Sometimes it has to be repeated. It will relieve for days and give a euthanasia, not a stupefaction as produced by morphine, benumbing the senses, but an actual comforting. *888*

SENEGA has sometimes cured pleuro-pneumonia when there was the extreme exhaustion of PHOSPHORUS and ARSENICUM. In such cases SENEGA has caused reaction; it has such weakness. Especially is it suited in the advanced cases of phthisis; it acts as a palliative. It does excellent patchwork without serious aggravation as it relates more especially to superficial conditions. It is not as deep acting as SULPH and SIL. We give such remedies only when we have a reasonable assurance that we can cure, when the patient is yet curable. But when we have given up all hope, then we pay more attention to the most painful parts; we pay more attention to the local symptoms, to the group which causes the most sufferings, and attempt to do patchwork. If the sufferings in the chest and exhaustion become most severe it is true that ARS will patch him up a little and make him feel more like life, and he will go on to the end with more comfort. If the pains in the chest are most severe such medicines as SENEGA or BRY will help him; if he is sore and feels as if bruised and he must move from side to side ARN will relieve; but these are not the remedies to go deep into the life and eradicate a deep seated disease like phthisis. Yet with these one may take a consumptive patient in comfort to the very grave, by simply patching him up and prescribing for his immediate sufferings. *916*

ARUM - The sneezing is like an ordinary coryza, with repeated chills over the body and aching in the bones as if the bones would break, like NUX, EUPATOR, ARN, RHUS, BRY and ARS that have aching all over during "cold". *180*

CROT-H - In PUERPERAL FEVER there is a continued oozing of black, offensive blood that will not coagulate; bleeding from every orifice of the body as well as from the uterus. Imagine a woman who is pregnant suffering from typhoid fever. She aborts and a low zymotic state comes on with the symptoms that I have described and with all the appearances as if she would bleed to death after the abortion. The blood will not coagulate and the flow continues. Or in a woman during a typhoid fever menstruation comes on. It is not a true menstrual flow, that is, it does not resemble the ordinary flow, because it is copious, dark and liquid, a continuous oozing with all the grave symptoms described, and especially the besotted countenance, the comatose state, the appearance as if she were intoxicated, lying as one dead. When aroused every muscle trembles; if the tongue is protruded it trembles, and there is inability to articulate. CROT-H may save her life. Would it be possible to think of graver states of sickness than such as are produced by the ophidia? When a physician sees these states of coming on he immediately thinks of a class of remedies that can cover such a state, remedies like BAPT, ARS, SEC and the OPHIDIA, and sometimes ARN, PHOS and PYR. *477*

ARSENICUM

Every experienced physician must have met with many cases where for a time he felt unable to cope with the case because of his inability to reach the constitutional state that underlies this continual taking of cold. So he puzzles for a long time, and prescribes on the immediate attack and palliates it. For instance, the immediate attack might look like BELL or BRY, FERRUM PHOS or ARS etc.; he treats that attack without taking into consideration the underlying constitutional state of the patient. It is quite a profitable business for one who has not much conscience and not much intelligence. But a conscientious physician feels worried and knows he is not doing what he ought to do by his patient, unless he reaches out for the remedy that touches the constitution. It is far more useful to keep people from taking colds than to cure cold. ***509***

It is peculiar that medicines come around on time with an exactitude. Diseases do the same thing, and we must see that it is also peculiar that they come with a regular cycle, a regular periodicity. We meet with headaches that come every 7 days, headaches that come once in every two weeks, and there are remedies that have 7 day aggravations and 14 day aggravations and 3 day aggravations, remedies that bring out their symptoms just in this form. Do not be surprised when your patient is perfectly under the influence of AUR if he has a characteristic aggravation every 21 days. There are quite a number of remedies having 14 day aggravations, eg. CHINA and ARS. Again there are autumnal aggravations, spring aggravations, winter aggravations, aggravations from cold weather, and aggravations in the summer from heat. Some remedies have both the latter. ***516***

That is one of the first things I observed, that outside of sycotics you will seldom find a cure for asthma. There is that peculiarity that runs through sycosis which gives you a hereditary disease, and asthma corresponds to that disease. Hence it is that SIL is one of the greatest cures for asthma; it does not cure every case, but when SIL corresponds to the symptoms you will be surprised how quickly it will eradicate it. While IPECAC, SPONG and ARS will correspond just as clearly to the supervening symptoms and to everything that you can find about the case, yet what will they do? They palliate; they repress the symptoms; but your asthma is no better off, your patient is not cured. ARS is one of the frequently indicated remedies for the relief of asthma; so also are BRY, IPECAC, SPONG and CARBO-VEG, but they do not cure; although surprisingly at times where a patient is sitting up, covered with a cold sweat, wants to be fanned by somebody on either side of the bed, dyspnoea is so distressing that it seems almost impossible for the patient to live longer, to get another breath, then CARBO VEG comes in and gives immediate relief and the patient will lie down and get a very good night's rest. But what is the result? On comes the asthma again the very next cold. NAT-S goes to the bottom of this kind of a case. ***793***

ARG-NIT - So marked is the aggravation from sugar that the nursing infant will get a green diarrhoea if the mother eats candy. Then is it astonishing that the baby can get a dynamised dose from the mother, when the dynamised dose can travel like lightning, and sugar takes all day to be digested and dynamised and fed as poison to the baby? I remember a case that I figured and figured on. The baby had MERCURIAL STOOLS, sure enough, they were grass green. Well, CHAM has grass green stools, and ARS and MERC and lots of remedies have grass green stools. Routinist that I was in those days I could not get anything but MERC out of it, and although the baby had gotten MERC, ARS and CHAM, there was no relief, until I found that the mother had been eating candy. When she was asked if she ate sweet things, sugar etc. she said, "Oh no." "Why, yes you do", said the husband, "I bring you home a pound of candy every day. What do you do with it?" "Oh, that was nothing" she replied. But the baby did not get well until it got ARG-NIT and the mother stopped eating sugar. ***140***

SPONG - Face distressed in croup; anxious; livid; pale and bloated; blue, pale with sunken eyes; red with anxious expression; alternating red and pale; cold sweat. These symptoms are the natural effects of difficult breathing, and are therefore not essential to the selection of a remedy. As primary symptoms they would probably indicate ARS, but when due to cardiac difficulties, they are unimportant. ***939***

SARS is suitable in low forms of chronic disease, especially in complex states resulting from mixed miasm; especially in cases of sycosis and syphilis; cases made complex by mercury, sycosis, syphilis and psora. Weakness stamps itself upon the whole economy, as in MERC, LACH and other remedies. The tissues become flabby, refuse to heal when injured, ulcerate from slight causes. After an injury an open sore remains and is indolent or becomes phagedenic and spreads like ARS, LACH and MERC COR. Weakness all over the body; a paralytic feeling. . ***904***

HEPAR competes with SILICA in syphilitic nasal catarrhs where the parts are phagedenic; HEPAR, MERC COR and ARS are the principal anti-syphilitics when there is phagedenic ulceration of the nose. Babies suffer from bloody nasal discharge. This is often CALC SUL. ***929***

THUJA - The skin looks unhealthy everywhere about the body and there is a copious sweat on first going to sleep like ARS. If you had only the waxiness such as ARS and THUJ produce you might prescribe ARS. ARS is often the acute and THUJ the chronic. You remember that ARS is usually a chronic remedy. A peculiar asthmatic condition is found in sycosis and ARS appears to be indicated for the symptoms, but it only relieves, it does not control the predisposition, it acts like ACON in acute diseases and only ameliorates for a moment. Asthmatic and many other sycotic conditions seem to call for ARS, but it will do nothing but palliate, the constitutionality is not reached by ARS, its fundamental symptoms are not similar. In syphilis and psora ARS acts a long time and eradicates the complaints, when similar to them, but it is not similar to sycosis. ARS does not go to the bottom of the trouble but THUJA and NAT SULPH will take up the work and cure. NAT SULPH and THUJA bring back the primitive manifestation that has been suppressed for years. ***996***

In a case confused by remedies think of CALC, ARS, SULPH, SEP and IPECAC. Never give CHINA or NAT MUR for irregular symptoms and stages. ***925***

In those complaints that should come to a crisis, if the patient goes into a state of exhaustion under remedies fairly well selected, you have an instance where AMM-C competes with ARS for the nervous prostration. ***100***

PULS has relief from motion. A few

remedies have relief from slow motion, and of these PULS and FERR are the most striking. A few remedies are relieved by hurried motion; want to move fast. Such are BROM and ARS. The ARS child cannot be carried fast enough. The PULS baby is content with moderate motion. Any motion that HEATS UP the PULS patient aggravates all complaints. *868*

Unlike ARS, running all through CADMIUM SULPH, he wants to be perfectly quiet; part of it is a state of indolence, part of it is an aversion to motion. He is worse from motion, which makes it like BRY. So we will see running all through CADMIUM SULPH the exhaustion of ARS and the aversion to motion of BRY. *304*

The burning of KALI CARB is like that of ARS. *625*

Anxiety and restlessness are words that prevail throughout all the conditions of TARENT-H. It is much like ARS. The anxiety is felt sometimes in the mind, sometimes in the whole body, sometimes in the limbs and stomach. Cardiac anxiety is a strong feature. *990*

TAR-H - The extreme restlessness of the limbs is like ARS and it is a deep acting medicine like ARS, and it sometimes has cured where ARS has failed although it seemed well selected. Anxiety, restlessness, constant motion of the arms, legs, trunk and head. Restlessness of the limbs in the evening, in bed before going to sleep, like ARS and LYC. *990*

A few days ago I saw a patient who could not lie down because of pain in both hypochondria; he had incessant vomiting, inflammatory rheumatism of the ankles, hands, arms and shoulders, he had purpuric spots on the arms and legs, he had inflammation of the stomach, and was a perfect museum of diseases. He had had PHOS and ARS and many remedies very high, all supposed to be well selected, but CADM SULPH put him to sleep in fifteen minutes. The point was that he wanted to keep perfectly still, and hence it was unlike ARS, although all the other symptoms were like ARS. That is a strong feature of CADM SULPH; he wants to keep as still as COLCH and BRY. For many years I have used it in such cases. I saw another case of cancer with coffee-ground vomit and CADM SULPH stopped her vomiting, and she ate quite well until she died 6 weeks later. The doctor in charge had given her ARS and PHOS and Morphine till she could take no more. *739*

TARENT-H - Restlessness of the lower limbs with constant desire to cry (ARS). *994*

TARENT-H - He is moving the legs constantly; heaviness in the legs, bruised pain in the legs; shooting pains in the right Tendo Achiles; he must walk the floor in the evening like ARS. It is much like ARS, going from chair to chair and from bed to bed, walking the floor. *994*

ARS has all the dropsical conditions of APIS and APOC. *125*

NIT-AC - Shocks on going to sleep (AGAR, ARG-M, ARS, NAT-M.) *801*

It is a strange thing to see a bright little girl of 8 or 9 years old taking on sadness, melancholy and commencing to talk of the future world and the angels and that she wants to die and go there, and she is sad and wants to read the Bible all day. That is a strange thing; and yet CALC has cured that. ARS has cured that state, and also LACH. They are a little inclined to be precocious and they have attended the Sunday school and have taken too seriously the things they have learned there. Children sad and unhappy and old people who take on a loathing of life, become weary of life. That is a good deal like AURUM. I explained that, and dwelt on it, that the highest love is love of life, and when an individual ceases to love his own life and is weary of it and wants to die he is on the borderland of insanity. In fact that is an insanity of the will...... ***319***

The MENTAL STATE of IODINE is that of anxiety, excitement, impulses, melancholy; he wants to do something, wants to hurry; he has impulses to kill. In this it is closely related to ARSENICUM and HEPAR. The ARS and HEPAR patients also have impulses to commit murder without being offended and without cause. The sensitiveness to heat will at once decide, for while IODINE is warm blooded, the ARS and HEPAR patients are always chilly. ***599***

If you watch an ARN patient in order to get the external manifestations of his state, you will see him turning and moving. You will at once ask yourself, "Why is he so restless?"; and if you compare remedies in your mind, you will say, "He is like RHUS TOX"; he stays in a place a little while, and then he moves. No matter if he is only semi-conscious, you will see him make a little turn, part way over, and then a little further over, and so on, until he is over on the other side. The question is why does he move so, why is he restless? It is an important matter to solve. We notice the awful ANXIETY of the ARS patient that keeps him moving all the time. We notice the PAINFUL UNEASINESS felt all over the body with the RHUS TOX patient, so that he cannot keep still. The ARN patient is so SORE that he can lie on one part only a little while, and then he must get off that part or on to the other side. So if we ask him, "Why do you move so?", he will tell us that the bed feels hard. That is one way of telling that the body is sore. A more intelligent individual will say it is because he is so sore and he feels as if bruised and beaten, and he wants to get into a new place. This state of soreness is present if it be a symptomatic typhoid, an intermittent fever, a remittent fever, or after an injury when he is really bruised all over. You get the same continual uneasiness and motion, moving every minute. He moves and thinks that now he will be comfortable, but he is comfortable only for a second. The soreness increases the longer he lies and becomes so great that he is forced to move. With RHUS TOX the longer he lies the more restless he grows, and the more he aches, until he feels as if he will fly if he does not move. With RHUS TOX the uneasiness passes off after moving and with ARN the soreness passes off if he gets into a new place. With ARS you see him moving about and look wild, and he is anxious, and this anxiety forces him to move, and he gets no rest, for he keeps going. The RHUS TOX and ARN patients get better from every little motion. ***144***

In BRY as in ARS there comes an anxious and uneasy feeling which compels him to move, but he is worse from motion, yet so uneasy and anxious that he must move, ... ***279***

IOD - Though mentally prostrated, he is compelled to keep busy to continue the work, which increases the prostration of mind. You tell a man who is threatened with softening of the brain from overwork, from anxiety and labour in literary work, "You must stop working, you must rest." "Why," he will say, "if I do I would die or go mad." Such a state comes under IODINE and ARSENICUM, but there is one grand distinction by which the remedies are seen to part company at once. The IODINE patient is warm blooded, wants a cool place to move in and to think in, and to work in, whereas the ARSENICUM wants heat, wants a warm room, wants to be warmly clothed and suffers from the cold. IODINE suffers from the heat. So that the anxiety and restlessness which are both of body and of mind in each remedy loom up before the mind as one, if the patient is a hot blooded patient we would never think of ARSENICUM; if a cold blooded and shivering patient we would never think of IODINE. *600*

IPECAC is sometimes as restless as ARS, but the IPECAC prostration comes by spells, whereas the ARS prostration is continuous. You will see IPECAC patients tossing over the bed as much as they do when they need RHUS, turning and tossing and moving the hands and feet, with restlessness........ *605*

BAR-C - Always borrowing trouble. Like CAUST, fear of something going to happen. Full of imaginations; imaginary cares and worries. Hatching up all sorts of complaints and grievances that may happen. A good deal like ARS. *224*

Let me give you a hint in ARS. In dipsomania the sinners who have been drinking a great many drinks in a day sometimes get to that state in which they must get up during the night for a drink or they will not be able to get up in the morning. In the morning the first two or three drinks will be thrown up, but the next one will stay down; they must take a number until one sticks. They have got to that state in which they must keep on taking it. If they sleep too long the first few drinks will not stay down in the morning until they have taken a number of drinks. You will see this in lawyers who do a great amount of work on stimulants. NUX, ARS and CAPS will do something for them if they will co-operate with you. *367*

SULPH, SIL and SANG have periodic weekly headaches. ARS has a headache every two weeks. Not that these remedies will not cure other headaches, for SANG has also a headache every 3 days. The majority of headaches coming every two weeks are cured by ARS, or greatly mitigated in broken down constitutions. The attempt to cure a chronic sick headache should be made before the senile decline. *901*

You will observe this about the AGAR eyes; as the patient looks at you there is a pendulum-like action of the eyes; they go back and forth all the time; they oscillate, though he tries his best to fix his look on you. This stops only during sleep. A few other medicines have cured this symptom - CIC, ARS, SULPH, PULS, but AGAR also produces and cures it. *44*

CINA - When the head symptoms are present, the milk or water gurgles down the oesophagus with a gurgling cluck. This is present in diarrhoea or vomiting with brain symptoms. ARS and CUPR are also prominent in gurgling down the oesophagus when swallowing. 437

AESC has a great DISTURBANCE OF DIGESTION, and we can see by these symptoms that we must class it with PHOS and FERR. As soon as the patient has swallowed the food, or a little while after, it becomes sour and he eructates it, until after a while he has emptied the stomach of its contents. Such is the state of PHOS, FERR, ARS, AESC and a few other medicines.

The CADMIUM SULPH nausea is distressing. Nauseated all the way down to the abdomen, like IPECAC, ANT-T and ARS. *305*

The ARS prostration and irritable stomach occur at the beginning of the fever, with heat and restlessness. CADMIUM SULPH comes in after the fever, and with his anxiety he wants to keep still. ARS has anxiety and wants to move from bed to bed and from chair to chair, and he fears death. In CADM SULPH he seems to say, "Don't speak to me, don't bother me, let me die in peace." ***305***

SEPIA - Aversion to food, to the smell of food cooking, like COLCH and ARS............ ***921***

SULPH AC - Vomiting of drunkards in the morning (compare ARS). ***978***

CAMPH - The pain in the stomach in gastritis is so violent that the anguish on the face is equal to that of ARS, a deathly anguish is felt in the stomach and he feels that he must die. ***357***

In CAMPH acute complaints there is violent thirst, in chronic complaints thirstlessness. It is the same in ARS, in the acute thirsty but in the chronic thirstless. ***358***

MERC has a well defined dysenteric condition. Slimy, bloody stools with much straining, he feels as if he could never finish, even when no more is passing, a "NEVER GET DONE" FEELING. This is the very opposite of NUX and RHUS in DYSENTERY. These are relieved if a little stool is passed, but MERC and SULPH will sit and strain, and all the salts of MERC have the same state. MERC COR has a more violent attack, with violent urging to stool and to urinate, and intense suffering, with burning in the parts and the passage of pure blood. MERC, IPECAC and ACON are frequently indicated in epidemic dysentery that comes in HOT weather, and IPECAC, DULC and MERC are frequently indicated in the dysentery of COLD weather. You should go to the bedside of a case of dysentery with your repertory or go home and send medicine. Your first prescription should cure in epidemic dysentery, and if you work cautiously you will cure every case. It is a very simple condition to cure, but a very bad thing to get mixed up. Do not give ARS just because it conforms to the dysenteric condition, for if it does not cure it will mix up the case. Hesitate about giving ARS in dysentery until you are perfectly sure it is indicated. ***738***

PULS - Most troublesome constipation with haemorrhoids; violent pains in the haemorrhoids, worse lying down, ameliorated from gentle motion, worse from the warmth of the bed, better moving about in the open air. She becomes so nervous in a room while at rest that the pains seem intensified and she must move about. "Haemorrhoids; painful, protruding, blind, with itching and stitches in anus." The aggravation from lying down in extremely painful haemorrhoids is contrasted with AMM-C which has violently painful haemorrhoids relieved by lying flat on the back. In violently painful haemorrhoids with intense burning, think of ARS and KALI CARB. In those with sticking, tearing pains, study AESC. Looking over a number of years I have been forced to use in these cases a remedy not yet fully proven. In painful haemorrhoids in a broken down constitution, where the whole disease seems to culminate in the haemorrhoids; bleeding, protruding; a mere touch almost causes a convulsion; it causes her to scream out at the top of her voice; it is so painful that she feels that death would be a relief; she lies in bed holding the nates far apart with her hands; after every stool she has 3 or 4 hours of intense suffering. In these cases look up the PAEONY. The haemorrhoids it cures look like the flowers of the plant, they are so inflamed, so red and bleeding; oozing; tender to touch; patient is so worn out with the pain. It has many times relieved the pain and cured these enormous haemorrhoidal tumours. I have cured them after they have been operated on, and all sorts of violence done to them, without relief. Do not go to this drug if you can find a remedy that covers ALL THE PATIENT. Many patients will not confess to any other symptoms, and some of these will suffer so much from the haemorrhoids that you will really need this remedy. *867*

The NOSE, the INNER CHEST and LUNGS furnish us with localities for much trouble. The patient has had pneumonia and it has gone on to the period of infiltration; you have taken the case in this advanced stage after BRY has overcome the threatening features, and now when the patient should rally he does not rally; he perspires all over and has a strange and singular consciousness that "there is something wrong in there, a load in there;" difficult breathing; flashes of heat yet not much fever; sometimes coldness alternating with flashes of heat. I have often heard them say, "There is a great load in there doctor, I cannot get rid of it." Upon examination you find there is hepatisation and now comes the time for such remedies as PHOS, LYC and SULPH, and SULPH leads them all. When BRY has been sufficient for the earlier symptoms or when ACON has cleared them up, there has been too much for these remedies to relieve, then hepatisation comes on. If this is confined to quite a small area it will keep up quite a chronic course, but SULPH will clear it up. If however it is a double pneumonia, or the hepatisation involves a considerable portion of the lung and the remedy given has not been sufficient and the case is advancing toward a fatal issue, it may be that all at once at two or three o'clock in the morning he begins to sink; his nose is pinched; his lips are drawn, he takes on a hippocratic countenance, is covered with cold sweat, he is too feeble in every part of his body to move, he only moves his head a little in a restless manner. Unless you are called at once and give him a dose of ARS he will die. You give the ARS and you have done well, but ARS has no ability to remove the results of inflammation. But though it cannot CURE that hepatised lung it acts as a vital stimulant; it warms up the patient and makes him feel he is going to get better; but, mark this, in 24 hours he will die unless you follow the ARS with the proper remedy. You must not wait upon your remedy too long in these cases. Just as soon as he rallies, and the reaction is at its highest pitch give him the antidote and natural follower of ARS, which is SULPH, and in 24 hours that patient will say, "I am getting better." As sure as you exist today it will do just that thing. There are times that you will see clearly that PHOS is the medicine to follow ARS with. If such a patient, rallying under ARS, goes into a fever, if a hot fever comes on with burning thirst and he cannot get enough ice-cold water, you must follow it with PHOS and it will do in that case what SULPH will do in the other. *974*

CANTH - Inflammation of the lungs, gangrenous type, prostration and the lung that is affected burns like fire and immediately he expectorates cadaverous smelling expectoration, thin, bloody, watery; it has come on in an astonishingly rapid manner, and in a little while he will die; the nose is contracted, there is the hippocratic countenance, and the urine is suppressed. I remember one patient who had just come out of a prolonged drunk. I left the patient in the evening in just such a state as I have described. He was drooling a bloody saliva from his mouth and he was dying. He had had this condition come on in one night from being nearly frozen in a drunk. It would be CANTH or death before morning, but by morning he was expectorating a rusty sputum and went on to make a good recovery. ARS has the burning in the lungs and he spits up black sputum, pneumonia signs are present, with the restlessness and anxiety, and other symptoms of ARS and ARS will stop it at once. These violent remedies are needed in those cases that will die.. *363*

Vomiting of pregnancy is not cured, although it may be temporarily relieved by IPECAC, as this is a medicine that corresponds merely to the nausea itself. In a large number of instances gagging and nausea are only second or third grade symptoms in the remedy that will cure. The condition really depends upon the constitutional state and the remedy that is to cure must be a constitutional remedy. SULPH, SEP and KALI CARB are among the remedies commonly indicated. Sometimes ARS is needed. Of course, if a pregnant woman has simply disordered her stomach and has vomited bile a few times the remedy might be IPECAC. When a pregnant woman has no constitutional symptoms at all, and upon examining the case you find nothing but the nausea, overwhelming deathly nausea with continuous vomiting day and night, a single dose of SYMPHORICARPUS RACEMOSA will help. That is prescribing upon very limited information and should only be done in circumscribed or one-sided cases. It is not a long acting remedy, it is not a constitutional remedy and acts very much like IPECAC. *633*

NIT-AC - SPREADING ULCERS, the ulcers discharge a brown, bloody water, offensive. Phagedenic ulcers (ARS, AUR-M-N, CAUST, MERC-C). *800*

DULC - Eruptions upon the scalp that look so much like crusta lactaea that DULC has been found a very useful medicine. Extreme soreness, itching, and the itching is not relieved by scratching, and the scratching goes on until bleeding and rawness take place. Eruptions that come out upon the face, upon the forehead, all over the nose, but especially upon the cheeks, which become completely covered with these crusts; eczema of infants. Children only a few weeks old break out with these scalp eruptions, and DULC is one of the medicines that you will need to know. It is about as frequently indicated as any of the medicines. SEPIA, ARS, GRAPH, DULC, PETR, SULPH and CALC are about equally indicated, but of these, in this climate at least, I think SEP is probably more frequently indicated. *507*

Now in ALUM it is very important to find out whether these crusts were produced by the scratching or whether the eruption came out as an itching eruption, for in ALUM at the beginning there in no eruption, but he scratches until the skin is off and then come the crusts. You must here prescribe not for the eruption, but for the itching of the skin without eruption. Now in MEZEREUM, ARSENICUM, DOLICHOS and ALUMINA the skin itches and he scratches until it bleeds, and then he gets relief. Of course, after this there is an apparent eruption because crusts form. As soon as the healing begins the itching begins and he is only relieved when the skin is raw. With the bleeding and moisture of the skin there is relief of the itching. Now some of the books do not make the distinction between itching without eruption and itching with eruption, and hence mostly all young doctors get to thinking that itching of the skin must always be associated with eruption, and make a mistake in figuring out what kind of an eruption it is. *71*

ALUM - Induration here and there so that

it favours lupus and epithelioma in one who is subject to these swellings and eruptions. ALUMINA and ALUMEN, like ARS, LACH, SULPH and CON are medicines that relate to these troubles. Some of these have made brilliant cures where there is infiltration. *71*

NAT-C throws out eruptions apon the knuckles and finger-tips; also the toes; vesicular eruptions open up and form ulcers on the joints or finger-tips. BORAX, SEP, ARS and NAT-C are the remedies most inclined to produce ulceration of the tips and knuckles of the fingers, and also the toes.......... *763*

Carbuncles that come upon the neck and upon the back begin with a pustule, and then several come, and they are surrounded by little pustules and papules and there is pitting upon pressure. For these carbuncles you will need to study particularly ARS, ANTHR, LACH, SEC and CROT-H. They are the medicines that have in their nature malignancy and manifestation............. *477*

When a patient has urticaria at the seashore ARS will cure in ARS cases and will often mitigate when it is the only symptom. *718*

TARENT-H has cured a dry, itching eczema of the extremities and other parts of the skin after ARS and SULPH have failed. *994*

DULC - In dry, teasing coughs that are winter "colds" that go away in the summer and return in the winter. PSOR has a dry, teasing winter cough. ARS has a winter cough.. *510*

ARUM - The sneezing is like an ordinary coryza, with repeated chills over the body and aching in the bones as if the bones would break, like NUX, EUPATOR, ARN, RHUS, BRY and ARS that have aching all over during "cold"... 180

PULS - When the hay fever comes on, all the other symptoms are better, she feels nothing except the hay fever, however all the symptoms interweave with each other. The NAT MUR symptoms will be worse in the morning and until toward noon, while in PULS they are worse in the evening, the nose filling up with thick, yellowish-green, ropy mucus, and when the nose has been cleared, a dry, burning, smarting feeling remains; if the room is warm at night, she cannot sleep. NAT MUR is a little like that in the smarting and inability to sleep at night in a warm room. In NAT MUR too the discharge may continue day and night. We have an acute class in which PULS is sometimes indicated - copious watery discharge which ends in sneezing. In the beginning we will think of CARBO-VEG, ARS, ALL-C, EUPH. With CARBO-VEG there is a watery discharge and the irritation extends into the chest, with hoarseness and rawness. In ALL-C we have one group of symptoms that points to this remedy. Excoriating discharge from the nose and bland discharge from the eyes; in the larynx, sensation as if hooks were there, and sometimes this extends below the larynx; this always means ALL-C; it is also worse in a warm room like PULS. The EUPH looks like ALL-C, only the discharge from the eyes is copious, watery and burning - the lachrymation burns the eyes and excoriates the cheeks; discharge from nose is bland like PULS. Sometimes this goes into the chest, then it is no longer EUPH. IOD is worse in a warm room; thick discharge from the nose which burns and excoriates and is yellowish-green; but there is one thing that differentiates it from all the others - the patient immediately begins to emaciate when the complaint comes on and is very hungry.

KALI HYDR with the thick yellowish discharge, worse in a warm room, there is a great amount of rawness and burning in the nose; external nose very sore to pressure; sensitiveness in the root of the nose; whole face aches and patient is very restless; wants to walk in the open air which does not fatigue him. ARS IOD; anxiety, restlessness and weakness; frequent sneezing and copious watery nasal discharge that burns the lip. Burning, watery discharge from the eyes like ARS. ARS wants to be very warm; wants hot water applied to the eyes; the only relief is from sniffing hot water up the nose. ARS IOD is worse in a warm room, and for days after sneezing the discharge thickens and becomes gluey, looking like THICK, YELLOW HONEY, this excoriates; much pain through the root of the nose and eyes; often rawness in the chest with dyspnoea. The remedies having the dyspnoea are ARSENIC, ARS IOD, IODINE, KALI HYDR and SABADILLA; these are the ones I have found most frequently indicated in the asthmatic forms of hay fever. If the complaint has been developed after being overheated about that time, you will find that SILICA, PULSATILLA and CARBO VEG must be carefully compared. There is another class of remedies having the stuffing up of the nose not relieved by the discharge. There is a constant desire to blow the nose, yet he gets no relief. This makes me think of LACH, KALI BI, PSOR, NAJA and STICTA. PSORINUM has the copious, watery, bland discharge from the nose, it may be excoriating, it has both. The stuffing up of the nose generally takes place in the open air; he is relieved in a warm, close room and by lying down; has some dyspnoea which is relieved by stretching the arms at right angles to the body. Hay fever is a psoric sickness. PSORINUM given in a single dose will so develop the symptoms that the case will be more clear. The attack is not the best thing to prescribe for. If it is too violent, a short acting remedy may be selected that will mitigate it. NUX VOMICA has a free, easy breathing in the open air, but when he goes into the warm room his nose stuffs up, which also occurs at night, though the water drips on the pillow yet he stuffs up like PULS, BRY and the IODINE preparations, ARS IOD and CYCLAMEN. Do not understand me to have given remedies for hay fever, we cannot lay down remedies for diseases. The whole constitution must be most carefully examined. ***863***

SABAD - HAY FEVER, when there is spasmodic sneezing, fluent coryza; nostrils stuffed up; inspirations through nose laboured; snoring; itching in the nose; profuse bleeding from the nose; bright red blood comes from the posterior nares and is expectorated; very sensitive to the smell of garlic; coryza with severe frontal pains and redness of the eyelids; violent sneezing; copious watery discharge from the nose. A peculiar kind of itching coming on in some hay fevers is an itching in the roof of the mouth, on the soft palate, and for relief the patient must draw the tongue back and forth over the soft palate with this coryza, sneezing etc. WYETHIA will cut this attack short. When the itching extends to the larynx and trachea with great irritability and sensitive to cold: NUX VOM. When the discharge burns a red streak over the upper lip and about the wings of the nose, with sneezing and profuse watery nasal discharge ARS. Copious acrid lachrymation, and copious bland flow from the nose with sneezing: EUPHRASIA. Copious bland watery discharge from the eyes and copious acrid watery discharge from the nose: ALLIUM CEPA. But these are not the constitutional remedies; they do not cure, but only palliate during the severe attacks. These symptoms are the outcome of the psoric constitution, and this constitution must be treated by antipsorics. Sometimes the hay fever is so severe that it seems to be the only manifestation of psora in the patient, but if it is restrained or stopped up by bad treatment he is not well during the whole year. Many a time the hay fever goes through the whole winter and only by constitutional upbuilding can it be mitigated. But with constitutional treatment each yearly attack is lighter, and at the end of treatment he is able to live in his own climate unaffected. He must not go to the mountains to mitigate it. If to any place, he should go where the affection would be worse, so that all its manifestations would be apparent. The hay fever will only be cured if the PATIENT is curable, but if not, if his condition is so broken down that he is incurable, his hay fever will not be cured. *894*

RUMEX is one of the most valuable palliatives in advanced phthisis; it will often carry a case through another winter. With RUMEX, PULSATILLA, SENEGA, ARS and NUX VOM you can patch up the last years of a phthisical patient. You will see ACETIC ACID recommended for the diarrhoea in phthisis. You had better let such conditions alone, unless they are very marked. If the diarrhoea is very exhausting use some simple medicine, like this one (RUMEX) to slack it up. But the phthisical patient is better off with a little diarrhoea, a loose morning stool. It is the same with the night sweats; if he does not have them he will have something more violent.The allopath stops the diarrhoea and night sweats and then has to feed morphine to his patient because of the consequent sufferings.The more you undertake to relieve these outward conditions, these vents, the more harm you will do the patient, and if you go on you will have to abandon your homoeopathy and give morphine, which is really a crime. You will remove the sore, bruised aching all over the body of a consumptive by ARN, and it will suit the cough and gagging and retching and make him sleep. Later PYR may be needed for the aching in the bones and distressing cough. You patch him up year after year. Sometimes ARS is the remedy, and it has to be more frequently repeated; sometimes it is LYC, PULS, PYR or ARN. These medicines help him along, and they have often to be changed, but finally the breakdown occurs, and these medicines are no longer suitable. An awful dyspnoea gradually creeps on the patient; there is craving for air; the breathing space is becoming diminished. Dropsy comes on in the extremities. The heart gives out; there is emaciation; the hippocratic countenance is seen; there is cold sweat, blue face, sinking. Even now we can palliate with TARENT-C. Sometimes it has to be repeated. It will relieve for days and give a euthanasia, not a stupefaction as produced by morphine, benumbing the senses, but an actual comforting. *888*

MAG CARB is especially useful if the history has been a tubercular one. Losing flesh and craving meat in those who are tubercular, or in those that are from tubercular parents. There are persons who have simply this tendency who go along year after year in this withered state, with the little hacking cough, not rousing up into much. Finally some favourable circumstance arises and the tuberculosis comes on rapidly after it has remained in a sluggish state for a long time. There are a few remedies more likely to be associated with that condition than any others — ARS, CALC, LYC, MAG CARB and TUB. They fit into this lingering state, this prelude to active phthisis. They sometimes set a patient thriving, but, mind you, these cases are hard cases to manage. They are difficult to find remedies for. Their trouble is so latent, the symptoms do not come out, and sometimes you will have to read between the lines. They are the one sided cases spoken of by Hahnemann. *716*

SENEGA has sometimes cured pleuro-pneumonia when there was the extreme exhaustion of PHOSPHORUS and ARSENICUM. In such cases SENEGA has caused reaction; it has such weakness. Especially is it suited in the advanced cases of phthisis; it acts as a palliative. It does excellent patchwork without serious aggravation as it relates more especially to superficial conditions. It is not as deep acting as SULPH and SIL. We give such remedies only when we have a reasonable assurance that we can cure, when the patient is yet curable. But when we have given up all hope, then we pay more attention to the most painful parts; we pay more attention to the local symptoms, to the group which causes the most suffering, and attempt to do patchwork. If the sufferings in the chest and the exhaustion become most severe it is true that ARS will patch him up a little and make him feel more like life, and he will go on to the end with more comfort. If the pains in the chest are most severe such medicines as SENEGA or BRY will help him; if he is sore and feels as if bruised and he must move from side to side ARN will relieve; but these are not the remedies to go deep into the life and eradicate a deep-seated disease like phthisis. Yet with these one may take a consumptive patient in comfort to the very grave, by simply patching him up and prescribing for his immediate sufferings. *916*

When treating a low form of continued fever with extreme prostration ARS, MUR-AC and PHOS-AC force themselves upon the mind. With ARS there has been the anxious restlessness; with PHOS-AC there has been the mental prostration and then the muscular weakness; and with MUR-AC the muscular weakness comes first, and there has been history of restlessness and the mind has been stronger than could be expected. With this great muscular exhaustion, with jaw hanging down and the patient sliding down in bed and soon the involuntary stool and urine, MUR-AC is forced upon the mind. Paralytic weakness is what it must be called. Soon the tongue is paralysed, as well as the sphincters of the bladder and rectum. It seems to be eminently fitted for the lowest forms of zymotic fever when the above symptoms are present. He finally becomes unconscious. There has been some restlessness, but nothing like ARS and RHUS TOX. He refuses to talk because it frets him to do so. PHOS-AC is slow answering questions because of exhaustion of mind which makes him unable to think. *752*

ANT-CRUD has all the prostration of typhoid, and it has the continued type of fever as well as the intermittent and remittent. The prostration is similar to ARS, but ARS has overwhelming fear of death, whereas this remedy has loathing of life; and so they both part company. ARS has overwhelming restlessness, this remedy is seldom restless. ARS has an immense thirst, this remedy is thirstless. So even though both these medicines have excessive exhaustion with continued fever, we see they have features dissimilar enough to make them wholly distinct. *105*

Is it any wonder that Hahnemann predicted that VERAT, CAMPH and CUPR would become remedies in the cure of cholera? he saw in their nature the ability to cure. He saw the similitude. In cases of this sort which are characterised by superabundance of cramps, CUPRUM is the simillimum. For those with coldness, blueness and scanty sweat, vomiting and purging, CAMPH is the remedy. These are called "dry cholera", they sink down and die without exhaustive discharges. In proportion as there are coldness, blueness and scanty discharges CAMPH is indicated. In proportion as copiousness, coldness, blueness are present VERAT is indicated. SEC has something of cholera in it. PODO has exhaustive stools; ARS anxious restlessness. ***1010***

It is not an uncommon thing for a malarial fever that has lingered a long time to be attended with swelling of the lower limbs. EUP-PER very strongly competes with NAT MUR, CHINA and ARS in such lingering malaria. When the symptoms have largely subsided and left only this state of anaemia and dropsy of the lower extremities, in the badly treated cases, it is very difficult to find what medicines to administer, and the course that the homoeopath must pursue is to go back and examine the patient to find the symptoms he had at the time of the intermittent fever, before he was meddled with. If now there is swelling of the extremities and yet symptoms to show you that he needed EUP PER in the beginning, EUP PER will still cure the dropsy of the extremities. It may bring back the chill, it may bring back an orderly state that you can prescribe on. If in the beginning he needed ARS, that remedy will bring back the chill, turn it right end to, and cure his symptoms. The trouble is that the symptoms were only suppressed, had not been cured. So the medicine he needed, but has never had for the chill, may be the medicine he needs now. Then think of EUP PER in dropsical swellings of the feet and ankles, and in gouty swellings also. The gouty swellings are all of an inflammatory character. Very commonly these are closely related to hydrarthrosis, and here EUP PER is to be compared with ARS. ***515***

SULPH is not so suitable in the cases that come on with rapidity and great violence, with vesicles and enormous blebs, but it suits those cases in which there is first an appearance of a mottled dusky red spot on the face, and a little distance from it another spot and then another, and these, as it were, all run together, and after a week or so it develops into a sluggish erysipelatous state, and the veins seem to be distended, and he is passing into a state towards unconsciousness. You will be astonished to see what SULPH will do in such a case, which comes slowly as if there were a lack of vitality to develop it, a slow, sluggish erysipelatous inflammation. Whereas if it be ARS, APIS or RHUS-TOX it spreads with rapidity. ARS and APIS burn like fire, and RHUS has blisters upon the erysipelatous patches. ***967***

ARSENICUM IODATUM

PULS - When the hay fever comes on, all the other symptoms are better, she feels nothing except the hay fever, however, all the symptoms interweave with each other. The NAT MUR symptoms will be worse in the morning and until toward noon, while in PULS they are worse in the evening, the nose filling up with thick, yellowish-green, ropy mucus, and when the nose has been cleared, a dry, burning, smarting feeling remains; if the room is warm at night she cannot sleep. NAT MUR is a little like that in the smarting and inability to sleep at night in a warm room. In NAT MUR too, the discharge may continue day and night. We have an acute class in which PULS is sometimes indicated - copious watery discharge which ends in sneezing. In the beginning we will think of CARBO-VEG, ARS, ALL-C, EUPH. With CARBO-VEG there is a watery discharge and the irritation extends into the chest, with hoarseness and rawness. In ALL-C we have one group of symptoms that points to this remedy. Excoriating discharge from the nose and bland discharge from the eyes; in the larynx, sensation as if hooks were there, and sometimes this extends below the larynx; this always means ALL-C; it is also worse in a warm room like PULS. The EUPH looks like ALL-C, only the discharge from the eyes is copious, watery and burning - the lachrymation burns the eyes and excoriates the cheeks; discharge from nose is bland like PULS. Sometimes this goes into the chest, then it is no longer EUPH. IOD is worse in a warm room; thick discharge from the nose which burns and excoriates and is yellowish-green; but there is one thing that differentiates it from all the others - the patient immediately begins to emaciate when the complaint comes on and is very hungry. KALI HYDR with the thick yellowish discharge, worse in a warm room, there is a great amount of rawness and burning in the nose; external nose very sore to pressure; sensitiveness in the root of the nose; whole face aches and patient is very restless; wants to walk in the open air which does not fatigue him. ARS IOD; anxiety, restlessness and weakness; frequent sneezing and copious watery nasal discharge that burns the lip. Burning, watery discharge from the eyes like ARS. ARS wants to be very warm; wants hot water applied to the eyes; the only relief is from sniffing hot water up the nose. ARS IOD is worse in a warm room and after days of sneezing the discharge thickens and becomes gluey, looking like THICK, YELLOW HONEY, this excoriates; much pain through the root of the nose and eyes; often rawness in the chest with dyspnoea. The remedies having the dyspnoea are ARSENIC, IODIDE OF ARSENIC, IODINE, KALI HYDR and SABADILLA; these are the ones I have found most frequently indicated in the asthmatic forms of hay fever. If the complaint has been developed after being overheated about that time, you will find that SILICA, PULSATILLA and CARBO VEG must be carefully compared. There is another class of remedies having the stuffing up of the nose not relieved by the discharge. There is a constant desire to blow the nose, yet he gets no relief. This makes me think of LACH, KALI BI, PSOR, NAJA and STICTA. PSORINUM has the copious, watery, bland discharge from the nose, it may be excoriating, it has both. The stuffing up of the nose generally takes place in the open air; he is relieved in a warm, close room and by lying down; has some dyspnoea which is relieved by stretching the arms at right angles to the body. Hay fever is a psoric sickness. PSORINUM given in a single dose will so develop the symptoms that the case will be more clear. The attack is not the best thing to prescribe for. If it is too violent, a short acting remedy may be selected that will mitigate it. NUX VOMICA has a free, easy breathing in the open air, but when he goes into the warm room his nose stuffs up, which also occurs at night, though the water drips on the pillow yet he stuffs up like PULS, BRY and the IODINE preparations, IODIDE OF ARSENIC and CYCLAMEN. Do not understand me to have given remedies for hay fever, we cannot lay down remedies for diseases. The whole constitution must be most carefully examined. ***863***

ARUM

BELL — The temperature I described among the generals as being so marked, so intense that you will carry it with you for hours after you have touched a BELL case. It differs wholly from the APIS case, which has a rough rash. BELL is smooth and shining. APIS wants to be cool, wants to be uncovered, BELL wants to be warm, wants a warm room; APIS has no thirst to speak of; in BELL it is the exception to have no thirst, generally thirsty for water, a little and often. The intense dryness of the mucous membranes and skin. Coldness of the extremities with hot head. In ARUM TRIPHYLLUM there is a constant picking of the mouth, with suppressed or scanty urine; pale surface, only here and there a little rash; the itching of the fingers, toes, nose and lips will lead you to prescribe ARUM. You remember the BAPT case, with that mental state where he is feeling all over the bed "to get the pieces together". On the other hand where there is no rash to speak of, now and then a patch enough to make a diagnosis, or the diagnosis is made from someone else having the disease in the family, the child is swallowing ice water, but vomiting it up when it gets warm in the stomach, who would not give PHOS? So it is at the bedside we pick out the distinguishing things and see that these remedies are not at all alike. *254*

The record of AIL in scarlet fever makes it worthy of further study; it ought to be reproved that we may have a fuller understanding of it. "Eruption plentiful, of a bluish tint. Typhoid scarlatina." "Eruption is slow to make its appearance, remains livid." "Body and limbs covered with an irregular patchy eruption of a very livid colour." Here you see but one type of scarlet fever. This low type of fever sometimes needs SULPH or PHOS or BELL or BAPT or LACH. That you may be able to distinguish one from another and keep the picture of each remedy clearly in mind requires a prolonged study of the Materia Medica. It is an easy matter to compare remedies for yourself after you have first studied each one separately. You can then bring out many comparisons, and especially in this case at the bedside. If you go to the bedside with a good knowledge of the generals of Materia Medica you will be surprised at the number of symptom pictures which will come into your mind, called up by the signs of the sickness. When you go to the bedside of scarlet fever you should not call to mind the names of these medicines which you may have heard recommended for scarlet fever; let the appearance of the patient bring to mind such remedies as appear like the patient, regardless of whether they have been associated with scarlet fever or not. When you see the rash perhaps you will say that looks like an ACON rash, but there is such scanty zymosis in the nature of ACON that it is no longer thought of. BELL is not suitable, for in that remedy the rash is shiny or smooth, the typical Sydenham rash. On the other hand you will say PULS has a measly rash, and often associated with a low form of fever, but not so low as the typhoid type, so PULS goes out of your mind. You now think of the remedies that are typical of all zymotic states; the prostration, the aggravation after sleep, general stupor and delirium, and almost at a glance you see LACH, the type of such forms of disease. Its picture comes into your mind speedily. You see another case of scarlet fever where there is a scanty rash, the child before you keeps picking the skin from the lips and nose, lies in a state of pallor and exhaustion, no rash to speak of, urine nearly suppressed; almost in a moment you think of ARUM TRIPH. It is the aspect of things which will call the remedy to mind. In another case you will have all the purple appearance I have spoken of in AIL; horrible foetor, a good deal of sore throat, and the child cannot get water cold enough, wants a stream of water running down the throat all the time; you may safely trust to PHOS. In these low types of sickness there is always something to tell the story, if you will only listen, study and wait long enough. *52*

ASAFOETIDA

MOSCH cures many hysterical girls who have come to adult age without ever learning what obedience means. They are self-willed, obstinate and selfish. When they have been encouraged to resort to crafty cunning to have every whim gratified from infancy to eighteen years of age, they become fit subjects for MOSCH, ASAF, IGN and VALER. *750*

STAPH - Nightly bone pains. ASAF, MERC, SIL. *948*

ASARUM

LAC-C - An oversensitive state prevails, a general hyperaesthesia of the skin and all parts. It makes women violently hysterical and causes all sorts of strange and apparently impossible symptoms. For example, a woman lay in bed for days with the fingers abducted and would go wild if they would touch each other. The fingers were not aggravated from hard pressure but she would scream if they touched. This state is difficult to cure outside of LAC-C and LACH. LACH has produced similar conditions. The sensitiveness of the abdomen so that the sheet cannot be permitted to touch the skin belongs to both. Another strange state is a peculiar vertigo, a condition when walking, in which she seems to be floating in mid-air, or when lying as if she were not on the bed. Other remedies have this. The sensation as if floating or not touching the bed, or sinking down, belongs to LACH. The sensation of gliding when walking is strong under ASARUM EUROPEUM. *675*

AURUM

It is peculiar that medicines come around on time with an exactitude. Diseases do the same thing, and we must see that it is also peculiar that they come with a regular cycle, a regular periodicity. We meet with headaches that come every 7 days, headaches that come once in every two weeks, and there are remedies that have 7 day aggravations and 14 day aggravations and 3 day aggravations, remedies that bring out their symptoms just in this form. Do not be surprised when your patient is perfectly under the influence of AUR if he has a characteristic aggravation every 21 days. There are quite a number of remedies having 14 day aggravations, eg. CHINA and ARS. Again there are autumnal aggravations, spring aggravations, winter aggravations, aggravations from cold weather, and aggravations in the summer from heat. Some remedies have both the latter. *516*

It is a strange thing to see a bright little girl of 8 or 9 years old taking on sadness, melancholy and commencing to talk of the future world and the angels and that she wants to die and go there, and she is sad and wants to read the Bible all day. That is a strange thing; and yet CALC has cured that. ARS has cured that state, and also LACH. They are a little inclined to be precocious, and they have attended the Sunday school and have taken too seriously the things they have learned there. Children sad and unhappy, and old people who take on a loathing of life, become weary of life. That is a good deal like AURUM. I explained that, and dwelt on it, that the highest love is love of life, and when an individual ceases to love his own life and is weary of it and wants to die he is on the borderland of insanity. In fact that is an insanity of the will...... ***319***

IGN has another thing - "thinks she has neglected some duty." That is very much like PULS, HELL and HYOS. Only AURUM believes that she has committed a great wrong. ***596***

When able to be about the HELL patient often appears to be sad, because she sits and says nothing, and seems to be in a woeful mood. But there is not that great lamentation, with walking the floor and wringing the hands that we find in AURUM. It is an apathetic state, she appears to be sad and melancholic, whereas perhaps she does little thinking. ***567***

CYCL - Sadness, as if she had wronged somebody (AUR). ***495***

ASAF - "Feeling as if the nose stopped high up, as if he could not breathe through it, with fulness of the head, while riding in a carriage." (AUR, AUR-M). ***185***

There is one class of patients you will find who will trouble you. Those cases that come into your office with puffed, venous, purple faces; they have an appearance of plethora; the face looks puffed, bloated and dropsical at times; it is a dark red, dusky face; such a face we shall cure sometimes with ASAFOETIDA. CARBO AN, AURUM, CARBO VEG and PULSATILLA are also related to this kind of face, but it is a very troublesome kind of face, it shows more or less cardiac disturbance and venous stasis. The venous side of the heart will often be involved, or about to be involved, when you have this kind of face. I never like to see them come into my office for they are hard cases to manage. ***183***

KALMIA - "Wandering rheumatic pains in the region of the heart." "When articular rheumatism has been treated externally and cardiac symptoms ensue." Rheumatism that goes from the lower to the upper limbs. Not uncommonly you will meet such things. These "rubbers" that go around the streets with a strong liniment and considerable magnetism frequently cause a rheumatism to leave the knee joint and, when it does that, the heart is likely to be the organ that suffers. Then KALMIA, AURUM, BRYONIA, RHUS-TOX, LEDUM, CALC, ABROTANUM and sometimes CACTUS are remedies that prove suitable for such cardiac affections. ***670***

AURUM MURIATICUM

ASAF — "Feeling as if the nose stopped high up, as if he could not breathe through it, with fulness of the head while riding in a carriage." (AUR, AUR-M). ***185***

AUR-M-N

CARBO AN — Chronic induration with enlargement of the uterus, which gradually grows from year to year (AUR-M-N). ***370***

NIT-AC — SPREADING ULCERS - The ulcers discharge a brown, bloody water, offensive. Phagedenic ulcers (ARS, AUR-M-N, CAUST, MERC-C). ***800***

BADIAGA

ARG NIT — Here is a striking feature. "Patient cannot lie on the RIGHT side because it brings on so much palpitation." We have plenty of remedies with palpitation worse from lying on the left side, but remedies with palpitation worse lying on the right side are rare (ALUMN, BAD, KALM, KALI NIT, LIL TIG, PLAT, SPONG). This is uncommon, strange, rare and peculiar. ***138***

BAPTISIA

PYR — The sore bruised condition is as marked as in ARN and BAPT; the aching in the bones like EUPATORIUM, the restlessness, ameliorated by motion and heat like RHUS. ***871***

MANG — Everywhere there is soreness to touch and soreness from jarring. The bones are sore from walking. ARN relieves only a day or two; but in MANG it is deep-seated and prolonged, and we would not think of ARN or BAPT, which would only give relief for a day or so. ***722***

PYR — Irritable. Delirium and confusion of mind about his body and limbs (BAPT). Sensation as if he covered the whole bed. Knew her head was on the pillow, but did not know where the rest of the body was. Feels when lying on one side she is one person, and another when turning on the other side. Sensation as though crowded with arms and legs. These symptoms are much like BAPTISIA, but if the temperature runs very high BAPT will not meet the condition so well as PYR. ***872***

In regard to the lips and the lower part of the face, that bloated, swollen condition, the sluggish circulation, a venous congestion or stasis will be found in BRY, making the aspect as one of long intoxicated. It is not so marked as in BAPT, and is not accompanied by so low a state, so advanced a stupor as in BAPT. ***284***

AIL — The countenance is purple and besotted, there eyes are congested and there is even bleeding from the eyes. There is an appearance of great prostration, but it is really stupefaction; he seems stupid and benumbed. If you look at the throat you see it is covered with little purple patches, intermingled with an oedematous appearance similar to that found in BAPT. ***49***

In cases of typhoid where there is the confusion like that found in BAPT and the heat too intense for that remedy, PYR should always be considered. ***871***

The record of AIL in scarlet fever makes it worthy of further study; it ought to be reproved that we may have a fuller understanding of it. "Eruption plentiful, of a bluish tint. Typhoid scarlatina." "Eruption is slow to make its appearance, remains livid." "Body and limbs covered with an irregular patchy eruption of a very livid colour." Here you see but one type of scarlet fever. This low type of fever sometimes needs SULPH or PHOS or BELL or BAPT or LACH. That you may be able to distinguish one from another and keep the picture of each remedy clearly in mind requires a prolonged study of the Materia Medica. It is an easy matter to compare remedies for yourself after you have first studied each one separately. You can then bring out many comparisons and especially in this case at the bedside. If you go to the bedside with a good knowledge of the generals of Materia

Medica you will be surprised at the number of symptom pictures which will come into your mind, called up by the signs of the sickness. When you go to the bedside of scarlet fever you should not call to mind the names of these medicines which you may have heard recommended for scarlet fever; let the appearance of the patient bring to mind such remedies as appear like the patient, regardless of whether they have been associated with scarlet fever or not. When you see the rash perhaps you will say that looks like an ACON rash, but there is such scanty zymosis in the nature of ACON that it is no longer thought of. BELL is not suitable, for in that remedy the rash is shiny or smooth, the typical Sydenham rash. On the other hand you will say PULS has a measly rash, and often associated with a low form of fever, but not so low as the typhoid type, so PULS goes out of your mind. You now think of the remedies that are typical of all zymotic states; the prostration, the aggravation after sleep, general stupor and delirium, and almost at a glance you see LACH, the type of such forms of disease. Its picture comes into your mind speedily. You see another case of scarlet fever where there is a scanty rash, the child before you keeps picking the skin from the lips and nose, lies in a state of pallor and exhaustion, no rash to speak of, urine nearly suppressed; almost in a moment you think of ARUM TRIPH. It is the aspect of things which will call the remedy to mind. In another case you will have all the purple appearance I have spoken of in AIL; horrible foetor, a good deal of sore throat, and the child cannot get water cold enough, wants a stream of water running down the throat all the time; you may safely trust to PHOS. In these low types of sickness there is always something to tell the story, if you will only listen, study and wait long enough. *52*

BARYTA CARBONICA

An adult takes on the ways of child, as a state of imbecility. This mental state is especially found under BARYTA CARB in adults who have never developed beyond childhood, who have always remained children. A person reasons like a child, talks like a child, whimpers like a child, cries like a child, wants to be petted like a child; so it is in BARYTA CARB. We find this state of mind in children who have developed epilepsy, but we do not prescribe this remedy on account of the epilepsy; the child has not developed properly, and the epilepsy is only one of the manifestations. The cause is far back, and is really the psoric condition. Thereby the mental state has not developed, the child has not grown into a man or woman in intellectual attainments or wisdom and remains as a whimpering, screaming child. This lack of development is found in BUFO and BARYTA CARB; they are related to each other in that the child-like state remains while the body grows old. We see in these medicines the fear and simplicity that belongs to the child; always sickly, deficient, never reaching adult fullness or growth, always a child. "How much like a child that woman appears." or "How much like a child that man is." We say that of some old people, they are so childish. The old routinists have said of those people who are prematurely old or who have taken on senility, that they need BARYTA CARB. BUFO also stands out in bold type for those prematurely senile; the man at fifty who acts like an old broken-down man of eighty; he has lost all he had 5 or 6 years ago, and has taken on a childish simplicity and innocence, an appearance of imbecility. This is when we think of BUFO. BARYTA CARB has hitherto been the leading one, but BUFO is very important also. *292*

If the head bones are slow in forming, or do not keep pace with the growth of the child, CALC PHOS is often called for. Where the child is losing flesh, slow learning to do things, slow learning to walk, or the legs are not strong enough to support the body, or it is behind in mental development, CALC PHOS is one to be examined (like BARYTA CARB, BORAX, PHOS AC, NAT-M, CALC-C). *334*

ZINC is not suitable in those who are naturally feeble-minded, when the child is in a state bordering on idiocy. BAR-C feeds such a mind. *1014*

If you have ever been going through a place where there are cobwebs and a little cobweb has strung across your face you will know what a peculiar sensation of crawling it produces, and you cannot leave it alone until it is removed. That sensation particularly belongs to ALUM, BORAX and BAR-C. *71*

ALUMEN cures young children growing up with enormously enlarged and very hard tonsils, in whom every cold settles in the throat. ALUMEN is one of the cognates of BAR-C, which has the same tendency. In one patient there will be one kind of constitution, and after thorough examining, it looks like BAR-C. You may have a different constitution in another patient, and after carefully examining it, see that it looks like ALUMEN; another you will see is SULPH; another, if you look into it carefully, you will find is CALC, and another CALC-IOD, and so on, among those remedies capable of bringing about the conditions described. If we can find symptoms which picture the constitutional state we have no trouble. When the symptoms have been well gathered the case is as good as cured; it is then easy to find a remedy.................... *62*

CALC-F — Large indurated tonsils will be cured after BAR-C has failed. *330*

CALC-P — Every cold settles in the tonsils (BARYTA CARB, ALUMEN). *336*

SIL — The parotids enlarge from every cold and get hard (BAR-C, CALC, SULPH)..... .... *928*

SIL likes ice cream, ice water and feels comfortable when it is in the stomach; it is sometimes impossible for him to drink hot fluids, they cause sweat about the face and head and cause hot flushes (BAR-C).... *931*

SIL — Enlarged abdomen in children and adults (BAR-C). *932*

BARYTA IODATA

BAR-C has cured various kinds of dim-sightedness, especially in those that have a hazy cornea, a slight opacity of the cornea (BAR IOD) so that things look hazy, "looking as through a fog, or through smoke." .. *225*

CALC has cured many cases of opacity of the cornea (BAR IOD)............................... *323*

BARYTA MURIATICA

BAR-C — Knots of lymphatic glands down the neck under the ears (BAR-M, TUB). *225*

BAR-C — There are a few remedies that have, in such high degree, this coarse rattling in the chest of old people, that it is well to emphasise it. BAR-C is one of them. SENEGA, AMMONIACUM and BARYTA MURIATICA should be compared. When there is coarse rattling in the chest all the time in an old person, an octogenarian, who is pretty comfortable in summer, but miserable all winter from the coarse rattling in the chest, and there are no other symptoms, AMMONIACUM will keep him comfortable. *226*

BELLADONNA

One of the most important things to decide when we are going into the mental state of a remedy is whether we shall use this remedy in hysteria, in the delirium of the various phases of fever, or in insanity, and to ascertain this we turn to that part of the proving which gives us the pace of the remedy. If we want to understand the delirium of BELL and BRY, to see which one would be suitable in a certain case, we turn to the febrile action of the remedy and see what the nature of that is; the pace tells us largely what kind of delirium, if we do not know from the delirium itself. So we will see that in BELL there is no continued fever, and as a remedy must in its very nature be adapted to the very nature of the disease, it would be useless to follow the many injunctions that are written in our books telling us to give BELL in the acute form of delirium in typhoid fever; but BRY has just that condition; hence we will see that BRY is useful in such cases which present symptoms similar to it; because the pace of the disease is similar to the pace of BRY, which has a continued fever. BELL has intermittent and remittent fever, and hence the acute delirium of BELL is similar to the acute delirium of remittent fever. Now to bring this point to bear, CALADIUM's fever is a continued fever; it has no great amount of fever in it, but it is a continued fever, we shall see that there is coma and stupor from fever, "delirium, unintelligible murmuring,", mental prostration. This remedy is suitable in low, murmuring, exhaustive cases of typhoid fever, cases that are running a very sluggish course; not a very active delirium, but muttering; a low form of semi-consciousness, very often coma or stupefaction like PHOS AC, a dazed mind. *307*

CALC is a medicine for CHRONIC SORE THROATS. The throat appearance itself is not always sufficient to prescribe on, but the complaints in the throat are those that come on in persons taking cold so frequently that the patient has not time to get over one before he goes into another, and this engrafts upon him a chronic sore throat. It may in the beginning be a BELL sore throat, which is quite likely, but before he gets over it he has taken another cold. Remember that this is a part of the CALC patient, that he takes cold so easily, he takes cold from every draught, from every exposure, and from damp weather. When getting over a BELL sore throat — about the time he thinks he is over it he takes a new cold. Perhaps it has been relieved two or three times with BELL, and then it settles down into a chronic state, and there are little red patches, perhaps little ulcers, in the throat. This extends all over. It extends to the roof of the mouth, with a sore tongue and a constant dry choking feeling in the pharynx, covering the tonsils and extending up into the posterior nares filling them with thick yellow mucus. Chronic inflammation. The uvula may be puffed, swollen. Parts swollen, red, tumid," but in patches. The throat very painful on swallowing, dry, choking feeling. *325*

In BRY the eyes are red and congested, he is listless, does not want to move, to speak, or to do anything, because all of these things are motion, are efforts and they make him worse. You will see that this is also true in BELL; it has all of this congestion and pressure. But remember BRY is slow, sluggish, passive and insidious in its approach and progress whereas in BELL the mental symptoms and everything in connection are marked by activity. *281*

The process of inflammation in BROM is slow; they are not that violent, rapid kind like we find in BELL and MERC. *271*

HYOS — Now to give you some idea as to the grading of this general type of insanity it should be compared with STRAM and BELL. You heard in the lecture on BELL that it is violent, its fever most intense. There is much excitement. In STRAM, when we reach that, you will see that his delirium, his insanity, is expressed in terms of extreme violence. These three run so close together that something can be brought out by associating them together. When considering HYOS in its mental state it is well to realise that it seldom has much fever in its insanity. It has a fever sometimes in the low form, but when HYOS is thought of in relation to the febrile state the intensity of the heat would be in this order: BELL, STRAM, HYOS. Now, BELL is very hot in its mental states, STRAM is most violent and active, murderously violent, is moderately hot in its fever, as a rule. HYOS has a low fever, sometimes none at all, with its insanity. When one comes to take into consideration the violence of its delirium, or the maniacal actions, then it changes the order. The order as to violence of conduct would be: STRAM, BELL, HYOS. That brings you to see that even when associated with those medicines that look most like it, it is at the bottom of the list. It goes as a passive medicine, while the upper ones are more active. *582*

Even early in the disease HELLEBORE lacks the wildness and acute delirium found in STRAMONIUM and BELLADONNA... *566*

In BELL especially, and also in many of those medicines that have this nature of cramping and constricting and contracting of circular fibres, there is convulsive tendency. The violent congestion of the brain in BELL will commonly be attended with cramps in the extremities and convulsions of the muscles all over, or in parts. Not so under CACT. Violent congestion, and he goes stupid under it. *299*

PSOR — Febrile state. Intermittents, bilious fever, fever from a cold. The patient is so hot that the hand under the covers feels as though in a steam bath and the sensation of heat causes one to draw it back. It is not the dry heat of BELL, yet it is as intense. It is a steam. He is covered with a boiling sweat in fevers. Head and body hot, and hot air beneath the covers, (OPIUM has this, but it is in a violent congestion to the head, an apoplectic condition). *856*

CACT has the violent congestion of the head found in BELL, but with BELL we have the intense heat of the body, fever heat, which is not found in CACT. In CACT it is only a moderate fever. The heat is in the upper part of the body, in the head and neck. Fulness of the neck; bloating of the neck. Feels as if the head would expand from the pressure of blood in the head, but without any great rise of temperature. It has fever, but it has these without fever. But with BELL, when you have these pulsations, the patient is immensely hot, and he burns all over. There is some burning in CACT, but not to be compared with BELL. *301*

CIC — Head hot and extremities cold, like BELL, in its convulsions. *435*

COCC — Extreme irritability of the nervous system. The least noise or jar is unbearable. You have that BELL is worse from a jar. So is COCC, and quite like BELL. COCC is also like BELL in its sleeplessness and other general conditions. *449*

COFF — "Neuralgic toothache entirely relieved by holding cold water in the mouth, returning as it becomes warm. Toothache during the menstrual period. Complaints of anaemic children during dentition." Those nervous, excitable children that talk to the mother and the nurse very rapidly with brilliant eyes, red face, cannot go to sleep. It will quiet the patient and actually favour the growth of the tooth in a painless manner. That is the description of a nervous child with many nervous brain and mental troubles. This child is extremely sensitive; it takes cold. The routine prescriber gives BELL to a child who has hot head, hot face, and throbbing carotids, and when it does not help he gives more BELL and increases the size of his dose until the child has a proving. He makes a BELL child out of it when COFF would have cured it. In most instances where BELL is indicated the child is sluggish and would like to sleep. With COFF there is excitement. ***457***

A feature of infancy is the following: Child may not have diarrhoea, may even be constipated, but it lies in bed and rolls the head in sleep. BELL and APIS roll head. APIS lies on back with the head on its side. Chewing motion of the jaws; sometimes a sucking; a grinding of the teeth in those who are old and have teeth; rolling the head from side to side; if you lift the eyelids you will find a strabismus. Provers felt as if the eyes were drawn inward. PODO has cured such a strabismus in congestion of the brain following a suddenly suppressed diarrhoea. ***851***

Children going into severe attacks of infantile fever may threaten convulsions, the head is hot and the body is cold. Most physicians will think of BELL, which has such cold extremities and such a hot head. Do not forget ARN, especially in those children who seem to have an aversion to being touched, and scream out every time the mother takes hold of the leg or arm. Look into the history a little and you will see that this is a soreness, and if you strip the child you may observe dusky spots, which give an added indication of ARN. ***148***

HYOS; Then again after he recovers from these low forms of disease there is quivering of the lids, and jerking of the lids, jerking of the muscles of the eye so the eyeball is unsteady. It moves from little spasms of the various muscles of the globe of the eye. All of these symptoms occur either along with the fever, of afterwards. The child goes into convulsions, or has periods of convulsions, where during the course of a week or ten days there have been from fifteen to fifty convulsions, and it may be that the convulsions have been remedied with BELL or CUPRUM or any one of a number of remedies, and afterwards these eye troubles, strabismus and disturbance of the vision. "An object looked at jumps." The letters jump, while reading. ***585***

After ACON follow well ARN and BELL. Sometimes it is true it will appear to you that ACON is capable of coping with all there is in the disease. But there seems to be a lingering something that holds on and such medicines as ARN and BELL and IP and BRY do have to come in to finish up the attack - or sometimes SULPH. Very commonly SIL. So we have to study the relations of medicines. ***30***

BRY has 3 pm aggravation, BELL will begin at 3 and run on towards midnight, but BRY will begin at 9 pm and run on through the night. ***278***

GLON — "Bad effects from having the hair cut." BELL is generally thought of for taking cold in the head from having the hair cut. "Bad effects from being exposed to the sun's rays." "Bad effects from sunstroke." ***553***

You will find some deep seated brain troubles that will try your patience. Some cases go slowly and gradually into unconsciousness; rolling of the head for days; eyes lustreless; body emaciated, involuntary discharges of faeces or urine in the bed; tongue dry and parched, so shrivelled that it looks like leather, lips also; face withered and each day looks older; paralysis of one hand or one foot, or it seems that the whole muscular system is paralysed. Screaming out in pain, although not so shrilly as in APIS. A dose of ZINC will sometimes bring this patient back to life. In a few days after the remedy there will be a jerking and a quivering in the parts that were motionless, or its action will be shown in a copious sweat, much vomiting; sudden arousing that is alarming, for it looks like a threatened sinking, but this is the beginning of reaction. Now, for days and nights while this little one is coming back to consciousness, the restoration of sensation in the parts is accompanied with the tormenting formication, tingling, prickling, creeping and crawling. The mother and the father and the neighbours will want something done for it, but if you antidote the case will return to where it was before. This suffering is but the awakening to life. It will go on in this way for a week or two and then will begin to show signs of falling back; it needs another dose of ZINC, which will again be followed by sweat, vomiting etc. You will see this in spinal meningitis. The early stage will be that of congestion and BELL may palliate, but with the onset of the symptoms enumerated above, ZINC is the only remedy that will cure. The BELL case will have flushed face, hot head, rolling of the head, flashing eyes, throbbing carotids. The BRY case will be docile, purple, stupid, sleepy, ameliorated by quiet. The HELL cases will exhibit but little fever; cold extremities, tossing of the head, dilated pupils, unconsciousness, can hardly be aroused; rolling head from side to side, but when the reflexes are abolished ZINC comes in. After the relief from GELS, BELL or BRY give ZINC. Rugged little fellows who hang on for weeks in this state, emaciating and unconscious. You must take the mother aside and inform her what will happen if the child returns to consciousness. If you do not, you may be turned out of the house. A person advanced in years cannot stand such an ordeal, but it is astonishing how the little ones can endure the prolonged congestion and inflammation. After scarlet fever and badly treated meningitis; tubercular meningitis. I have carried these severe forms of brain disease through on PHOS which has a picture somewhat like that of ZINC. There is no record of recovery from tubercular meningitis, but a homoeopath can cure some of these cases, though it may take two or three months to go down and come up out of it, with two or three relapses. ***1015***

As a convulsive medicine IPECAC is not well enough known. Convulsions in pregnancy. Convulsions in whooping cough; frightful spasms affecting the whole of the left side, followed by paralysis; clonic and tonic spasms of children and hysterical women. Tetanus, rigidity of the body, with flushed redness of the face. These are strong features of IPECAC, and they have not been sufficiently dwelt upon, and the remedy is not sufficiently known as having these states so prominently. Medicines like BELL are more frequently spoken of in the books and in treatises on spasms, yet IPECAC is just as important a remedy to be studied in relation to spasms and its action on the spine. ***609***

STRAM — In cerebral congestions the delirium subsides into unconsciousness; the patient has the appearance of profound intoxication; pupils dilated or contracted (in BELL they are dilated). ***950***

STRAM is useful in mania that has existed for some time; attacks of mania coming on in paroxysms, appearing with more or less suddenness so that a single attack would look like BELL, but the history differentiates. BELL would be hardly more than a palliative in the first attack, and the second exhibition of it would do nothing. *949*

Another thing running through HYOS in insanity and in the delirium of fevers is a fear of water, fear of running water. Of course, hydrophobia, which is named because of that symptom being a striking feature, has fear of water, but some remedies also have that fear of water. "Anxiety on hearing running water. A fear of water." That runs through BELL, HYOS, CANTH and, of course, the nosode HYDROPHOBINUM (LYSSIN). STRAM has the fear of anything that might look like water, shining objects, fire, looking glass. Fear of things that have in any manner whatsoever the resemblance to fluids. HYDROPHOBINUM (LYSSIN) has cured "involuntary urination on hearing running water." It has cured a chronic diarrhoea when that symptom was present. *583*

COLOC — The faceache is especially important, because COLOC is one of the most frequently indicated remedies for neuralgia of this region. There are three remedies which are indicated in faceache more often than any others, BELL, MAG PHOS and COLOC. The BELL pains are as violent as any, and are accompanied by red face, flashing eyes, hot head and great sensitiveness of the part to touch. In COLOC the pains come in waves, are better from heat, from pressure, worse if anything during rest, and are brought on by excitement or vexation. They are generally on the left side; while those of BELL are on the right, and are caused by cold. MAG PHOS has tearing pains that shoot like lightning along the nerves and are relieved by heat and pressure. *466*

SULPH — Long and tedious right-sided neuralgias. Persistent neuralgias in those that live in a malarial climate, when the short acting remedies given for the neuralgia, such as BELL and NUX-V have only for a short time mitigated the suffering. If upon studying the whole case you find he turns out to be a SULPH patient, SULPH will permanently cure the neuralgias. *966*

RUTA — "Eyes feel hot like balls of fire." To use RUTA for a pure inflammation when the eyes feel hot would be a failure. EUPHRASIA, BELL and ACON are used in simple inflammations from a cold, and the anti-psorics where the case is chronic. But if a woman strains her eyes from long SEWING ON FINE WORK, and the balls feel like fire, she needs RUTA. ACON if after exposure to cold winds there is inflammation with lachrymation, and the eyes look like raw beef. *891*

SIL is full of throat symptoms but is seldom indicated in acute forms because its pace is too slow; it comes on after there has been a series of colds, such colds as are ameliorated a number of times by BELL or other acute remedies, but still continue to settle in the tonsils and in the glands of the neck. SIL breaks up the tendency. There is a catarrhal state in the throat that is roused up by every cold into an increased flux, with hoarseness, settling back into the chronic state again; chronic catarrhs of the pharynx. It competes with NAT MUR in inveterate sore throat. *930*

The CALC voice is that of painless hoarseness. The vocal cords are tired and cannot endure strain; almost a paralytic weakness. Sometimes a copious flow of mucus from the larynx. Much irritation in the larynx, but weakness. Not that burning and rawness that we find in BELL and PHOS, but painless hoarseness. In PHOS it is painful, in BELL it is very painful. He cannot speak without pain. But in CALC he wonders why he has so much trouble with the larynx, because he has no feeling in it. ***327***

PHOS, BELL and RUMEX have soreness of the larynx, sore to touch, but the BROM soreness is commonly below the larynx and in the throat pit as well. ***275***

BAR-C — Children with enlarged tonsils, and with enlarged glands elsewhere, somewhat dwarfish intellectually, slow to learn - BAR-C will cure the enlarged tonsils. But these, you see, are constitutional symptoms. You are not selecting the remedy purely on enlarged tonsils. "Inflammation of the tonsils." The inflammation is not so violent as that which comes on in BELL, it does not come on in a night, it does not go on rapidly to suppuration; but it is a very sore throat, has come on slowly and after many days of exposure and there is gradual growth and development, while that of BELL comes on with great rapidity. HEPAR is also rapid and goes on to suppuration. There is a remedy for inflammation of the tonsils where the ear is involved and is ameliorated by heat that very few use, but it is of great value; it is CHAM and it is especially indicated if the patient is irritable. The pain is ameliorated by heat and comes on with great violence. It might be mistaken for a BELL inflammation, but CHAM cures it permanently......... ***227***

CYCL — Desires lemonade (NIT AC, BELL, SAB)... ***496***

One may not practice long before he will find a CHEL patient, sitting up in bed with high fever, bending forward upon his elbows, holding himself perfectly still, for this medicine has as much aggravation from motion as BRY. All of the pains are extremely aggravated from motion. This patient is sitting with a pain that transfixes him; he cannot stir, he cannot move without the pain shooting through him like a knife. The next day you will see that his skin is growing yellow. If you see him in the beginning CHEL will relieve him and you will prevent that pneumonia. It is not uncommon in children and it is extremely common in adults. Do not get confused with BRY. Both are violently worse from motion. BRY wants to lie on the painful side, or wants to lie on the back if the pneumonia is mostly in the posterior part of the right lung. In CHEL he is worse from touch and motion. BELL has that extremely painful tearing rending of the right lung with pleurisy, but in BELL one cannot touch the right side, cannot press it, but must lie on the other side, and he cannot move. Cannot stand a jar of the bed because of the extreme sensitiveness to motion. I mention all three in this particular way because they have some things in common, but the remedies are different............. ***426***

PULS — Most troublesome cases of prolapsus. It competes with SEP, BELL, NAT MUR, NUX-V and SEC; all of these are remedies with great relaxation, bearing down; some have even cured procidentia. ***870***

SQUIL — Dry cough at 11 pm, worse from cold water and cold air (RUMEX). BELL has cough at 11 pm, worse from uncovering, red face, congestion in head. LACH has cough soon after going to sleep, which may be 11 pm. ***942***

Until PHYT was known there was but one remedy for the old cicatrices in the mammary gland. Women who were confined years before, had abscesses of the breast which were poulticed and lanced, had a cicatrix left, and now in the present confinement they have trouble; inflammation in the old cicatrices; ulceration which eats off the lacteal glands or turns the ducts aside and twists them; high inflammation; throbbing and pain; milk bloody. GRAPH was the old routine remedy, but PHYT is a better remedy and suits the concomitants oftener. The symptoms usually found in an inflamed breast after confinement are: aching in the back and bone pains; fever and shivering. PHYT has these and falls into the very nature of the case. GRAPH has it only in a limited way. If there is high fever; congestion to the head; throbbing carotids; much redness, and the redness radiates from the nipple, BELL is the remedy. When the entire gland is as heavy as a stone, and hard, and the patient is sensitive to motion and touch, BRY. MERC when the general symptoms agree. HEP and SIL after suppuration is inevitable, especially when the only comfort is obtained from heat. HEPAR when there is extreme pain and soreness, irritability and this relief from heat; it limits the suppuration and opens the part without pain. *837*

Then we have SEPTICAEMIC CONDITIONS, with purulent lochia or suppression of the lochia. You may go to a case in which, on the third day, there has been a chill, the lochia has been suppressed, the woman has a high temperature and is covered from head to foot in sweat. As you put your hand under the covers you feel steam come up from the body so that you want to take your hand away; it is so hot. She is dazed and is sensitive over the whole abdomen. You know now the meaning of suppression of the lochia; you have a PUERPERAL FEVER on hand. STUDY CLOSELY FOR SULPHUR instead of hunting around among ACON, BRY, BELL, OP etc. With these you will make a total failure in most instances, but SULPH fits into just such a state and has cured many cases of puerperal fever. If it is but a milk fever or mammary indisposition and the chill is only acute, then your short acting remedies will do very well and even ACON has been useful, but when it is a case of septicaemia SULPH goes to the very root of it. When the feet burn, when there is a hungry feeling in the stomach, the night aggravation with sinking and exhaustion, and when throughout the body there is a sensation of steam rising or hot flushes one after another, you must give SULPH. Now, on the other hand, if in such a case, with the hot sweat and other general features, you have one rigor following another in rapid succession, and no end to them, you cannot get out of the case without LYC, which goes as deeply into the case as SULPH. When there is a continuous intermingling of little chillinesses and little quiverings throughout the body and the pulse has lost its proper relationship to the temperature, PYR must be administered. If there is a purplish appearance of the body, cold sweat all over, if there are remittent or intermittent chills, with thirst during the chill and at no other time and the face is red during the chill, you must give FERRUM, as no other remedy looks just like that. When one side of the body is hot and the other side is cold, and you find the woman in a tearful state, trembling with fear, nervous excitement and restlessness, give PULS, which also has a septic state and is sufficient to overcome the septic condition. In these deep seated septic states somewhere from beginning to end SULPH will most likely be wanted. You may see in the earlier stages of that septic state a number of BRY symptoms, but BRY cannot take hold of that case. Remember that in a septic state you want to get ahead of it in the first 24 hours, you do not want to let it run on, and if BRY has only mitigated it in its beginning then it is too late for SULPH. Go to SULPH at once. Now another thing, even if you have made a mistake in giving SULPH, and you find it does not take hold of the case, it always simplifies it, does good and never spoils it. It gives you a good basis to begin on. It goes to the bottom and simplifies the matter and, if you have mental and nervous symptoms left, still you have overcome that violent septic state which must be met at once, and the remaining symptoms in many instances are simple. SULPH is a general remedy to begin with in those cases where the symptoms are not perfectly clear for another. *972*

In an ABORTION you may have selected BELL, which was suitable while the woman was aborting, and it may have overcome the present state, or you may have selected APIS or SABINA, which was suitable for the early state, and it either postpones or checks the haemarrhage for the time or hurries the expulsion of the foetus; but the haemorrhage starts in again and with its return we have prolonged tribulation. In many of these cases we can do nothing until we put the patient on SULPH. If the symptoms are masked, SULPH stands very high. When BELL has been given you will often have to follow it with SULPH. SABIN, which has the most violent gushing haemorrhage in abortions, very commonly needs to be followed by SULPH. In such haemorrhagic affections, i.e. in a prolonged recurring haemorrhage, a chronic condition, not in the first or most exciting time, not in the time of the earliest gushing, there are two very frequently indicated remedies, viz SULPH and PSOR. The flow keeps coming back in spite of ordinary remedies, and in spite of remedies selected upon this group of symptoms related to the pelvis. *971*

In many instances we go to a haemorrhage and the pelvic symptoms are prominent and all other symptoms are clouded; there is a gushing flow, the blood is hot, etc. and there are only a few symptoms; but the next time you see the woman she is quiet enough to give other symptoms, and in the course of a few days more symptoms come out, as the haemorrhagic state is an outcome of the chronic condition. This is unlike measles. You do not have to look into the chronic state until the measles or scarlet fever or smallpox is finished; these are acute miasms. But the haemorrhage is part of her constitutional state, it is not a miasm; and hence when it is violent, calling for a remedy, probably the best adapted will be the short acting remedies, such as BELL or even ACON; but then look into the constitutional state, for it is likely some remedy will have to follow the ACON or BELL, and commonly it is SULPH, the acute remedy being suitable to the violent action and then followed by its complementary medicine. *971*

CIC was the old remedy for tetanus and spasms caused by splinters in the skin or under the nails, competing with BELL. At the present day we find the most frequently indicated remedies for injuries to nerves are LEDUM and HYPERICUM. *433*

BELLIS PERENNIS

PHOS — Glands enlarge, especially after contusions, like BELLIS...................... *825*

BENZOIC ACID

BERB is changeable like BENZ-AC. These two remedies run very much together, yet their symptoms are wholly unlike. *261*

BERBERIS

SIL has also cured fistulous openings. Patients who have a tendency to phthisis are subject to abscesses about the region of the rectum that break inside or out and form complete or incomplete openings. These seem to take the place of what would otherwise come, and if healed by operation or other external means, the tendency is to end in chest trouble, either in the form of a fixed catarrh or tubercular infiltrations. SIL is one of the remedies that turns the constitution into order and in one to five years the opening ceases to be necessary and it will heal. Surgeons heal it up at once and for a time the patient is comfortable, but in a few years he breaks down. CAUST, BERB, CALC, CALC PHOS, GRAPH, SULPH etc. are suitable in such cases. SIL here follows THUJ well. *932*

BORAX

NAT-C — Music causes a tendency to suicide, melancholy, weeping and trepidation; playing the piano is so exhausting that she must lie down; music causes great sadness which increases to a religious insanity. This is true of all the SODIUMS, but especially of NAT-C; aggravation from the slam of a door, a pistol shot, which causes a headache and complaints in general, aggravated from music. *763*

NAT-C throws out eruptions upon the knuckles and finger-tips; also the toes; vesicular eruptions open up and form ulcers on the joints or finger-tips. BORAX, SEP, ARS and NAT-C are the remedies most inclined to produce ulceration of the tips and knuckles of the fingers, and also the toes. *763*

We say sometimes that CALC CARB is late in learning to walk, but BARYTA CARB is also late learning to walk, although it has an entirely different cause. To express it in a common, old-fashioned way, BARYTA CARB is late learning how to walk even with pretty good limbs. CALC has miserable, weakly limbs, flabby muscles, poor bones, and hence he is late learning to walk. "Late walking" is CALC. "Late learning to walk" is BARYTA CARB. It competes also with BORAX and NAT MUR. All three of these medicines have a peculiar kind of tardiness in the development of the brain, so that they are late learning to do things; late in developing. *221*

If the head bones are slow in forming, or do not keep pace with the growth of the child, CALC PHOS is often called for. Where the child is losing flesh, slow learning to do things, slow learning to walk, or the legs are not strong enough to support the body, or it is behind in mental development, CALC PHOS is one to be examined, (like BARYTA CARB, BORAX, PHOS AC, NAT-M, CALC-C). *334*

NAT-C — A nervous, cold baby, easily startled like the BORAX baby. So are the NATRUM babies in general. *765*

KALI PHOS; Night terrors in children (BORAX). *653*

LYC — While the abdomen is distended he is so nervous that he cannot endure any noise. The noise of the crackling of paper, ringing of bells or slamming of doors goes right through him and causes fainting, like ANT-CRUD, BORAX and NAT-MUR...704

CIS — He feels as if paralysed after mental exertion and mental excitement increases his sufferings, like CALC and BORAX. If he is compelled to fast headache comes on, and like LYC, the headache will be relieved after eating. *444*

If you have ever been going through a place where there are cobwebs and a little cobweb has strung across your face you will know what a peculiar sensation of crawling it produces, and you cannot leave it alone until it is removed. That sensation particularly belongs to ALUM, BORAX and BAR-C. *71*

BROMIUM

PULS has relief from motion. A few remedies have relief from slow motion, and of these PULS and FERR are the most striking. A few remedies are relieved by hurried motion; want to move fast. Such are BROM and ARS. The ARS child cannot be carried fast enough. The PULS baby is content with moderate motion. Any motion that HEATS UP the PULS patient aggravates all complaints. *868*

BRYONIA

Every experienced physician must have met with many cases where for a time he felt unable to cope with the case because of his inability to reach the constitutional state that underlies this continual taking of cold. So he puzzles for a long time, and prescribes on the immediate attack and palliates it. For instance the immediate attack might look like BELL or BRY, FERRUM PHOS or ARS etc.; he treats that attack without taking into consideration the underlying constitutional state of the patient. It is quite a profitable business for one who has not much conscience and not much intelligence. But a conscientious physician feels worried and knows he is not doing what he ought to do by his patient, unless he reaches out for the remedy that touches the constitution. It is far more useful to keep people from taking colds than to cure cold. *509*

Get the pace, the periodicity of remedies. Some remedies have a continued fever, some a remittent, others an intermittent fever. In ACON, BELL and BRY we have 3 different paces, 3 different motions, 3 different forms of velocity; so in SULPH, GRAPH, NAT-M, CARBO-V - a different form, a different development. Some would not hesitate in a continued fever to give BELL, but its complaints come on in great haste, with great violence and have nothing in their nature like a continued fever. This is not like typhoid. BELL and ACON have no manifestations of typhoid, even if the symptoms are present. Be sure that the remedy has not only the group of symptoms, but also the nature of the case. The typhoid case has a likeness in BRY or RHUS, but not in BELL. We owe no obedience to man, not even to our parents, after we are old enough to think for ourselves. We owe obedience to truth. *769*

CUPR; Repression or driving in of eruptions, attended with diarrhoea and convulsions, sometimes only convulsions. We note a case of measles or scarlet fever with a rash that has been suppressed by a chill or exposure to wind and convulsions have come on. That belongs to ZINC and CUPRUM, sometimes to BRY, but to ZINC and CUPR particularly. *492*

One may not practice long before he will find a CHEL patient, sitting up in bed with high fever, bending forward upon his elbows, holding himself perfectly still, for this medicine has as much aggravation from motion as BRY. All of the pains are extremely aggravated from motion. This patient is sitting with a pain that transfixes him; he cannot stir, he cannot move without the pain shooting through him like a knife. The next day you will see that his skin is growing yellow. If you see him in the beginning CHEL will relieve him and you will prevent that pneumonia. It is not uncommon in children and it is extremely common in adults. Do not get confused with BRY. Both are violently worse from motion. BRY wants to lie on the painful side, or wants to lie on the back if the pneumonia is mostly in the posterior part of the right lung. In CHEL he is worse from touch and motion. BELL has that extremely painful tearing rending of the right lung with pleurisy, but in BELL one cannot touch the right side, cannot press it, but must lie on the other side, and he cannot move. Cannot stand a jar of the bed because of the extreme sensitiveness to motion. I mention all three in this particular way because they have some things in common, but the remedies are different. ***426***

After ACON follow well ARN and BELL. Sometimes it is true it will appear to you that ACON is capable of coping with all there is in the disease. But there seems to be a lingering something that holds on, and such medicines as ARN and BELL and IP and BRY do have to come in to finish up the attack - or sometimes SULPH. Very commonly SIL. So we have to study the relations of medicines. ***30***

ANT TART — Such medicines as IPECAC and BRY come in for the first period and your impression is, when administering these medicines, that they will be sufficient for the whole case, and they will be, except in those states wherein this weakness is present from the beginning, or there is a lack of ability to react sufficiently from your remedy to recover under it. Then comes in a second remedy and this is the time when ANT-T begins its operation. ***110***

GELS is only a short acting remedy, though slow in its beginning. In this it is like BRY. BRY complaints come on slowly, and hence it is suitable for fevers coming on in the southern climates (of USA) but it also has sudden violent complaints, though not to the extent we find in BELL. ***544***

The disinclination and aversion to the slightest motion is common in BELL, and as strong in BELL as BRY. ***252***

Unlike ARS, running all through CADMIUM SULPH, he wants to be perfectly quiet; part of it is a state of indolence, part of it is an aversion to motion. He is worse from motion, which makes it like BRY. So we will see running all through CADMIUM SULPH the exhaustion of ARS and the aversion to motion of BRY. ***304***

All the complaints of COLCH are aggravated from motion. The painful complaints, the head complaints, the bowel complaints, the liver complaints, the stomach complaints are all worse from motion. Such an aggravation from motion that he dreads to move. About as marked as we find in BRY. Aversion to motion and aggravation from motion... ***460***

With GELS the child will lie as still as in BRY but there is more congestion to the head; there is the dark red face and duskiness like BRY. Running through the febrile complaints of GELS, in the spinal meningitis, in congestion of the brain, in intermittents or remittents that change to a continued fever, and even in a cold when the patient is sneezing and has a hot face and red eyes, there is one grand feature, viz. a feeling of great weight and tiredness in the entire body and limbs. The head cannot be lifted from the pillow, so tired and heavy is it, and there is such a great weight in the limbs. The BRY patient lies quietly because if he moves the pains are worse. He has an aversion to motion because he is conscious that it would cause an increase of suffering. ***545***

That is a strong feature of CADM SULPH; he wants to keep as still as COLCH and BRY. *739*

RAN-B is as sensitive to motion as BRY, and to the cold damp weather as DULC..... *874*

BRY may be confused with RUMEX in aggravation from motion and from talking but BRY is not so sensitive to cold air, is often relieved from cold air and worse in a warm room; the complaints subside if the room becomes cool. *888*

EUP-PER — Painful soreness in the eyeballs, like BRY and GELS. The eyeballs are very sensitive to touch and sore to pressure; feels as if he had been struck a blow in the eye; sore, bruised pain in the eye. *515*

CAPS is useful in perplexing and troublesome chronic hoarseness. He has had a cold and remedies for the acute condition have been given, perhaps two or three remedies, ACON, BRY, HEP, PHOS, but all at once you wake up to the fact of his chronic constitutional state of hoarseness. He is rotund, chilly, red-faced, and the hoarseness disappears under CAPS. It is the same with the cough. After making several blunders you wake up and see that it is a CAPS case and that you have never yet gotten at the root of the trouble. This shows the importance of getting at the things general first. If there is much acute suffering, of course you must give an acute remedy, but if the patient has delayed recovery and convalescence is slow the next remedy should be the remedy for the patient. Sometimes it is SULPH, PHOS, LYC and sometimes it is CAPS. If the patient has a good constitutional state he will get over the cold on the acute remedy, but the old gouty, rheumatic, flabby patients need a constitutional remedy. *367*

Healthy bile dissolves gall-stones in the sac; healthy urine does the same to a stone in the pelvis of the kidney. NUX runs close to BRY in abdominal complaints with marked yellowness of the skin. BRY is worse from motion and not better from heat - NUX is both and is more suited to portal congestion, the neuralgias etc.; is worse from the slightest pressure (COLOC is better from the slightest pressure - MAG P is better from pressure and heat). BRY, indicated more in peritonitis, lies with limbs drawn up. Haemorrhoids, portal congestion, cutting pains in rectum causing urging to stool. CUPR has cutting pains from front to back as if transfixed. Abdomen sunken in NUX, while in CALC and SEP it is engorged. INULA resembles NUX; has colic with urging to stool and to urinate. *808*

NUX-V — Tendency to jaundice in all the febrile states. Sclerotics become yellow. Skin becomes very yellow. Old intermittents with yellow skin. Runs close to BRY in abdominal complaints with jaundice. *807*

PULS has dribbling of urine, dribbles on the slightest provocation. She must keep her mind continually on it, or she will lose her urine. As soon as she goes to sleep it flows away. Little, mild, gentle, florid, plethoric, warm-blooded girls, who kick the covers off at night and have nocturnal enuresis. Yellow, sallow, sickly girls who lose their urine in their first sleep call for SEP. Losing the urine in the first sleep is looked upon as a strong symptom, but you can figure it out, and hence it is NOT SO. All those cases that have to make an effort to hold the urine during the day lose it in their first sleep; for then the mind is taken off it, and as soon as the mind is taken off it the urine dribbles. CAUST and SEP are remedies looked upon as curing involuntary urination during the first sleep, but I have cured it with many other remedies. A man past middle age flooded the bed at night as soon as he went to sleep. The medicines which have this are limited, and he had had them all. I found I must figure it out on another basis. I ascertained that when moving about at his work he had no difficulty in holding the urine, but when he sat down he had to make an effort to control it. At the time this condition developed he had been in Atlantic City and had bathed much in the ocean. Here were the aggravation and amelioration of RHUS, and RHUS cured him. Few would think of BRY in urinary trouble. When he moves the urine dribbles, when he walks it flows. He is relieved only by keeping quiet. BRY is aggravated by motion; RHUS is relieved by motion. *868*

The NOSE, the INNER CHEST and LUNGS furnish us with localities for much trouble. The patient has had pneumonia and it has gone on to the period of infiltration; you have taken the case in this advanced stage after BRY has overcome the threatening features, and now when the patient should rally he does not rally; he perspires all over and has a strange and singular consciousness that "there is something wrong in there, a load in there;" difficult breathing; flashes of heat yet not much fever; sometimes coldness alternating with flashes of heat. I have often heard them say, "There is a great load in there, doctor, I cannot get rid of it." Upon examination you find there is hepatisation and now comes the time for such remedies as PHOS, LYC and SULPH, and SULPH leads them all. When BRY has been sufficient for the earlier symptoms or when ACON has cleared them up, there has been too much for these remedies to relieve, then hepatisation comes on. If this is confined to only a small area it will keep up quite a chronic course, but SULPH will clear it up. If however it is a double pneumonia, or the hepatisation involves a considerable portion of the lung and the remedy given has not been sufficient and the case is advancing toward a fatal issue, it may be that all at once at two or three o'clock in the morning he begins to sink; his nose is pinched; his lips are drawn, he takes on a hippocratic countenance, is covered with cold sweat, he is too feeble in every part of his body to move, he only moves his head a little in a restless manner. Unless you are called at once and give him a dose of ARS he will die. You give the ARS and you have done well, but ARS has no ability to remove the results of inflammation. But though it cannot CURE that hepatised lung it acts as a vital stimulant; it warms up the patient and makes him feel he is going to get better; but, mark this, in 24 hours he will die unless you follow the ARS with the proper remedy. You must not wait upon your remedy too long in these cases. Just as soon as he rallies, and the reaction is at its highest pitch, give him the antidote and natural follower of ARS, which is SULPH, and in 24 hours the patient will say, "I am getting better." As sure as you exist today, it will do just that thing. There are times when you will see clearly that PHOS is the medicine to follow ARS with. If such a patient rallying under ARS goes into a fever, if a hot fever comes on with burning thirst and he cannot get enough ice-cold water, you must follow it with PHOS and it will do in that case what SULPH will do in the other. *974*

NAT-S has a cough with a sensation of "all-goneness" in the chest. In this it competes with BRY; both hold the chest when coughing. BRY holds the chest because he feels as if it would fly to pieces; there is such a soreness that he feels the necessity of steadying his chest. The complaints of BRY are relieved by pressure. NAT-S has this same desire to hold the chest; but in NAT-S the muco-pus that is expectorated is thick, ropy and yellowish-green, looking like pus - purulent - and there is an "all-gone", empty feeling in the chest. He feels a sense of weakness there; that his lungs are all gone, that he must die in a few days with consumption or some other failing like that, and that it is coming on in a short time. BRY corresponds more to the irritable states with the cough, where there is great rawness, great constriction, great sense of tearing in the chest; burning in the chest; while NAT-S corresponds to a case that has been going on for perhaps a week; every cough brings up a mouthful of purulent sputa with a desire to press upon the chest to relieve the weakness; NAT-S is then your remedy. *792*

BELL — The chest is so painful that the child dreads the cough and screams. By the child's cry we know that it is going to have a coughing spell. Just like BRY, HEPAR and PHOS which have that feature more than any other remedies. *251*

EUP PER has a dry, hacking, teasing cough, that seems to rack the whole frame, as if it would break him up, it is so sore, and he is so much disturbed by motion. A great amount of tribulation is found in the respiratory tract, in the bronchial tubes. We find a cough in capillary bronchitis that shakes the whole frame, analogous to BRY and PHOS. The subject is extremely sensitive to the cold air, as much so as in NUX VOM. NUX has aching in the bones as if they would break; he wants the room hot, and wants to be covered with clothing, which relieves; often the slightest lifting of the covers increases the chilliness, which is true also of EUP PER, so they run close together. In NUX we have the dreadful irritability of temper; in EUP PER we have overwhelming sadness. The NUX patient is not likely to say much about dying; he is too irritable to go into the next world; not so with EUP PER, he is full of sadness. *515*

EUPH — The cough, considered by itself, furnishes a very rare group of symptoms. Cough with copious expectoration along with or following coryza. Difficult respiration ameliorated at night while lying down. Worse in the morning when moving about, with copious expectoration. Violent cough from tickling in the larynx. No cough at night causes the remedy to resemble BRY and MANG. *517*

NUX-V — Cough; burning in the air passages; all the mucous membranes in a state of irritation; nasal tone to voice; sore throat; tickling cough. Dry, teasing cough with great soreness of the chest, like BRY, the head feels as if it would split. *806*

STANNUM is frequently indicated in cases where the routinist would prescribe BRY etc. in low potencies to loosen up the cough. *944*

KALMIA — "Wandering rheumatic pains in the region of the heart." "When articular rheumatism has been treated externally and cardiac symptoms ensue." Rheumatism that goes from the lower to the upper limbs. Not uncommonly you will meet such things. These "rubbers" that go around the streets with a strong liniment and considerable magnetism frequently cause a rheumatism to leave the knee joint and, when it does that, the heart is likely to be the organ that suffers. Then KALMIA, AURUM, BRYONIA, RHUS-TOX, LEDUM, CALC, ABROTANUM and sometimes CACTUS are remedies that prove suitable for such cardiac affections. *670*

Until PHYT was known there was but one remedy for the old cicatrices in the mammary gland. Women who were confined years before, had abscesses of the breast which were poulticed and lanced had a cicatrix left, and now in the present confinement they have trouble; inflammation in the old cicatrices; ulceration which eats off the lacteal glands or turns the ducts aside and twists them; high inflammation; throbbing and pain; milk bloody. GRAPH was the old routine remedy, but PHYT is a better remedy and suits the concomitants oftener. The symptoms usually found in an inflamed breast after confinement are: aching in the back and bone pains; fever and shivering. PHYT has these and falls into the very nature of the case. GRAPH has it only in a limited way. If there is high fever; congestion to the head; throbbing carotids; much redness, and the redness radiates from the nipple, BELL is the remedy. When the entire gland is as heavy as a stone, and hard, and the patient is sensitive to motion and touch, BRY. MERC when the general symptoms agree. HEP and SIL after suppuration is inevitable, especially when the only comfort is obtained from heat. HEPAR when there is extreme pain and soreness, irritability and this relief from heat; it limits the suppuration and opens the part without pain. *837*

SENECIO AUREUS — The whole urinary tract is painful and subject to bleeding. But bleeding especially in the absence of the menstrual flow is the feature of this remedy. Wherever there is an inflammatory spot or catarrhal condition of the mucous membrane, it will bleed in case the menstrual flow does not appear. We have other medicines having the symptoms of vicarious haemorrhage, such as HAMAMELIS, PHOS and BRY, but SENECIO has this condition strikingly, and is one of the newer remedies for such condition. *913*

Do not forget the symptoms of ARN in appendicitis. You do not need to run for the surgeon in every case of appendicitis if you know BRY, RHUS TOX, BELL, ARN and similar remedies. The homoeopathic remedy will cure these cases, and if you know it you need never run after the surgeon except in recurrent cases. *147*

ARUM — The sneezing is like an ordinary coryza, with repeated chills over the body and aching in the bones as if the bones would break, like NUX, EUPATOR, ARN, RHUS, BRY and ARS that have aching all over during "cold". *180*

BORAX has cured pleurisy that very much resembled BRY, especially on the right side like BRY; stitching or darting pains from without inward as if through the upper right lung posteriorly; the stitching pains might make you think of BRY. *270*

ABROT has cured pleurisy where BRY, which seemed indicated, had failed. *17*

A violent attack of pleurisy associated with pneumonia, too deep and too vicious for BRY, often finds its remedy in SENEGA. SEN is a sort of cross between BRY and RHUS TOX. The violent symptoms are those of BRY, yet it is worse from rest, unlike BRY. The symptoms of SENEGA are not so much like RHUS TOX but it has an amelioration of RHUS-T, better from motion, the pains being worse when at rest. The chest pains, rheumatic pains and inflammatory pains are worse during rest, but the cough is made worse from motion and the asthmatic troubles are made worse from the slightest motion. *914*

PULS — When the hay fever comes on, all the other symptoms are better, she feels nothing except the hay fever, however, all the symptoms interweave with each other. The NAT MUR symptoms will be worse in the morning and until toward noon, while in PULS they are worse in the evening, the nose filling up with thick, yellowish-green, ropy mucus, and when the nose has been cleared a dry, burning, smarting feeling remains; if the room is warm at night she cannot sleep. NAT MUR is a little like that in the smarting and inability to sleep at night in a warm room. In NAT MUR too the discharge may continue day and night. We have an acute class in which PULS is sometimes indicated - copious watery discharge which ends in sneezing. In the beginning we will think of CARBO-VEG, ARS, ALL-C, EUPH. With CARBO-VEG there is a watery discharge and the irritation extends into the chest, with hoarseness and rawness. In ALL-C we have one group of symptoms that points to this remedy. Excoriating discharge from the nose and bland discharge from the eyes; in the larynx, sensation as if hooks were there, and sometimes this extends below the larynx; this always means ALL-C; it is also worse in a warm room like PULS. The EUPH looks like ALL-C, only the discharge from the eyes is copious, watery and burning - the lachrymation burns the eyes and excoriates the cheeks; discharge from nose is bland like PULS. Sometimes this goes into the chest, then it is no longer EUPH. IOD is worse in a warm room; thick discharge from the nose which burns and excoriates and is yellowish-green; but there is one thing that differentiates it from all the others - the patient immediately begins to emaciate when the complaint comes on and is very hungry. KALI HYDR with the thick yellowish discharge, worse in a warm room, there is a great amount of rawness and burning in the nose; external nose very sore to pressure; sensitiveness in the root of the nose; whole face aches and patient is very restless; wants to walk in the open air which does not fatigue him. ARS IOD; anxiety, restlessness and weakness; frequent sneezing and copious watery nasal discharge that burns the lip. Burning, watery discharge from the eyes like ARS. ARS wants to be very warm; wants hot water applied to the eyes; the only relief is from sniffing hot water up the nose. ARS IOD is worse in a warm room and for days after sneezing the discharge thickens and becomes gluey, looking like THICK, YELLOW HONEY, this excoriates; much pain through the root of the nose and eyes; often rawness in the chest with dyspnoea. The remedies having the dyspnoea are ARSENIC, IODIDE OF ARSENIC, IODINE, KALI HYDR and SABADILLA; these are the ones I have found most frequently indicated in the asthmatic forms of hay fever. If the complaint has been developed after being overheated at about that time, you will find that SILICA, PULSATILLA and CARBO VEG must be carefully compared. There is another class of remedies having the stuffing up of the nose not relieved by the discharge. There is a constant desire to blow the nose, yet he gets no relief. This makes me think of LACH, KALI BI, PSOR, NAJA and STICTA. PSORINUM has the copious, watery, bland discharge from the nose, it may be excoriating, it has both. The stuffing up of the nose generally takes place in the open air; he is relieved in a warm, close room and by lying down; has some dyspnoea which is relieved by stretching the arms at right angles to the body. Hay fever is a psoric sickness. PSORINUM given in a single dose will so develop the symptoms that the case will be more clear. The attack is not the best thing to prescribe for. If it is too violent, a short acting remedy may be selected that will mitigate it. NUX VOMICA has a free, easy breathing in the open air, but when he goes into the warm room his nose stuffs up, which also occurs at night, though the water drips on the pillow yet he stuffs up like PULS, BRY and the IODINE preparations, IODIDE OF ARSENIC and CYCLAMEN. Do not understand me to have given remedies for hay fever, we cannot lay down remedies for diseases. The whole constitution must be most carefully examined........................ ***863***

Sometimes the scarlet fever patient will go into convulsions because the rash fails to come out. APIS is sometimes a suitable remedy and must be compared with BRY, CUPRUM and ZINC.......................... ***120***

CACTUS

STANNUM — The pain sometimes begins at sunrise, increases until noon and gradually diminishes, and ceases with sunset. On the other hand, it may begin at any time, as often at 10 am. and increasing for 10 or 20 minutes, then gradually decrease until gone. A few other remedies have these sun headaches. KALM has a similar headache, not so regularly increasing and diminishing, but especially worse at noon. CACT has a sun headache. NAT MUR has never been known to cause it, but has cured it, especially when beginning at 10 am., and worse from 2 to 3 pm. SANG has headache coming and going with the sun. *942*

LYC — If he goes beyond his dinner hour a sick headache will come on. He must eat with regularity or he will have the headache he is subject to. This is somewhat like a CACTUS headache. CACTUS has a congestive headache which becomes extremely violent with flushed face if he does not eat at the regular time. One distinguishing feature is that with the LYC headache if he eats something the headache is better, while the CACTUS headache is worse from eating. *706*

GELS — There are cardiac nervous affections like DIGITALIS, CACTUS and SEPIA. SEPIA is not known to be as great a heart remedy as CACTUS, but it has cured many cases of heart troubles. *545*

KALMIA — "Wandering rheumatic pains in the region of the heart". "When articular rheumatism has been treated externally and cardiac symptoms ensue". Rheumatism that goes from the lower to the upper limbs. Not uncommonly you will meet such things. These "rubbers" that go around the streets with a strong liniment and considerable magnetism frequently cause a rheumatism to leave the knee joint and, when it does that, the heart is likely to be the organ that suffers. Then KALMIA, AURUM, BRYONIA, RHUS-TOX, LEDUM, CALC, ABROTANUM and sometimes CACTUS are remedies that prove suitable for such cardiac affections. *670*

There is a dry, hacking cough with sweating in the palms of the hands that is cured by NAJA. The cardiac cases are often attended by a dry, hacking cough, a cough with every little exertion. It is not a catarrhal state, nor is it tubercular. The heart beats slowly and will not be urged to work, and a cough comes on from exertion. CACTUS also has a cardiac cough. *756*

CALADIUM

LEDUM counteracts the effects of whiskey and takes away the appetite for whiskey. LEDUM is to whiskey what CALADIUM is to the smoking habit. You can break patients from the habit of smoking so that they go to the other extreme and have an aversion to it. *698*

CALCAREA CARBONICA

CIS is an anti-psoric, a deep-acting remedy. It runs very close to CALC, but is milder in its action. It has the same exhaustion from exertion, dyspnoea, sweating and coldness that we find in CALC. What will forcibly call your attention to a remedy will be the curing of a bad and typical case. I remember the first time my attention was called to CIS. I had put it on my list to study from time to time and had come to the conclusion that it was only a side issue until a young lady nineteen years of age fell under my observation. The glands of the neck were large and hard, the parotids especially; she had foetid otorrhoea; her eyes were inflamed and suppurating; there were fissures at the corners of the eyes; her lips were cracked and bleeding, and she had salt rheum at the ends of the fingers. I could not make CALC fit the patient, but after much study this little remedy seemed to be just what I needed, and although she had had an immense amount of homoeopathy, good and bad, this remedy cured. *443*

When the homoeopathic remedy is really and truly able to cure the diseased condition it will hold the case, so that when the symptoms come back again the same remedy will be indicated, only a changed potency perhaps will be necessary. The same remedy is often called for; but it is an indication for TUB when at every coming back of the case it calls for a new remedy. CALC breaks up the case once, and the next time it comes back it calls for something else, and it keeps turning around. Perhaps a number of times it calls for the same remedy again. Changing about. That very changing and unsatisfied symptom image is a strong indication for TUB. *1005*

At the present day it is fashionable to use the cautery to make local applications to stop leucorrhoea and other discharges and to heal up ulcers. Now when these external conditions go there is an anaemic condition established in the economy, the patient becomes waxy and pallid, sickly looking, and these catarrhal discharges come on as a relief because of the suppression of some other condition. For instance, since the suppression of a leucorrhoea the woman has had a thick, bloody or watery discharge from the nose. ARS is frequently suitable to the constitution when an ulcer has been dried up by salves, or an old ear discharge has been stopped by the outward application of powders. The doctor thinks he has done a clever thing in stopping such discharges, but he has only succeeded in damming up the secretions which are really a relief to the patient. Such medicines as SULPH, CALC and ARS are suitable for the catarrhal conditions that come from these suppressions in broken down constitutions. *159*

BELL is not suitable for those recurrent complaints even though the single attack should be mitigated with BELL. Take any of these attacks, whether they are convulsions or headaches or congestion of the brain, they are running down and become excitable and take on congestive headaches, go right to bed and roll the head. You treat those with BELL, the attack is relieved. Take notice, I start out by saying this is only one of a series. You may not know it. This may be the first one. You reduce that one, and when that same exposure comes again, that same attack comes back, but BELL does less this time than it did before. After 2 or 3 attacks BELL will do no more and you are worse off than you were before. When it has broken the first one the physician should see that this is one of a series, and that BELL is not suitable. Often it is a case that needs CALC. I say often and not always. All the symptoms should be examined between attacks so that the child may be elevated above these attacks because the acute remedy will do no more than suit the first, second or third at most. It has not the depth of action. It has not the length of action. It does not affect the economy profoundly enough. It passes away after a few days, has to be frequently repeated. The patient should be followed up and watched in these recurrent spasmodic and periodical complaints. *253*

MAG CARB is especially useful if the history has been a tubercular one. Losing flesh and craving meat in those who are tubercular, or in those that are from tubercular parents. There are persons who have simply this tendency who go along year after year in this withered state with the little hacking cough, not rousing up into much. Finally some favourable circumstance arises and the tuberculosis comes on rapidly after it has remained in a sluggish state for a long time. There are a few remedies more likely to be associated with that condition than any others - ARS, CALC, LYC, MAG CARB and TUB. They fit into this lingering state, this prelude to active phthisis. They sometimes set a patient thriving, but mind you, these cases are hard cases to manage. They are difficult to find remedies for. Their trouble is so latent, the symptoms do not come out, and sometimes you will have to read between the lines. They are the one sided cases spoken of by Hahnemann. ***716***

When patients are under constitutional remedies, they need caution about certain kinds of food that are known to disagree with their constitutional remedy. A BRYONIA patient is often made sick from eating sauerkraut, from vegetable salads, chicken salad, etc. so that you need not be surprised, after administering a dose of BRY for a constitutional state, to have your patient come in and say that she has been made very ill from eating some of these things. It is well to caution persons who are under the influence of PULS to avoid the use of fat foods, because very often they will upset the action of the remedy. It is well to say to patients who are under LYC, "See that you do not eat oysters while taking this medicine." These medicines are known to produce states in the stomach inimical to certain kinds of foods; certain remedies have violently inimical relation to acids, lemons etc. If you do not particularly mention the fact, and say, "You must not touch vinegar or lemons; nor take lemon juice while taking this medicine." you will have the remedy spoiled, and then wonder why it is. Homoeopathy will rule out such things as are inimical to the remedies and inimical to patients in general, or do not agree with a particular constitution. To have an iron-clad rule is not correct practice; the only iron-clad rule is to be sure that the remedy is similar to the patient when you administer it, and the things he is to have are to be in agreement with that remedy. It is not an uncommon thing for a patient who has been under the influence of RHUS TOX, and has been doing well up to a certain time, after he has taken a bath, to have his symptoms return in the form of a RHUS state; the action of the remedy stops right there. He must of course take a bath, and yet it is true that some constitutional cases under RHUS must stop taking their ordinary bath in order to keep themselves under the influence of RHUS. It is the same with CALCAREA - a bath will often stop the action. I only speak of these things to impress upon you the importance of feeding and treating your patient in accordance with the remedy; in accordance with principle and not by rule; do not have one list of foods for your patients; do not have a list of things for everybody. There is no such thing in homoeopathy. ***286***

Persons who are always grinding kaolin and the various products that are used in the manufacture of china and the workers in stone especially require CALC and SIL, but those who work in the coal mines often require SULPH. ***960***

In a case confused by remedies think of CALC, ARS, SULPH, SEP and IPECAC. Never give CHINA or NAT MUR for irregular symptoms and stages. ***925***

The relationship between TUB and CALC is very close. They are interchangeable; that is, the one may be indicated for a while, and then the other. They are both deep acting remedies - also SIL is closely related to TUB, on the same plane of action, going deep into the life in a similar way; CALC, TUB, SIL and the SILICATES. ***1003***

"Every cold he takes ends in asthma" calls for DULC, but very often the fag-end of that attack will remain and the physician has to give a deep-acting remedy. After DULC has done all it can do SULPH comes in as its complementary remedy. CALC has a similar relationship to DULC. ***973***

RUMEX is not so deep as SULPH, but it is an anti-psoric. It is limited however to the early stages, will carry a chronic case so far, but it will require to be followed by another anti-psoric. CALC follows it well. ***887***

CAPS — In those constitutions in which the face looks rosy, but it is cold and not warm, and upon close examination the face is seen to be studded with a fine system of capillaries. Plump and round, with no endurance, a false plethora like CALC. ***364***

CHIN ARS — Relaxed and flabby (CALC). ***428***

SIL — Complementary to CALC, PULS, THUJA. ***935***

After the abuse of BELL, CALC comes in as one of the natural antidotes. ***256***

Nowadays we frequently find the dry hacking cough in the hands of doctors who have given too much LACH. LACH is commonly given to oversensitive women; and it produces many of these conditions; it sometimes cures great troubles but leaves behind a dry, hacking cough that stops her from sleeping. Sometimes it comes on after the first sleep, which is commonly around 11 o'clock; a dry, hacking cough from lying down. BELL will cure this old effect of LACH, the nervous state, the excitability and the cough. BELL will be suitable as an antidote to LACH, that is for its acute symptoms. CALC is an antidote for the more chronic effects of LACH. ***256***

A high potency of ARN is most satisfactory in bruises and when no decided contraindication is present ARN is the first remedy; but for the weakness of tendons that follows such a condition ARN is not always sufficient, and then RHUS TOX is its natural follower. If the weakness and tenderness remain in the joints, follow the RHUS with CALC. One of course will not give these remedies all on the same day, and not in the same glass, but will wait until all the good has been gotten out of the ARN before following with RHUS. It is quite a common thing for aching and restlessness and weakness to come into a part that has been injured, and RHUS is then a suitable remedy; and it is quite common for a joint that has been badly treated to remain sore and weak, and then CALC comes in as a natural follower of the RHUS. Now and then we have to resort to CAUST, STAPH and other remedies, because of some peculiar feature of the case, but these remedies are all related more or less to ARN, RHUS and CALC. For another class of injuries compare LED and HYPER. ***146***

RUTA — "Pain and lameness in the ankles after a sprain or dislocation." "Lameness after sprains, especially of the wrists and ankles." Immediately after a sprain, for the inflammatory state you will most likely need to give ARN, and RHUS will probably follow. But when nodules form in the tendons as a result of the strain RUTA is called for. RUTA is a great remedy for a mere sprain; it has all the soreness and weakness of tendons. ARN, RHUS and CALC are often necessary in a routine way when there is absence of all symptoms except the strain alone. ***891***

Now when a man arrives at the state when

he wants to go somewhere else, that he wants to go away from home, that he is disturbed at home, that everything annoys him at home, that he no longer loves his children as he once did, he needs FL-AC. "Feeling of indifference to those he loves best." The SEPIA state is like this, but SEP is more frequently indicated in women. The woman will say, "Doctor, there is one thing I regret very much, and that is, I do not seem to enjoy my children, my home, my companions, my husband and my friends. There is a sort of alienation." Such is the way it is told when it is SEPIA. In the man it is more commonly FL-AC, in the woman more commonly SEPIA, but this need not necessarily be so. SEPIA corresponds more closely to the condition of the uterus and ovaries, and such conditions as the woman alone can have. (Compare CALC.) *540*

In contrast with HEPAR (although HEPAR is a form of CALC) CALC CARB has no such tearing down nature in it. It does not establish inflammation around foreign bodies and tend to suppurate them out, but causes a fibrous deposit around bullets and other foreign substances in the flesh. It causes tubercular deposits to harden and contract and become encysted. *577*

AGAR — The brain seems to be developed tardily. Children are late in learning to talk and walk, thus combining the features of two remedies, NAT MUR which has the symptom "late learning to talk" and CALC CARB which has the symptom "late learning to walk". It will be noticed in CALC that this is due to a weakness of bone. In AGAR it is due to a mental defect, a slowly developing mind. *42*

We say sometimes that CALC CARB is late learning to walk, but BARYTA CARB is also late learning to walk, although it has an entirely different cause. To express it in a common, old-fashioned way, BARYTA CARB is late learning to walk even with pretty good limbs. CALC has miserable, weakly limbs, flabby muscles, poor bones, and hence he is late learning to walk. "Late walking" is CALC. "Late learning to walk" is BARYTA CARB. It competes also with BORAX and NAT MUR. All three of these medicines have a peculiar kind of tardiness in the development of the brain, so that they are late learning to do things; late in developing. *221*

BAR-C — You will have patients to treat, where this slow development manifests itself in girls 18 to 25 years of age, who do the things they did when they were children, and say things as they said them when they were children. "Childish manner of doing things, and childish behaviour. Playing with dolls and saying foolish things." They have not come into womanhood. They are late in taking on the activities and uses of the woman. They lack the prudence of the woman. They have not become circumspect, and say things just as a boy or just as a little girl would say them. That is the dwarfishness of the mind. To appreciate that late development, and to see it in BARYTA CARB from all of its symptoms and peculiar features, leads to such remedies as GRAPH, SULPH and CALC, but nothing compared to this remedy. *221*

BAR-C — The infant looks like a little old person, like the state we find in NAT MUR and CALC. *226*

If the head bones are slow in forming, or do not keep pace with the growth of the child, CALC PHOS is often called for. Where the child is losing flesh, slow learning to do things, slow learning to walk, or the legs are not strong enough to support the body, or it is behind in mental development, CALC PHOS is one to be examined, (like

BARYTA CARB, BORAX, PHOS AC, NAT-M, CALC-C). *334*

If the infant does not develop properly, if the bones do not grow and there is a slow closing of the fontanelles, CALC may be the remedy and SULPH is next in importance for such slow growth. *957*

CIS — He feels as if paralysed after mental exertion, and mental excitement increases his sufferings, like CALC and BORAX. If he is compelled to fast headache comes on, and like LYC, the headache will be relieved after eating. *444*

The desire to travel, that cosmopolitan condition of the mind belongs so strongly to the one who needs TUB. It comes out so often in clinical experience, is found so often in the CALCAREAS and especially in CALC PHOS, always wanting to go somewhere. *1003*

AUR — "In upper dark section of field of vision occasional showers of bright, star-like bodies." In CALCAREA there is a queer symptom; he sees a sudden flash arise from the lower portion of the field of vision; it shoots up, divides and then he sees stars in every direction. It is the appearance you will see sometimes in the shooting off of one those rockets that explode and come down in a shower. That has been observed in CALCAREA. *198*

VERAT — Head feels as if packed with ice, as if ice lay on the vertex and occiput (CALC). *1011*

DULC — Eruptions upon the scalp that look so much like crusta lactaea that DULC has been found a very useful medicine. Extreme soreness, itching, and the itching is not relieved by scratching, and the scratching goes on until bleeding and rawness take place. Eruptions that come out upon the face, upon the forehead, all over the nose, but especially on the cheeks, which become completely covered with these crusts; eczema of infants. Children only a few weeks old break out with these scalp eruptions, and DULC is one of the medicines that you will need to know. It is about as frequently indicated as any of the medicines. SEPIA, ARS, GRAPH, DULC, PETR, SULPH and CALC are about equally indicated, but of these, in this climate at least, I think SEP is probably more frequently indicated. *507*

PSOR — Increased growth of hair on the face; a fuzz (NAT-M, SULPH, CALC). *856*

SIL — The parotids enlarge from every cold and get hard, (BAR-C, CALC, SULPH). *928*

ALUMEN cures young children growing up with enormously enlarged and very hard tonsils, in whom every cold settles in the throat. ALUMEN is one of the cognates of BAR-C, which has the same tendency. In one patient there will be one kind of constitution, and after thoroughly examining, it looks like BAR-C. You may have a different constitution in another patient, and after carefully examining it, see that it looks like ALUMEN; another you will see is SULPH; another, if you look into it carefully, you will find is CALC, and another, CALC-IOD, and so on among those remedies capable of bringing about the conditions described. If we can find symptoms which picture the constitutional state we have no trouble. When the symptoms have been well gathered the case is as good as cured; it is then easy to find a remedy. *62*

LAC-C — Sore throat beginning and ending with the menstrual period. MAG CARB has sore throat before the menstrual period and CALC has cured sore throat when menstruating. *677*

MEZ — Sensation of goneness, fear, apprehension, faintness in the stomach, as if something would happen; every shock, pain and hearing bad news, cause this apprehensive, hungry, faint, weak, all-gone feeling in the pit of the stomach. It comes on when the doorbell rings, if the patient is expecting the postman, while waiting at the depot for the arrival of a friend, or the departure of the cars; on being introduced to someone, he experiences a thrill beginning in the stomach, is "frightened in the stomach". CALC, KALI-C, PHOS and MEZ have this. These "solar plexus" individuals often have a deep-cracked tongue and are hard to cure. *748*

PODO — Vomiting, greenish, profuse, watery, vomits everything; vomiting of milk (CALC, AETH - the latter sometimes retains water). *850*

The SULPHUR patient emaciates, and a peculiar feature is the EMACIATION OF THE LIMBS WITH DISTENDED ABDOMEN. The abdomen is tumid, with rumbling, burning and soreness, and with the distended abdomen there is emaciation of all other parts. The muscles of the neck, back, thorax and limbs wither, and the muscles of the abdomen are also wasted, but there is much distension of the abdomen itself. This condition of affairs is found in marasmus. You will find a similar state under CALC; and in women needing CALC you will notice great enlargement, distension and hardness of the abdomen with shrivelling of all other parts of the body. *956*

SIL has also cured fistulous openings. Patients who have a tendency to phthisis are subject to abscesses about the region of the rectum that break inside or out and form complete or incomplete openings. These seem to take the place of what would otherwise come, and if healed by operation or other external means, the tendency is to end in chest trouble, either in the form of a fixed catarrh or tubercular infiltrations. SIL is one of the remedies that turns the constitution into order and in one to five years the opening ceases to be necessary and it will heal. Surgeons heal it up at once and for a time the patient is comfortable, but in a few years he breaks down. CAUST, BERB, CALC, CALC PHOS, GRAPH, SULPH etc. are suitable in such cases. SIL here follows THUJ well. *932*

PODO — A child who should have a coloured stool has instead a white one like chalk (CALC). *851*

NIT AC — Every exertion brings on uterine haemorrhage (CALC). *800*

SEPIA comes in when the woman ought to menstruate when the child ceases to nurse; sometimes the child dies and menses ought to be re-established but do not appear, and the mother runs down, pines away; SEPIA will re-establish the flow. CALC is the opposite; the menses come on while the child is nursing. Thick, greenish, acrid or milky leucorrhoea. Leucorrhoea in little girls. *924*

In SIL there is a very easy flow of blood from the uterus; a haemorrhagic flow comes on before the menses from excitement, and especially when nursing; when the child is put to the breast a flow of blood starts. Notice the distinction between CALC and SIL. CALC has a tendency to flow during lactation, but not when the child is put to the breast. *933*

MANG — In women past the turn of life, every little while there will come a little haemorrhage, a little watery flow. Anaemic old ladies, with a little watery flow from the uterus. We have had in the past to rely mostly on CALC for the old ladies with haemorrhage of the uterus. **725**

KALMIA — "Wandering rheumatic pains in the region of the heart". "When articular rheumatism has been treated externally and cardiac symptoms ensue". Rheumatism that goes from the lower to the upper limbs. Not uncommonly you will meet such things. These "rubbers" that go around the streets with a strong liniment and considerable magnetism frequently cause a rheumatism to leave the knee joint and, when it does that, the heart is likely to be the organ that suffers. Then KALMIA, AURUM, BRYONIA, RHUS-TOX, LEDUM, CALC, ABROTANUM and sometimes CACTUS are remedies that prove suitable for such cardiac affections. ***670***

When the case is of sycotic origin, small or large white gelatinous polypi form in the larynx and they are sore, causing loss of voice or cracked voice. When they cause choking or uneasiness HEPAR is one of the remedies. HEPAR, CALC, ARG NIT and NIT AC and sometimes THUJA are the remedies related to such a condition. . ***575***

AMBR GR — "Listening to music brings on congestion to head." Music aggravates his cough. Think of one commencing to cough simply because he hears music! What a strange thing that is! CALC has such sensitiveness that the stroke of the piano is painful in parts, especially in the larynx. ***94***

Like LYC and CALC when suitably administered in old gouty conditions, not when there is much organic change present, SULPH will keep the rheumatic state in the joints and extremities. ***958***

ZINC — Aching in the dorsal, lumbar and sacral regions, better from walking and worse rising from a seat. (In RHUS the aching is in the sacral region and better when walking and coming on while sitting. CALC, RHUS, PHOS, SULPH and SEP have this in the highest degree. ZINC occupies a lower grade in the aggravation when rising from a seat, as do PETR and LEDUM.)... .... ***1014***

APOC — "Hydrocephalus, with great stupor." That is the last stage of it where there is great prostration, loss of flesh, stiffness of all the limbs, with dropsical swellings. Many times in hydrocephalus pains shoot along the nerves and attack the joints. Then it is that such remedies as APIS and CALC and APOC take hold with wonderful depth. The first permanent and substantial indication that the remedy is working in a hydrocephaloid case is that it increases the flow of urine, which has been scanty all the time. For hydrocephalus study TUB. ***125***

SIL — Slow recovery after pneumonia (LYC, SULPH, PHOS, SIL, CALC). Flushes, rattling in the chest. Flushes in the face during the day (SULPH, SEP, LACH), rattling in the chest like ANT TART, flushes like SULPH and LYC. ***934***

SIL — Phthisis; thick, yellow, green, foetid sputa, more pronounced coldness than CALC, and head sweat; pains in the lungs, sore lungs, stitches. ***934***

Some of our most stubborn cases of intermittent fever will relapse and continue relapsing, even when such remedies as SIL and CALC and the deeper acting remedies have been indicated, have acted well, have broken the fever, and in a few weeks, from exposure to cold, from sitting in a draft, from being fatigued, from mental exertion, from overeating and disordering the stomach this ague has returned. Any of these circumstances will bring back these stubborn cases of intermittent fever when TUB is needed. ***1001***

CALCAREA ARSENICOSUM

The desire to travel, that cosmopolitan condition of the mind belongs so strongly to the one who needs TUB. It comes out so often in clinical experience, is found so often in the CALCAREAS and especially CALC PHOS, always wanting to go somewhere. *1003*

CALCAREA FLUORATA

The desire to travel, that cosmopolitan condition of the mind belongs so strongly to the one who needs TUB. It comes out so often in clinical experience, is found so often in the CALCAREAS and especially CALC PHOS, always wanting to go somewhere. *1003*

CALCAREA IODATA

The desire to travel, that cosmopolitan condition of the mind belongs so strongly to the one who needs TUB. It comes out so often in clinical experience, is found so often in the CALCAREAS and especially CALC PHOS, always wanting to go somewhere. *1003*

ALUMEN cures young children growing up with enormously enlarged and very hard tonsils, in whom every cold settles in the throat. ALUMEN is one of the cognates of BAR-C, which has the same tendency. In one patient there will be one kind of constitution, and after thoroughly examining, it looks like BAR-C. · You may have a different constitution in another patient, and after carefully examining it, see that it looks like ALUMEN; another you will see is SULPH; another, if you look into it carefully, you will find is CALC, and another CALC-IOD, and so on among those remedies capable of bringing about the conditions described. If we can find symptoms which picture the constitutional state we have no trouble. When the symptoms have been well gathered the case is as good as cured; it is then easy to find a remedy. 62

CALCAREA PHOSPHORICA

RUMEX — Every cold seems to affect the joints. This is a marked feature of CALC PHOS; every change to cold is felt in the joints; from bathing and getting chilled afterwards. *887*

The desire to travel, that cosmopolitan condition of the mind belongs so strongly to the one who needs TUB. It comes out so often in clinical experience, is found so often in the CALCAREAS and especially CALC PHOS, always wanting to go somewhere. *1003*

The weight of the hat is a very common aggravation in headaches in schoolchildren. The little ones work all day in a hot stuffy room and feel better in the open air, but the weight of the hat is an encumbrance in GLONOINE as in NIT-AC and CALC PHOS. *550*

LYC is also suitable for girls at puberty when the time for the first menstrual flow to appear has come, but it does not come. She goes on to 15, 16, 17 or 18 without development, the breasts do not enlarge, the ovaries do not perform their functions. When the symptoms agree LYC establishes a reaction, the breasts begin to grow, the womanly bearing begins to come and the child becomes a woman. It has a wonderful power for developing, and in that respect it is very much like CALC PHOS....................... *712*

PULS — Flow slow in being established and then scarcely more than a leucorrhoea. Menstruation that has been painful since puberty in plethoric girls. I have seen PULS cure a great many girls of 16 to 18 years old. The mother comes to me saying her daughter has suffered since her first menses; she went in swimming, or got her feet wet, and has suffered since. The doctor says the parts are undeveloped and she must be operated on. PULS has established a normal flow in a few months. Now I will give you a contrast in another remedy. Scrawny girls who are sensitive to cold, have also taken a bath at the time the first menses should appear, or have got the feet wet, and the flow is partially suppressed, or has come on with an inflammation; a state of undevelopment is established, a stenosis; horrible menstrual colic; bearing down pains, as if everything would escape into the world, doubling the patient up; ameliorated by heat and aggravated by cold. CALC PHOS is the remedy. *869*

PSOR — Horribly offensive discharge from the nose; gluey discharge from the nose; offensive like MERC, SIL, CALC-P, HEPAR. *853*

KALI BICH — Catarrhal conditions of the larynx and trachea are worse in winter especially in the cold damp weather, like CALC PHOS, when the snow melts. .. *618*

SIL has also cured fistulous openings. Patients who have a tendency to phthisis are subject to abscesses about the region of the rectum that break inside or out and form complete or incomplete openings. These seem to take the place of what would otherwise come, and if healed by operation or other external means, the tendency is to end in chest trouble, either in the form of a fixed catarrh or tubercular infiltrations. SIL is one of the remedies that turns the constitution into order and in one to five years the opening ceases to be necessary and it will heal. Surgeons heal it up at once and for a time the patient is comfortable, but in a few years he breaks down. CAUST, BERB, CALC, CALC PHOS, GRAPH, SULPH etc. are suitable in such cases. SIL here follows THUJ well.. *932*

CALCAREA SULPHURICA

HEPAR is worse at night and in the morning. And when ACON has apparently controlled, but the croup returns the next morning, HEPAR comes in. Or if it comes on again the next evening with rattling HEPAR will also be suitable. Dry, with no rattling is SPONG. If the child wants to be covered, or says that it is chilly, HEPAR. If it says the room is too warm and kicks the covers off, it needs CALC SUL. *938*

The desire to travel, that cosmopolitan condition of the mind belongs so strongly to the one who needs TUB. It comes out so often in clinical experience, is found so often in the CALCAREAS and especially CALC PHOS, always wanting to go somewhere....... *1003*

HEPAR competes with SILICA in syphilitic nasal catarrhs where the parts are phagedenic; HEPAR, MERC COR and ARS are the principal anti-syphilitics when there is phagedenic ulceration of the nose. Babies suffer from bloody nasal discharge. This is often CALC SUL................................ *929*

CALCAREA SILICATA

The relationship between TUB and CALC is very close. They are interchangeable; that is, the one may be indicated for a while, and then the other. They are both deep acting remedies - also SIL is related to TUB, on the same plane of action, going deep into the life in a similar way; CALC, TUB, SIL and the SILICATES. *1003*

The desire to travel, that cosmopolitan condition of the mind belongs so strongly to the one who needs TUB. It comes out so often in clinical experience, is found so often in the CALCAREAS and especially CALC PHOS, always wanting to go somewhere. *1003*

CALENDULA

When tetanus comes on from punctured wounds in the palms or soles or in other parts, think of HYPERICUM, or when you have a punctured wound to treat, give LEDUM at once and you will prevent tetanus. When the fingernails have been torn, or the nerves in sentient parts like the ends of the fingers have been torn and lacerated, HYPERICUM becomes the remedy. For the bruising of various parts, and when the patient feels as if bruised all over, no matter how extensively he is bruised, ARNICA is generally the remedy. It may be said, for punctured wounds study LEDUM; for lacerated wounds of sentient nerves study HYPERICUM; for bruises study ARNICA; for open lacerations and cuts study CALENDULA. The conditions that come from the external ought to be remedied to a great extent by external means. A solution of CALENDULA is excellent in conditions that come from the external, and it should be applied externally. When you have lacerated wounds or cuts with knives or other sharp instruments, apply CALENDULA, because the injury is external without internal effects. The symptoms that arise from internal cause, treat with internal remedies, and symptoms that arise from external cause, when all that there is of the case is external, treat locally; in other words, for local causes use local means, and for internal or dynamic causes use internal means. Let internal wrongs be treated by the homoeopathic remedy and external or local conditions be treated by such soothing dressings as are most comfortable. Always protect surfaces that are exposed, raw and bleeding with something of a bland and superficial character. Wounds must be dressed with as simple a means as possible, and there is no simpler dressing than CALENDULA, 1 part to 4 or 6 of water. The tincture will smart too much. Your open wounds will granulate most beautifully under CALENDULA, and you will have no constitutional effects. When the constitutional state is orderly and there is an open injury let the constitution alone, but put on some soothing application externally. In doing this there is no law to govern the action of the physician. Air is an irritant to a raw part and will keep up an unnecessary discharge of pus, even from a perfectly healthy sore. CALENDULA will keep it protected. The sides of a cut must be drawn together, and if it is perfectly tight it will heal itself by first intention. If it does not, then you may know there is a constitutional condition that you must ferret out and find a remedy for. Local treatment must then be suspended. These remedies that I have mentioned, to a great extent cover the management of wounds, and it is simple. Anyone has sense enough to draw together and close up a yawning wound, and to properly dress it. The muscles that naturally draw a wound open have to be overcome by stitches or by strappings. They do not belong to prescribing, they belong to the surgeon. *696*

CAMPHOR

Medicines having much trouble with the veins are often disturbed by hot bathing, weakness after a hot bath, weakness in warm weather, aversion to heat and desire for cold. It is the state of PULS. The PULS veins contract in cold weather and the shrivelling up makes the patient feel better, but the veins fill and become engorged in the warm air and after a hot bath. A tepid bath sometimes makes a PULS patient feel better, but a Turkish bath is generally distressing. Many of the complaints of AESC are of this sort; AESC often feels better in cold air. The symptoms of AESC are often brought out by temperature, especially the little stinging pains. It is characteristic of these superficial pains that they are nearly always ameliorated by heat, while the deeper affections are nearly always ameliorated by cold. Now in PULS, the stinging pains in the scalp and those over the body, here and there, are often ameliorated by the local application of heat, while the patient himself wants to be in the cold; in the same way AESC stinging pains are better from heat, while the patient is often better from cold, although at times he is aggravated from cold damp weather in rheumatic and venous conditions. Again in SECALE we see that the little sharp pains that follow the course of the nerves are better from heat, but the patient himself wants to be in the cold air, or to be uncovered, except for the spot of pain, which he wants kept warm. We notice the same thing running through CAMPH; during the twinges of pain he wants the windows closed and wants hot applications; but as soon as the pain is over he wants the windows up and desires to be uncovered so that he can breathe. These are general things that are to be observed in analysing symptoms............................... ***38***

LAUR should be compared with CAMPH, AMM-C and SECALE.......................... 694

STRAM — During spasms, covered with cold sweat; sometimes almost as cold as ice; cold sweat in mania; this feature is equalled only by CAMPHOR.................................. ***949***

SEC — Chronic diarrhoea, exhaustive, watery discharges, cholera. It is related to CAMPHOR. Scrawny people take cholera, skin cold and blue; better from cold. Violent and continued thirst........................... ***909***

Is it any wonder that Hahnemann predicted that VERAT, CAMPH and CUPR would become remedies in the cure of cholera; he saw in their nature the ability to cure. He saw the similitude. In cases of this sort which are characterised by superabundance of cramps, CUPRUM is the simillimum. For those with coldness, blueness and scanty sweat, vomiting and purging, CAMPH is the remedy. These are called "dry cholera", they sink down and die without exhaustive discharges. In proportion as there are coldness, blueness and scanty discharges CAMPH is indicated. In proportion as copiousness, coldness and blueness are present, VERAT is indicated. SEC has something of cholera in it. PODO has exhaustive stools; ARS anxious restlessness.......................... ***1010***

CANNABIS INDICA

SQUIL — Quite similar to CANN IND or GELS in brain affections, but SQUIL has not many brain affections nor many febrile complaints. PHOS has inflammation of the brain and when the dangerous turn comes this increase of urine is a bad sign. ***941***

CANNABIS SATIVA

In the urethral disease of sycotic character THUJA leads all other remedies. In the non-sycotic variety CANN SAT is sufficient, but those cases that have proved to be sycotic CANN SAT left uncured, it ameliorated the burning during and after urination and the thick yellowish-green discharge, but some other remedy always had to follow when they were shown to be sycotic. It is not so with THUJA, because it is capable of finishing the case. *1000*

When a debilitated subject, one suffering from bone and cartilaginous troubles, contracts gonorrhoea, with it he will have an enormous swelling of the prepuce, and nothing seems to act on it. FL-AC will cure oedema of the prepuce with gonorrhoea in such a subject. CANN SAT has the same symptom, but it is especially useful in robust cases. *538*

PULS — Tumefaction about the penis. Foreskin dropsical (NIT-AC, FL-AC, CANN SAT). *869*

CANTHARIS

In the CAMPHOR mental state there is anxiety and extreme fear; fear of persons, of strange spheres, of the dark, the dark is filled with imaginary spectres, he dare not get out of bed in the dark; everything that moves is a spectre and the inanimate objects of the room become alive and terrify him. Frenzy. Coupled with this there is kidney and urinary trouble like that of CANTHARIS and because of this similarity the two remedies are both complementary and antidotal to each other. If a woman has poisoned herself with CANTH and there is present the frenzy and excitement CAMPH will act as antidote. *355*

At times in the beginning of a gonorrhoea this condition of priapism and intense uncontrollable sexual desire with swelling of the prepuce is overcome by FL-AC. There are times when this priapism demands CANTH, but that remedy differs wholly in its nature from this. *541*

Another thing running through HYOS in insanity and in the delirium of fevers is a fear of water, fear of running water. Of course, hydrophobia, which is named because of that symptom being a striking feature, has fear of water, but some remedies also have that fear of water. "Anxiety on hearing running water. A fear of water." That runs through BELL, HYOS, CANTH and, of course, the nosode HYDROPHOBINUM (LYSSIN). STRAM the fear of anything that might look like water, shining objects, fire, looking glass. Fear of things that have in any manner whatsoever the resemblance to and sound of fluids. HYDROPHOBINUM (LYSSIN) has cured "involuntary urination/defecation on hearing running water." It has cured a chronic diarrhoea when that symptom was present. *583*

CAMPH — I once knew a French woman who had an insane desire to keep her boys always at home with her, and she thought she could accomplish this if she could only keep them away from the girls; and to destroy their sexual desire she kept a bag of camphor under their pillows. All of them were made impotent. But in some provers it establishes sexual erethism. It has this like CANTH. *358*

APIS — The whole urinary tract is irritated, very much like CANTH, and these two medicines antidote each other. If you are called to a child that has been drugged with crude *Apis,* you can generally antidote it with CANTH. If you go to a woman who has taken CANTH for vicious purposes, you can very often overcome it with APIS. The violent frenzy that has been brought on by CANTH will be overcome by APIS. The smarting, burning and stinging along the urinary tract will be found under APIS. ***121***

The CAMPH urine is bloody and comes by drops like CANTH. ***357***

CAPSICUM

CADM SULPH — Every time he takes cold water, which he craves, goose-flesh comes out, a creeping or horripilation like CAPS. ***305***

CARBOLIC ACID

But you meet one who is sensitive to the sting of the honey bee, and if he gets one little sting in one place in his body, he comes down with nausea and anxiety that makes him feel that he is dying, and in about ten minutes he is covered with urticaria from head to foot; he stings and burns and wants to be bathed in cold water; he fears that he will die if something is not done to mitigate his suffering, rolls and tosses as if he would tear himself to pieces. I have seen all these symptoms come on after APIS. The antidote for that is CARB-AC. I have seen CARB-AC administered in that state and the patient described the sensation of the CARB-AC going down his throat as a cooling comfort. He says, "Why doctor, I can feel that dose go to the ends of my fingers." When you administer an antidote under such circumstances, listen to what your patient says. When you get the true natural antidote, and at times when you get the true curative medicine in a case, no matter how high the potency is, the patient will say, "I feel that to the roots of my hair and to the ends of my toes." Such is the feeling it gives when the true antidotal medicine goes to the innermost portions of his economy, and that is the way we want to get our medicines always, to be guided by the symptoms of our patient that they will tell us what medicines to administer, and when the medicine is administered its highest reaction is of that sort. ***118***

CARBO ANIMALIS

CRAVING FOR AIR IS STRONG IN THE CARBONS, yet often easily chilled and just as EASILY OVERHEATED, and complaints that come on from being overheated are related to the CARBONS. 554

BAR-C — A sensation of weight in the brow with headaches as if the forehead was pressing down over the eyes. Like CARBO VEG, CARBO AN and NATR MUR. ... ***225***

There is one class of patients you will find who will trouble you. Those cases that come into your office with puffed, venous, purple faces; they have an appearance of plethora; the face looks puffed, bloated and dropsical at times; it is a dark red, dusky face; such a face we shall cure sometimes with ASAFOETIDA. CARBO AN, AURUM, CARBO VEG and PULSATILLA are also related to this kind of face, but it is a very troublesome kind of face, it shows more or less cardiac disturbance and venous stasis. The venous side of the heart will often be involved, or about to be involved, when you have this kind of face. I never like to see them come into my office for they are hard cases to manage. *183*

Separation of the gums from the teeth. The teeth get loose. We hear about "the teeth rattling in his mouth". The CARBONS produce just such a state, a settling away and absorbing of the gums. They get spongy and bleed easily and hence looseness of the teeth with bleeding of the gums, which are very sensitive. *376*

CIS — Burning, bruised pain in the coccyx, worse from touch. That is like CARBO AN in which the coccyx burns when pressed on, especially after a slight injury in a nervous woman. 445

Slight irritation or inflammation at the lower end of the [spinal] cord; it feels lacerated and sore, and never passes over until the results of the injury right in the spot have been removed. Such injuries, if taken early, can be cured by HYPERICUM. It is in the remedy. These injuries have been cured in after years by CARBO AN, SIL and THUJA, and other remedies as indicated. *591*

GRAPH has restrained the growth of cancer of the cervix uteri, when there was burning and putrid bloody discharge, in this it resembles CARBO AN. 558

CARBONEUM SULPHURICUM

The CARBONS affect the veins more or less, relaxing and paralysing. *368*

CRAVING FOR AIR IS STRONG IN THE CARBONS, yet often easily chilled and just as EASILY OVERHEATED, and complaints that come on from being overheated are related to the CARBONS. *554*

Separation of the gums from the teeth. The teeth get loose. We hear about "the teeth rattling in his mouth". The CARBONS produce just such a state, a settling away and absorbing of the gums. They get spongy and bleed easily and hence looseness of the teeth with bleeding of the gums, which are very sensitive. 376

CARBO VEGETABILIS

That is one of the first things I observed, that outside of sycotics you will seldom find a cure for asthma. There is that peculiarity that runs through sycosis which gives you a hereditary disease, and asthma corresponds to that disease. Hence it is that SIL is one of the greatest cures for asthma; it does not cure every case, but when SIL corresponds to the symptoms you will be surprised how quickly it will eradicate it. While IPECAC, SPONG and ARS will correspond just as clearly to the supervening symptoms and to everything that you can find about the case, yet what will they do? They palliate; they repress the symptoms; but your asthma is no better off, your patient is not cured. ARS is one of the frequently indicated remedies for the relief of asthma; so also are BRY, IPECAC, SPONG and CARBO-VEG, but they do not cure; though they relieve surprisingly at times. Where a patient is sitting up, covered with a cold sweat, wants to be fanned by somebody on either side of the bed, dyspnoea is so distressing that it seems almost impossible for the patient to live longer, to get another breath, then CARBO VEG comes in and gives immediate relief and the patient will lie down and get a very good night's rest. But what is the result? On comes the asthma again the very next cold. NAT-S goes down to the bottom of this kind of a case. ***793***

Think of KALI CARB when after troubles like measles, a catarrhal state is left behind due to lack of reaction, the psoric sequelae. The cough following measles is very often a KALI CARB cough. KALI CARB, SULPH, CARBO VEG and DROSERA are perhaps more frequently indicated than other medicines in such coughs as follow pneumonia or measles. ***635***

GRAPH — From eruptions, catarrhal discharges, menstrual flow, ulcers, breath and perspiration there is marked offensiveness (like CARBO VEG, PSORINUM, KALI PHOS, KALI ARS). ***553***

CRAVING FOR AIR IS STRONG IN THE CARBONS, yet often easily chilled and just as EASILY OVERHEATED, and complaints that come on from being overheated are related to the CARBONS. ***554***

The CARBONS affect the veins more or less, relaxing and paralysing. ***368***

PETR is not so closely related to SIL as it is to GRAPH and CARBO VEG, which are carbonaceous substances, and all carbonaceous products affect the back of the head. "Pain from occiput over head to forehead and eyes, with transitory blindness; he gets stiff; loses consciousness". "Circumscribed pain in the occiput, aggravated on shaking the head." PETR, unlike CARBO VEG, has oversensitiveness of the senses, hearing, touch and smell. ***818***

Like CARBO VEG, CARBONEUM SULPHURATUM is a most useful remedy in COLLAPSE. Marked venous stasis in organs and parts. ***387***

DIG — Constant desire to take a deep breath. When he goes to sleep the breath seems to fade away, then he wakes up with a gasp. LACH, PHOS, CARBO VEG and some other remedies have that; remedies that affect the cerebellum particularly, producing a congestion of the cerebellum. ***500***

SPONG — Wakens at night in great fear, and it is some time before he can rationalise his surroundings, (AESC, LYC, SAMB, LACH, PHOS, CARBO VEG). ***938***

BAR-C — A sensation of weight in the brow with headaches as if the forehead was pressing down over the eyes. Like CARBO VEG, CARBO AN and NATR MUR. ***225***

SIL — Weight in the occiput as if it would be drawn back, with a rush of blood to the head, like CARBO VEG and SEPIA. .. ***927***

There is one class of patients you will find who will trouble you. Those cases that come into your office with puffed, venous, purple faces; they have an appearance of plethora; the face looks puffed, bloated and dropsical at times; it is a dark red, dusky face; such a face we shall cure sometimes with ASAFOETIDA. CARBO AN, AURUM, CARBO VEG and PULSATILLA are also related to this kind of face, but it is a very troublesome kind of face, it shows more or less cardiac disturbance and venous stasis. The venous side of the heart will often be involved, or about to be involved, when you have this kind of face. I never like to see them come into my office for they are hard cases to manage. ***183***

"Eructations relieve." "Flatulence passes upwards in quantities." Frequent eructations. Eructations do not always relieve. It is more like CHINA in its eructations. The eructations of CARBO VEG relieve for some time and he feels better. This is the way with CARBO VEG; he is distended almost to bursting and he cannot get up any wind, but finally after much pain and distension it wells up in empty eructations and then he gets relief. With CHINA he is distended and every little while getting up gas, but with no relief. It does not seem to help and sometimes patients will say they seem to get worse after it. So it is with ARG NIT at times. It evidently has both. *140*

CHINA — Flatulent distension almost to bursting. There are constant eructations, loud and strong, and yet no relief, so extensive is the flatulence. In CARBO VEG after belching a little there is relief. LYC has both. *442*

GRAPH — Flatulence is just as marked as in CARBO VEG, and the relief from belching is just as great. *557*

KALI IOD has all the flatulence and belching of CARBO VEG and LYC. *640*

RUMEX — Very flatulent, full of flatulent pains; pains relieved (CARBO VEG) by belching and passing flatus. *887*

Inflammation of the parotid (mumps) changing to testes or mammae is generally cured by CARBO VEG or PULS, but ABROT has cured when these remedies have failed. *17*

CAMPH — The air as it leaves the chest feels like that from a cellar, like CARBO VEG and VERAT. *256*

SQILLA — has a loose morning cough and a dry evening cough (ALUM, CARBO-VEG, PHOS-AC, SEP, STRAM, PULS). *941*

Retching in an effort to expectorate is usually controlled by CARBO VEG, but SIL has it. *931*

GRAPH — Hoarseness in the evening (like CARBO VEG). *558*

You remember, when we were going over the symptoms of CARBO VEG I told you that the hoarseness was worse in the evening. Now observe that the hoarseness of CAUST is worse in the morning. He gets up in the morning with a hoarse voice; if it is an ordinary case, after moving about and expectorating a little mucus, it is better....... *403*

GRAPH has cured deep seated spinal complaints, and in such cases the patient delights to lie heavily covered in a cold draft from an open window. It is easy to see in this the resemblance to CARBO VEG, which often cures when the patient wants to be fanned. *554*

HYPERICUM — After a surgical operation, where there has been much cutting, a great state of prostration, coldness, oozing of blood, almost cold breath, of course the Materia Medica man, if there is one around, will say, "Why, give him CARBO VEG, of course." Yes, you will, but it will not help him. It may disappoint you. But if you are a surgeon, know your surgical therapeutics better than a Materia Medica man, you will say, "No, STRONTIUM CARB is what I want." It relieves that congestion all over the body; he gets warm and has a comfortable night. STRONTIUM CARB is the CARBO VEG of the surgeon. 592

When the hay fever comes on, all the other symptoms are better, she feels nothing except the hay fever, however, all the symptoms interweave with each other. The NAT MUR symptoms will be worse in the morning and until toward noon, while in PULS they are worse in the evening, the nose filling up with thick, yellowish-green, ropy mucus, and when the nose has been cleared a dry, burning, smarting feeling remains; if the room is warm at night she cannot sleep. NAT MUR is a little like that in the smarting and inability to sleep at night in a warm room. In NAT MUR too the discharge may continue day and night. We have an acute class in which PULS is sometimes indicated - copious watery discharge which ends in sneezing. In the beginning we will think of CARBO-VEG, ARS, ALL-C, EUPH. With CARBO-VEG there is a watery discharge and the irritation extends into the chest, with hoarseness and rawness. In ALL-C we have one group of symptoms that points to this remedy. Excoriating discharge from the nose and bland discharge from the eyes; in the larynx, sensation as if hooks were there, and sometimes this extends below the larynx; this always means ALL-C; it is also worse in a warm room like PULS. The EUPH looks like ALL-C, only the discharge from the eyes is copious, watery and burning - the lachrymation burns the eyes and excoriates the cheeks; discharge from nose is bland like PULS. Sometimes this goes into the chest, then it is no longer EUPH. IOD is worse in a warm room; thick discharge from the nose which burns and excoriates and is yellowish-green; but there is one thing that differentiates it from all the others - the patient immediately begins to emaciate when the complaint comes on and is very hungry. KALI HYDR with the thick yellowish discharge, worse in a warm room, there is a great amount of rawness and burning in the nose; external nose very sore to pressure; sensitiveness in the root of the nose; whole face aches and patient is very restless; wants to walk in the open air which does not fatigue him. ARS IOD; anxiety, restlessness and weakness; frequent sneezing and copious watery nasal discharge that burns the lip. Burning, watery discharge from the eyes like ARS. ARS wants to be very warm; wants hot water applied to the eyes; the only relief is from sniffing hot water up the nose. ARS IOD is worse in a warm room, and for days after sneezing, the discharge thickens and becomes gluey, looking like THICK, YELLOW HONEY, this excoriates; much pain through the root of the nose and eyes; often rawness in the chest with dyspnoea. The remedies having the dyspnoea are ARSENIC, IODIDE OF ARSENIC, IODINE, KALI HYDR and SABADILLA; these are the ones I have found most frequently indicated in the asthmatic forms of hay fever. If the complaint has been developed after being overheated at about that time, you will find that SILICA, PULSATILLA and CARBO VEG must be carefully compared. There is another class of remedies having the stuffing up of the nose not relieved by the discharge. There is a constant desire to blow the nose, yet he gets no relief. This makes me think of LACH, KALI BI, PSOR, NAJA and STICTA. PSORINUM has the copious, watery, bland discharge from the nose, it may be excoriating, it has both. The stuffing up of the nose generally takes place in the open air; he is relieved in a warm, close room and by lying down; has some dyspnoea which is relieved by stretching the arms at right angles to the body. Hay fever is a psoric sickness. PSORINUM given in a single dose will so develop the symptoms that the case will be more clear. The attack is not the best thing to prescribe for. If it is too violent, a short acting remedy may be selected that will mitigate it. NUX VOMICA has a free, easy breathing in the open air, but when he goes into the warm room his nose stuffs up, which also occurs at night, though the water drips on the pillow yet he stuffs up like PULS, BRY and the IODINE preparations, IODIDE OF ARSENIC and CYCLAMEN. Do not understand me to have given remedies for hay fever, we cannot lay down remedies for diseases. The whole constitution must be most carefully examined...................... ***863***

At times a case of yellow fever gets along fairly well, but a draft causes a slight cold, and on comes sudden prostration, black vomit, death. In that state CADM SULPH competes with CARBO VEG, which used to be the main remedy in the hands of good prescribers. *306*

CAULOPHYLLUM

CIMIC should be compared with CAUL. 34

CAUSTICUM

As you might suppose, ALUM has fissures; you would naturally expect this when you consider what kind of mucous membranes and tissues this patient manufactures. He suffers greatly from constipation, he does much straining, the mucous membrane is thickened and swollen and hence we have a fissure. When you see a remedy manufacturing and producing such a state upon the economy, growing that kind of mucous membrane that would favour fissures, you do not have to wait until you have cured a fissure with that remedy to find out if it will suit the case. You do not have to resort to the repertory to see what this remedy has done in fissure. From your general knowledge of the medicine you will see that it ought to cure the patient, as it produces such a condition of the mucous membrane and skin as would naturally be found in one who has a fissure. The skin indurates and ulcerates and becomes clumsy and unhealthy and constipation is produced, and so, after studying the remedy in that way, you are not surprised if it cures a fissure. If you look into the nature of NIT-AC, CAUST and GRAPH you will see why they have had a wonderful record for curing fissure. That is the way to study your Materia Medica; see what it does to the man himself, to his organs and tissues. *73*

CADMIUM SULPH has numbness of parts - the nose, one hand; numbness in spots. In this it is similar to CAUST. *305*

In psoric cases complicated with syphilis and mercury and other violent drugs we find use for GUAIACUM, the most neglected remedy. It is closely related to CAUSTICUM, SULPHUR and TUBERCULINUM............ *562*

In some of these cases of brain syphilis SULPH and CAUST have caused prolonged suffering and weakness. SYPH will act favourably. *987*

FL-AC follows SIL as naturally as SIL follows PULS. They exist in threes. There are other remedies that exist in threes but the most common ones you will think of will be SULPH, CALC, LYC; SULPH, SARS, SEP; COLOC, CAUST, STAPH, which often follow each other and rotate in this way. Do not let these facts make you give a routine remedy unless symptoms agree, but it helps to remember that remedies are somewhat similar. *539*

KALI BICH — Sensitive to cold winds. CAUST, it will be remembered, is sensitive to cold dry winds. The KALIS generally are sensitive to cold, dry weather. *618*

BAR-C — Always borrowing trouble. Like CAUST, fear of something going to happen. Full of imaginations; imaginary cares and worries. Hatching up all sorts of complaints and grievances that may happen. A good deal like ARS. *224*

KALI PHOS — Paralysis of one side of the face, like CAUST. *649*

SIL has cured fistulous openings. Patients who have a tendency to phthisis are subject to abscesses about the region of the rectum, that break inside or out and form complete or incomplete openings. These seem to take the place of what would otherwise come, and if healed by operation or other external means, the tendency is to end in chest trouble, either in the form of a fixed catarrh or tubercular infiltrations. SIL is one of the remedies that turns the constitution into order and in one to five years the opening ceases to be necessary and it will heal. Surgeons heal it up at once, and for a time the patient is comfortable, but in a few years he breaks down. CAUST, BERB, CALC, CALC PHOS, GRAPH, SULPH etc. are suitable in such cases. SIL here follows THUJ well. ***932***

BELL — When becoming old, or chilled, or in very cold air, women lose their urine, like DULCAMARA and CAUSTICUM. ***247***

HYOS — "Paralysis of the bladder after labour, so that the urine remains in the bladder, with no desire to urinate." The routine remedy for retention of urine after labour is CAUST. CAUST, like RHUS, is a great remedy for the effects of strain upon muscles and parts, and the violent effort that the woman passes through in expelling the child from the womb in many instances leaves all the pelvic muscles tired, relaxed, paralysed. ***586***

PULS has dribbling of urine, dribbles on the slightest provocation. She must keep her mind continually on it, or she will lose her urine. As soon as she goes to sleep it flows away. Little, mild, gentle, florid, plethoric, warm-blooded girls, who kick the covers off at night and have nocturnal enuresis. Yellow, sallow, sickly girls who lose their urine in their first sleep call for SEP. Losing the urine in the first sleep is looked upon as a strong symptom, but you can figure it out, and hence it is NOT so. All those cases that have to make an effort to hold the urine during the day lose it in their first sleep; for then the mind is taken off it, and as soon as the mind is taken off it the urine dribbles. CAUST and SEP are remedies looked upon as curing involuntary urination during the first sleep, but I have cured it with many other remedies. A man past middle age flooded the bed at night as soon as he went to sleep. The medicines which have this are limited, and he had had them all. I found I must figure it out on another basis. I ascertained that when moving about at his work he had no difficulty in holding the urine, but when he sat down he had to make an effort to control it. At the time this condition developed he had been in Atlantic City and had bathed much in the ocean. Here were the aggravation and amelioration of RHUS, and RHUS cured him. Few would think of BRY in urinary trouble. When he moves the urine dribbles, when he walks it flows. He is relieved only by keeping quiet. BRY is aggravated by motion; RHUS is relieved by motion. ***868***

SENEGA — The rattling in the chest is as marked as in ANT-T, the tenacious mucus is as copious, as gluey and stringy as in KALI BICH, so much is this the case that he can get it only part way up and with a spasmodic effort he swallows it, like SPONG and CAUST. ***914***

SPONG — At times, after great dyspnoea, white tough mucus forms in the air passages, difficult to expectorate; it comes up and often has to be swallowed (ARN, CAUST, LACH, KALI-C, KALI-S, NUX-MOSCH, SEP, STAPH). ***939***

RUMEX — Hoarse; cannot speak because the vocal cords are covered with tough mucus. Chronic cases have often been cured. PHOS has this hoarseness, but especially aphonia relieved by hemming up a little mucus from the vocal cords. The CAUST hoarseness is due to a weakness of the vocal cords. PHOS has an inflammatory state and the continual accumulation of mucus impedes speech. RUMEX has the accumulation of tough, gelatinous, gluey mucus and he continually scrapes the larynx............ *886*

NIT-AC — SPREADING ULCERS. The ulcers discharge a brown, bloody water, offensive. Phagedenic ulcers (ARS, AUR-M-N, CAUST, MERC-C). *800*

KALI BICH — Gouty conditions are as common in this remedy as they are in the other KALIS. It is especially like CAUST with its cracking in the joints. *617*

CENCHRIS

CROT-H — I once had the privilege of tracing up a dog that had been bitten by the CENCH and had survived. It was bitten in the region of the neck, and in that region a large abscess formed every spring as long as that dog lived, until old age, when he died of that disease. *474*

Give AMM-C not as an antidote per se, but when indicated in blood-poisoning and animal bites with zymosis, with a tendency to black liquid bleeding, as in ELAPS. Running through the snake poisons there is a tendancy to bleeding of black blood that will not coagulate.. *99*

In PUERPERAL FEVER there is a continued oozing of black, offensive blood that will not coagulate; bleeding from every orifice of the body as well as from the uterus. Imagine a woman who is pregnant suffering from typhoid fever. She aborts and a low zymotic state comes on with the symptoms that I have described and with all the appearances as if she would bleed to death after the abortion. The blood will not coagulate and the flow continues. Or in a woman during a typhoid fever menstruation comes on. It is not a true menstrual flow, that is, it does not resemble the ordinary flow, because it is copious, dark and liquid, a continuous oozing with all the grave symptoms described, and especially the besotted countenance, the comatose state, the appearance as if she were intoxicated, lying as one dead. When aroused every muscle trembles; if the tongue is protruded it trembles, and there is inability to articulate. CROT-H may save her life. Would it be possible to think of graver states of sickness than such as are produced by the ophidia? When a physician sees these states coming on he immediately thinks of a class of remedies that can cover such a state, remedies like BAPT, ARS, SEC and the OPHIDIA, and sometimes ARN, PHOS and PYR. *477*

CHAMOMILLA

ARG-NIT — So marked is the aggravation from sugar that the nursing infant will get a green diarrhoea if the mother eats candy. Then is it astonishing that the baby can get a dynamised dose from the mother, when the dynamised dose can travel like lightning, and sugar takes all day to be digested and dynamised and fed as poison to the baby? I remember a case that I figured and figured on. The baby had MERCURIAL STOOLS, sure enough, they were grass green. Well CHAM has grass green stools, and ARS and MERC and lots of remedies have grass green stools. Routinist that I was in those days I could not get anything but MERC out of it, and although the baby had gotten MERC, ARS and CHAM, there was no relief, there was no relief until I found that the mother had been eating candy. When she was asked if she ate sweet things, sugar etc. she said, "Oh no." "Why, yes you do", said the husband, "I bring you home a pound of candy every day. What do you do with it?" "Oh, that was nothing", she replied. But the baby did not get well until it got ARG-NIT and the mother stopped eating sugar. *140*

The aggravation of the CHAM patients, who are also extremely irritable, is at 9 am. Sometimes we go to the bedside and can hardly distinguish between BRY and CHAM because they are both so spunky, but the CHAM baby is worse at 9 am., the BRY baby is worse at 9 pm. *278*

BELL has in its nature all the sensitiveness to pain. It is a part of the general sensorium; the whole bodily state is intensified. The CHAM patient is oversensitive to pain but we do not need to sympathise with the CHAM patient, he will fight it out himself. But you will pity the BELL patient, the PULS patient, the NIT-AC patient. *239*

When coffee furnishes a crutch, it is a sure sign that drinking it must be stopped. So it is with tea or any beverage. Such persons sometimes become sensitive to coffee and they drink it in great quantities; the face becomes red; headaches come on, and other symptoms of COFFEA. Stopping the coffee brings out quite a proving, and you have to study CHAM and NUX VOM for an antidote. In all these remedies you get opposite effects. *458*

In BRY there is a keynote which really applies to a dozen or more remedies, "he wants something and he knows not what." It is a very important symptom of BRY. It is a symptom that calls for BRY only when the rest of the symptoms agree. You go to a child who is being carried in the arms of the nurse and wants one toy after another; you give him the toy he wants and he does not want it and throws it right back at you. When that case is looked into thoroughly it may be covered by KREOSOTE. Another is never satisfied with anything and rejects everything he asks for; you look into that case and it may be covered by CHAM. *278*

This SLUGGISH state of mind then is the state of BRY, not an excitable state as in COFF, NUX VOM, IGN, but sluggish, aggravated from motion, aggravated from being talked to, wants to lie still in bed, very great irritability, which is as extreme as that found in NUX or CHAM. *278*

SEPIA — The cough is a violent one. Cough during first sleep (LACH. In irritable children CHAM). *919*

STAPH — "Chronic diarrhoea or dysentery of weakly, sickly children after anger; after being punished, after emotions." (COLOC and CHAM). *946*

BAR-C — There is a remedy for inflammation of the tonsils where the ear is involved and is ameliorated by heat, that very few use, but it is of great value; it is CHAM, and it is especially indicated if the patient is irritable. The pain is ameliorated by heat and comes on with great violence. It might be mistaken for a BELL inflammation, but CHAM cures it permanently. *227*

CHELIDONIUM

The patient has been taking mercury all his life and his liver is enlarged, and his joints are enlarged. He goes to every doctor, with an endeavour to get relief from his distressing sufferings. Mercury and disease are so mixed up that a great turmoil will result from your first prescription. He will go through these stages of violence and periodical attacks. You will have to know such medicines as AURUM, CHELIDONIUM and

STAPHISAGRIA to get this patient over these awful attacks which he is obliged to go through. *196*

CHINA

The more chronic the complaint is, the longer is its cycle, so that we will find the more acute and sharp troubles in which ARS is suitable will have every other day aggravations and every 4th day aggravations; but as the trouble becomes chronic and deep-seated, it takes on the 7th day aggravation, and in the psoric manifestations of a long lingering, deep seated kind there is a 14th day aggravation. This appearing in cycles is common to a good many remedies, but is especially marked in CHINA and ARS. These two remedies are similar to each other in many respects, and they are quite similar in their general nature to the manifestations that often occur in malaria. It is true, however, that ARS is more frequently indicated than CHINA. In every epidemic of malarial fever that I have gone through I have found ARS symptoms more common than those of CHINA. *154*

NAT MUR is one of the greatest malarial remedies, but it is full of order like CHINA, SEP is full of disorder. In a case confused by remedies think of CALC, ARS, SULPH, SEP and IPECAC. Never give CHINA or NAT MUR for irregular symptoms and stages. *925*

CYCL — Complaints after weaning (CHINA). *497*

Another grand feature of FERRUM is that, like CHINA, it has complaints from loss of animal fluids; from prolonged haemorrhage, with weakness remaining a long time. There is no repair, no assimilation. *527*

CALC SIL — The muscles, tendons and joints are weak and easily strained. The weakness is much like ARS or CHINA, or as though from loss of fluids. *338*

PHOS AC — From the beginning the mental state has been most marked, and finally comes the muscular weakness, which increases until the jaw drops and it seems that the patient must die of exhaustion. Such states of weakness may come on from haemorrhages (CHINA was the routine remedy among the older homoeopaths). It checks the haemorrhage and causes a rally, prevents the dropsy. *821*

CYCL — Thinks she is alone in the world and persecuted by everyone (CHINA). *495*

COFF — So full of ideas that she lies awake nights making plans, thinking of a thousand things; utterly unable to banish the thoughts that flood the mind; hears the clocks on distant steeples, as do OP, CHINA and NUX VOM. *457*

When persons have bled out and have become waxy and pale the routinist thinks of CHINA, but when there has been no bleeding and this same state is present from breaking down of the blood corpuscles MANG is to be thought of. *724*

MAG CARB and CHINA, when no other symptoms are present, are prominent remedies among affections of the teeth during pregnancy. *714*

ARG NIT — "Eructations relieve", "Flatulence passes upwards in quantities" Frequent eructations. Eructations do not always relieve. It is more like CHINA in its eructations. The eructations of CARBO VEG relieve for some time and he feels better. This is the way with CARBO VEG; he is distended almost to bursting and he cannot get up any wind, but finally after much pain and distension it wells up in empty eructations and then he gets relief. With CHINA he is distended and every little while getting up gas, but with no relief. It does not seem to help and sometimes patients will say they seem to get worse after it. So it is with ARG NIT at times. It evidently has both. . *140*

KALI-BICH — Diarrhoea after beer, like ALOE, CHINA, GAMBOGIA, LYC, MUR-AC and SULPH. *621*

Suppose a woman should come to you who has been suffering from haemorrhage, from prolonged oozing, who is pallid and weak and distended with flatulence, with much belching and passing of gas, and the more she passes the worse she feels, and she has the symptoms of straining a long time to pass a soft stool, tremendous effort with inactivity of the rectum. You could do nothing but give her CHINA. You may have twenty remedies all possessing a certain symptom, but if you have a few real decided things that you can say about the patient, the manner in which he does business, the manner in which disease affects the entire man, then you have something to individualise by. You have seen the ALUM patient, the CHINA patient and the NUX-M patient. The sole duty of the physician is to treat the sick, which means to study the PATIENT HIMSELF until an idea of the sickness is obtained........... *68*

Great straining at stool belongs to many remedies but especially to ALUMINA, ALUMEN, CHINA, NAT MUR, NUX VOM, NUX MOSCH, and SIL. *932*

PODO — Painless stools, in which compare CHINA, which has stools coming on at night and after eating. *848*

APOC will cause the patient to bleed so copiously that she becomes anaemic from uterine haemorrhage; and then will follow dropsy. The old practitioners were in the habit of giving CHINA in most instances in which dropsy followed a haemorrhage. It was so generally useful and so commonly relieved that they seldom used any other remedy. But APOC is also a remedy for dropsy following haemorrhage. Many times it will fit the symptoms clearly in dropsy following haemorrhage. *127*

It is not an uncommon thing for a malarial fever that has lingered a long time to be attended with swelling of the lower limbs. EUP-PER very strongly competes with NAT MUR, CHINA and ARS in such lingering malaria. *515*

PSOR — Involuntary stool at night (CHINA has a black, profuse, watery stool at night and after meals.) In PSOR we find the haste of SULPH, the flatulence of OLEAN and ALOE, and difficulty of expelling a soft stool like ALUM, CHINA and NUX-M. *855*

CICUTA VIROSA

Twitching and jerking of the eyes. You will observe this about the AGAR eyes; as the patient looks at you there is a pendulum-like action of the eyes; they go back and forth all the time; they oscillate, though he tries his best to fix his look on you. This stops only during sleep. A few other medicines have cured this eye symptom - CIC, ARS, SULPH, PULS. *44*

CIMICIFUGA

PODO — Great soreness of the abdomen before and during the menstrual period (APIS, CIMIC, VESPA, LACH, but these are not so likely to have diarrhoea and, if so, it is not as copious). *849*

ZINC has a striking symptom; no matter what the violent symptoms are, pain in the ovaries, in the uterus, hysterical excitement; as soon as the menstrual flow appears there is relief. Violent pains in the ovaries relieved by the flow. This is a great contrast to CIMIC, which has nervous excitement and hysteria during the flow, and the more copious it is, the more violent are the pains. The LACH and ZINC symptoms are worse before and better with the flow, but in the former the pains all return when the flow slackens up again. CIMIC has at times an intermittent flow, the pain ceasing with each intermission, returning when the flow again appears. *1016*

KALI CARB — It is a severe labour, a prolonged labour; the uterus appears to be weak, and the pains are feeble; they are all in the back and do not go to the centre of operation as they should. Now this same kind of a pain may deceive you in taking another form. The pains begin in the back, appear to go to the uterus and then run up the back, which would turn you aside entirely from the KALI CARB pain into a pain that would indicate GELS. Sometimes these pains are so severe that they appear to prevent rather than encourage the contractions of the uterus; when the contractions of the uterus cease and the woman screams out with pain in each side of the abdomen rather than in the centre, in the region where the broad ligament ought to be, and wants her hips rubbed, CIMIC will make the pains regular. *634*

CINA

ARUM is one of the most striking medicines as an illustration of the keynote system, that is, with those who prescribe on one symptom and give this medicine whenever the patient bores his nose or picks his lips, notwithstanding that CINA bores the nose and picks the lips. CINA has more of the congestive and nerve symptoms. *180*

IGN — The child is cold and pale, and has a fixed staring look, like CINA. *594*

SEPIA — Sensation of a lump in the throat (like LACH but it is better from swallowing.) The same in worm troubles indicates CINA. *921*

COCCULUS

CON — Inability to stand any physical effort without great exhaustion. Gradually growing paralytic weakness, somewhat as described in COCC. *468*

The vertigo most common in CON is that which comes on while LYING IN BED ROLLING THE EYES or TURNING THE EYES. This is somewhat as it is in COCC, not as to vertigo alone, but the general slowed down condition of the muscles. *470*

COLCH — The stomach and bowel symptoms are very decided. This is very like COCC. Absolutely unable to touch food. Nausea, gagging, retching at the bare mention of food in his presence. The thought and smell of food bring on nausea and vomiting. With all these low forms of disease, these states described, we can see that this kind of weakness is little different from the COCC weakness. *461*

Post-diphtheritic paralysis is a serious condition and only a few remedies can cure it. CAUST is one of them. LACH and COCC are also important. *401*

COCCUS CACTI

CUPR — The cough is brought on sometimes by inhaling cold air, but stopped by drinking cold water, like COCC-C. *493*

A patient much debilitated with bronchial catarrh; susceptible to cold, to every change in weather, from change to damp weather, to every draft, to change of clothing; always taking new "cold". There is burning in the chest behind the sternum; thick, tough, ropy expectoration; spasmodic cough, and every cough ends in belching; eructations of gas, empty eructations. If to the burning in the chest, the severe pains in the larynx and trachea while talking and cough ending in belching, you add heat in the palms and soles, SANG will patch him up and mitigate the trouble. Many such cases get SULPH, but to their destruction. There is a class of remedies that suits these phthisical patients better than SULPH, SIL and GRAPH; such remedies as PULS, SANG, SENECIO GRACILIS and COCCUS CACTI, which will palliate, mitigate his sufferings and may even build him up so that he could take a medium potency of a deep remedy...... *900*

COFFEA

If you have administered ACON in too many doses or given it too strong and your patient is slow in recovering from the attack, or your patient has taken ACON himself unwisely, then COFFEA or NUX will often put the patient in a better condition................ *31*

OP — There is also a sensation of bodily well being; great happiness; great state of confidence in the first few hours of the drug. Hence complaints from sudden joy, anger, shame, sudden fright. COFF has a similar state of beatitude. It is both a physical and mental beatitude in OP. OP and COFF are related; they antidote each other. *813*

GRATIOLA is a great remedy for nervous prostration; marked lassitude, with mental and bodily weakness. It is closely related to COFFEA and NUX VOMICA and especially useful for the weakness of will and neuralgic pains in coffee drinkers. *560*

There are some remedies that correspond to extreme irritation in very sensitive natures; like HEPAR where she faints with the pain; like NITRIC ACID who cannot bear the noise of vehicles going along the street, because it creates such violent sufferings; like COFFEA where footsteps aggravate all the complaints; he was so sensitive to pain that the noise of one entering the door when he was on the third floor aggravated his sufferings intensely, though no one else could hear it. In NUX VOMICA even the sound of footsteps increases the pain all over the body. BELL has in its nature all this sensitiveness to pain. It is a part of the general sensorium; the whole bodily state is intensified..................... *239*

The sluggish state of mind is the state of BRY, not an excitable state as in COFF, NUX VOM, IGN, but sluggish, aggravated from motion, aggravated from being talked to, wants to lie still in bed, very great irritability, which is as extreme as that found in NUX or CHAM.............................. *278*

FERR PHOS — His ideas are abundant and there is unusual clearness of mind (COFF). *532*

STAPH — Crawling etc. in the female external genitals, COFF, PLAT, PETROL, APIS, TARENT HISP. *947*

COLCHICUM

That is a strong feature of CADM SULPH; he wants to keep as still as COLCH and BRY. *739*

SEPIA — Aversion to food, to the smell of food cooking, like COLCH and ARS. .. *921*

SEP — The acute diarrhoeas and dysenteries with jelly-like stools are more in keeping with KALI BICH and COLCH. *922*

COLOCYNTH

All recurrent troubles, those that come periodically, or after eating certain articles, or from exposure, or with a periodicity that belongs to time - all these states are chronic, they are not acute troubles. They are simply a small portion of a chronic miasm, a side view, and all such cases must have a constitutional remedy sooner or later. You can, it is true, relieve a violent pain at the first visit, but then you must look deeper and prevent your patient having more trouble. Otherwise if you should give BELL or COLOC or any medicine that simply fits the colic the trouble will come back again; you have not cured your patient; you have only palliated. *630*

KALI CARB — Colic, with cutting, tearing pains, doubling him up, coming on every little while. Tremendous flatulence. When the attack of colic is on it might remind you of COLOCYNTH or of some other of the acute remedies that cure colic in 2 or 3 minutes, but you will find that these acute remedies that relieve colic so speedily when given the second or third time do not produce so marked an effect. You will find it necessary to hunt for an anti-psoric, a remedy that will control the whole case. In the study of the colic alone during its attacks you only get a one sided view of the case and after the colic is over (say after the colic has been cured by COLOC) you now study the patient and go over the case and behold, all the symptoms are covered by KALI CARB. *630*

STAPH — "Chronic diarrhoea or dysentery of weakly, sickly children after anger; after being punished, after emotions." (COLOC and CHAM). STAPH and COLOC resemble each other. In both, eating and drinking cause griping and stool, both have colic as if stones were squeezing; STAPH in the intestines, head and testes, COLOC in the intestines and ovaries; both are worse from anger. CAUST, COLOC and STAPH follow each other like SULPH, CALC and LYC. *946*

STANN — Colic better from pressure, lying on the stomach (COLOC, CUPR). *944*

BELL has violent colic, intense cramping pain in children. Face red and hot; pain relieved only by bending forward. The mother finds that by holding the child on her hand it will relieve the colic. That is like COLOCYNTH; but COLOCYNTH is without much fever, without much thirst, a pain in one spot, an intense colic in the abdomen ameliorated by doubling up, ameliorated by bending across something hard, that is COLOCYNTH. In that instance COLOCYNTH can be prescribed on that one group of symtoms. *246*

MAG PHOS — Pain at the pit of the stomach. Spasms of the stomach with clean tongue. Colic ameliorated by doubling up, like COLOC, and ameliorated by heat. The colic is not so markedly relieved by heat in COLOC but is relieved by pressure. ... *721*

CONIUM

CON has sweat on closing the eyes. These were the points used by keynote prescribers, and sometimes good results were obtained. I remember once curing an organic stricture which had been dilated but was no better. The patient described his symptoms and the stricture was all he could think of. I did not see his remedy and gave everything without relief. One day however he told me he could not close his eyes to go to sleep without having a profuse sweat. I gave him CON on that keynote alone but it cured him of the sweat and the stricture, brought back an old gonorrhoeal discharge and resorption of the inflammatory material took place. A scientific prescriber would not do that; but when he heard that symptom he would not know it was in the nature of CON to have the stricture, and in another case he would see that CON did not suit, and he would know when and when not to give it. ***717***

SIL — Begins to sweat as soon as he falls asleep (PULS, CON). ***934***

There is great exhaustion in RUTA. The legs give out on rising from a chair, the patient totters and makes several efforts on rising from a seat. Routinists give PHOS and CON for this. RUTA and PHOS both have violent unquenchable thirst for ice-cold water. Compare PHOS and CON because of the weakness through the hips and thighs. ***890***

BAR-M is the natural complement of CONIUM in glandular affections and it [BAR-M] is very similar, but much deeper acting. ***230***

BAR-M — Complaints of the eyes and head through exertion of vision, much like CONIUM. 230

GRAT — Violent palpitation after stool (CONIUM). ***561***

STAPH — Meibomian tumours (CON, THUJA). ***946***

NUX-V — Pressure and sense of weakness in the left inguinal ring - hence cures hernia in babies (LYC, right side). ARN relieves soreness etc. CON also - it competes with NUX in sense of goneness in the groin.. .... ***809***

CROTALUS HORRIDUS

Give AMM-C not as an antidote PER SE, but when indicated in blood-poisoning and animal bites with zymosis, with a tendency to black liquid bleeding, as in ELAPS. Running through the snake poisons there is a tendency to bleeding of black blood that will not coagulate. ***99***

KALI BICH — There is pain in the liver, hard, contracting pain extending to the shoulder, resembling CROT-H. ***621***

On inflamed surfaces NAJA produces greyish exudations. It does not partake so extensively of this character as do LACH and CROT. There is only a shadow of the septic in NAJA, but it is extensive in LACH and extremely marked in CROT. NAJA is not as subject to haemorrhage as either LACH or CROT. 755

CROTON TIGLIUM

Here I might speak of several remedies which relate to the RHUS poison. There are many vesicular remedies that look like RHUS and all of them you will have to use more or less in their antidotal relations to each other, but it is well to be sure in a given case which one of them produced the poison. CROTON TIG, RHUS, RANUNCULUS, ANAC and CLEM at times look so alike that I am unable to tell them apart by their eruptions. They are all similar enough to each other to become universal antidotes. The others are all deeper acting than RHUS. ***446***

CUPRUM

CUPRUM is so sensitive all over. It has sensitive skin, sensitive polypi, everything sensitive; and it is so sensitive in its reaction that when it is needed partially indicated remedies will not work, because the patient is so oversensitive to everything that everything overacts. The smallest dose, the mildest dose, the simplest dose overacts and everything aggravates. Odours aggravate, well selected remedies disturb instead of cure. CUPRUM tones down, relieves that sensitivity and well selected remedies will then act curatively and long. CUPRUM lacks it in that state of high congestion - it is not like BELL in that. CUPRUM does not have that sensibility along with the active fever and congestion, the throbbing and disturbance of the circulation, but it has it in a chronic state. Women and children are so sensitive that they get no sympathy - and it is not suitable for hysterical ones either, but those that are not able to control themselves perfectly. Such is CUPRUM. ***239***

Sometimes the scarlet fever patient will go into convulsions because the rash fails to come out. APIS is sometimes a suitable remedy and must be compared with BRY, CUPRUM and ZINC. ***120***

CIC — The convulsions spread from above downwards, and thus it is the opposite of CUPR. The convulsions of CUPR spread from the extremities to the centre; ie, the little convulsions, merely cramps, are first felt in the fingers, and then in the hands and later in the chest and whole body. In CIC the little convulsions of the head, eyes and throat spread down the back to the extremities with violent contortions. ***433***

HYOS — Then again after he recovers from these low forms of disease there is quivering of the lids, and jerking of the lids, jerking of the muscles of the eye so the eyeball is unsteady. It moves from little spasms of the various muscles of the globe of the eye. All of these symptoms occur either along with the fever, of afterwards. The child goes into convulsions, or has periods of convulsions, where during the course of a week or ten days there have been from fifteen to fifty convulsions, and it may be that the convulsions have been remedied with BELL or CUPRUM or any one of a number of remedies, and afterwards these eye troubles, strabismus and disturbance of the vision. ***585***

CIC — Convulsive action about the eyes; pupils dilated and insensible; patient lies fixed in one place, with staring, fixed, glassy, upturned eyes, like CUPR. ***435***

DROS — Ordinarily the face is pale and sunken, with heat of the face and cold extremities, except when coughing, at which time the face becomes red, congested and purple like BELL and CUPR.............. ***502***

CINA — When the head symptoms are present, the milk or water gurgles down the oesophagus with a gurgling click. This is present in diarrhoea or vomiting with brain symptoms. ARS and CUPR are also prominent in gurgling down the oesophagus when swallowing. ***437***

STANN — Colic better from pressure, lying on the stomach (COLOC, CUPR). *944*

CURARE

CURARE is analogous to the symptoms of ALUM. I wish we had a finer proving of it, but it is rich with a great many things similar to ALUM and PLUMB and especially in the weakness of the hands and fingers of pianists. An old player will say that after she has been playing for some time her fingers slow down. The weakness seems to be in the extensors. Lack of ability to lift the fingers; the lifting motion is lost. CUR to a great extent overcomes that, causes quickness to that lifting power of the fingers. But this remedy also runs through in a general way such paretic conditions; while CUR is especially related to a paralytic condition of the extensors more than the flexors, the paralysis in ALUM is of both flexors and extensors. *72*

PLUMB — The paralysis begins in the extensors, so that we have wrist-drop. He cannot raise or lift anything with the hand. Extension is difficult. This occurs in piano players; they cannot lift their fingers sufficiently rapid to keep up the pace, while flexion is alright. CURARE is another remedy which corresponds to this state in piano players; a paralysis from overexertion of the extensor muscles. When the muscles become fatigued from playing fixed exercises, scales etc. for hours at a time, when the player has to do the same things over and over again, RHUS comes in, but it is an acute remedy and only holds for a short time. It is especially a RHUS condition when certain muscles become overused and the patient takes cold and a weakness sets in; after a cold bath or plunge the muscles take on paresis; getting wet when tired brings on the RHUS state. For the chronic state which follows, PLUMB and sometimes CURARE will be indicated. *845*

CYCLAMEN

PULS — A striking feature is, when the menstrual flow is present there is milk in the breasts. In girls at puberty - milk in the breasts; a premature establishment of milk. In non-pregnant women, milk in the breasts (CYCL, MERC)................................... *870*

NUX VOMICA has a free, easy breathing in the open air, but when he goes into the warm room his nose stuffs up, which also occurs at night, though the water drips on the pillow yet he stuffs up like PULS, BRY and the IODINE preparations, IODIDE OF ARSENIC and CYCLAMEN. *864*

DIGITALIS

In severe liver and heart affections the stomach is not able to keep up assimilation; palpitation, great weakness, liver congested, white stool. DIG comes in here with its deathly sinking not better by eating. In SEPIA this symptom is associated with loss of affections, the lump in the rectum with the constipation, etc. *922*

LYC — Awful "goneness" or weakness in the stomach, not relieved by eating (DIGIT).. .... *711*

LAUR — Emptiness in the stomach after eating (DIG) as if he were still hungry.... .... *694*

DOLICHOS

In ALUM at the beginning there in no eruption, but he scratches until the skin is off and then come the crusts. You must here prescribe not for the eruption, but for the itching of the skin without the eruption. Now in MEZEREUM, ARSENICUM, DOLICHOS and ALUMINA the skin itches and he scratches until it bleeds, and then he gets relief. Of course, after this there is an apparent eruption, because crusts form. As soon as the healing begins the itching begins and he is only relieved when the skin is raw. With the bleeding and moisture of the skin there is relief of the itching.. ***71***

DROSERA

STANNUM — Paralytic symptoms; writer's cramp; women who cannot let go of the broom. (DROS cures most cases.) ***944***

Think of KALI CARB when after troubles like measles, a catarrhal state is left behind due to lack of reaction, the psoric sequelae. The cough following measles is very often a KALI CARB cough. KALI CARB, SULPH, CARBO VEG and DROSERA are perhaps more frequently indicated than other medicines in such coughs as follow pneumonia or measles. ***635***

DULCAMARA

RAN-B is as sensitive to motion as BRY, and to the cold damp weather as DULC..... ***874***

MANG — Sore bones, burning in the soles, arthritic enlargements, painful periosteum, sore joints. It has not rapid inflammatory rheumatism, like PULS and BELL, but tenderness of the joints with not much swelling and aggravation from damp weather, like RHOD, RHUS and DULC. ***726***

A strong feature running through MANG is similar to DULC in that it is worse from cold, cold air and cold, damp weather......... ***724***

CALC — Diarrhoea that can't be stopped, because every time he gets a cold it renews the diarrhoea. When it is an acute attack DULC often relieves it, but when it has recurred several times DULC can no longer relieve it, and CALC then becomes one of the remedies. ***326***

SULPH — Every "cold" in some patients settles in the bladder. This is like DULC, and when DULC will no longer hold, or when it has been suitable in earlier stages, SULPH follows it well.. ***970***

MERC, IPECAC and ACON are frequently indicated in epidemic dysentery that comes in HOT weather, and IPECAC, DULC and MERC are frequently indicated in the dysentery of COLD weather..................... ***738***

MAG CARB — "Stools green, like scum on a frog pond; sour, frothy; with white floating lumps like tallow, bloody, mucous." Floating like lumps of tallow is more characteristic of PHOS, and many times DULC has cured it. ***715***

CIMIC — Tendency to take cold and thereby she takes on sensitiveness in the glands and larger organs, such as the liver and uterus. Complaints in these organs come on from damp, cold weather (DULC) and from being chilled. ***31***

BELL — When becoming old, or chilled, or

in very cold air, women lose their urine, like DULCAMARA and CAUSTICUM........ *247*

PULS — Urinary troubles worse when getting chilled (DULC)........................ *868*

MANG — Every spell of cold rouses up a bronchitis, like DULC *726*

ELAPS

CROT-H — There is some reason to think that this will be more or less a heart remedy from the cardiac weakness it produces. But the other snake poisons like NAJA, LACH and ELAPS have had more clinical application than this one *477*

CROT-H — In PUERPERAL FEVER there is a continued oozing of black, offensive blood that will not coagulate; bleeding from every orifice of the body as well as from the uterus. Imagine a woman who is pregnant suffering from typhoid fever. She aborts and a low zymotic state comes on with the symptoms that I have described and with all the appearances as if she would bleed to death after the abortion. The blood will not coagulate and the flow continues. Or in a woman during a typhoid fever menstruation comes on. It is not a true menstrual flow, that is, it does not resemble the ordinary flow, because it is copious, dark and liquid, a continuous oozing with all the grave symptoms described, and especially the besotted countenance, the comatose state, the appearance as if she were intoxicated, lying as one dead. When aroused every muscle trembles; if the tongue is protruded it trembles, and there is inability to articulate. CROT-H may save her life. Would it be possible to think of graver states sickness than such as are produced by the ophidia? When a physician sees these states coming on he immediately thinks of a class of remedies that can cover such a state, remedies like BAPT, ARS, SEC and the OPHIDIA, and sometimes ARN, PHOS and PYR.. *477*

EUPATORIUM PERFOLIATUM

ARUM — The sneezing is like an ordinary coryza, with repeated chills over the body and aching in the bones as if the bones would break, like NUX, EUPATOR, ARN, RHUS, BRY and ARS that have aching all over during "cold". *180*

PYR — The aching in the bones like EUPATORIUM.................................... *871*

EUPHRASIA

MANG — The cough is ameliorated from lying down. Most coughs are worse from lying down and few remedies have amelioration from lying. In EUPH there is a cough coming from coryza, especially acute coryza in vigorous persons, and the cough is better while lying... *726*

RUTA — "Eyes feel hot like balls of fire." To use RUTA for a pure inflammation when the eyes feel hot would be a failure. EUPHRASIA, BELL and ACON are used in simple inflammation from a cold, and the anti-psorics when the case is chronic. But if a woman strains her eyes from long SEWING ON FINE WORK, and the balls feel like fire, she needs RUTA. *891*

ZINC and EUPH are closely related in eye troubles.. *1016*

MEASLES when they come out with that purplish colour very often require SULPH. SULPH is a great remedy in measles. A routinist can do pretty well in this disease with PULS and SULPH, occasionally requiring ACON and EUPH. *960*

SABAD - HAY FEVER when there is spasmodic sneezing, fluent coryza; nostrils stuffed up; inspirations through nose laboured; snoring; itching in the nose; profuse bleeding from the nose; bright red blood comes from the posterior nares and is expectorated; very sensitive to the smell of garlic; coryza with severe frontal pains and redness of the eyelids; violent sneezing; copious discharge from the nose. Copious acrid lachrymation, and copious bland flow from the nose with sneezing: EUPHRASIA. *894*

PULS — When the hay fever comes on, all the other symptoms are better, she feels nothing except the hay fever, however all the symptoms interweave with each other. We have an acute class in which PULS is sometimes indicated - copious watery discharge which ends in sneezing. In the beginning we will think of CARBO-VEG. In ALL-C we have excoriating discharge from the nose and bland discharge from the eyes; in the larynx, sensation as if hooks were there, and sometimes this extends below the larynx; this always means ALL-C; it is also worse in a warm room like PULS. The EUPH looks like ALL-C, only the discharge from the eyes is copious, watery and burning - the lachrymation burns the eyes and excoriates the cheeks; discharge from nose is bland like PULS. Sometimes this goes into the chest, then it is no longer EUPH. *863*

FERRUM METALLICUM

FERR PHOS — Many symptoms are worse lying in bed and from rest, and ameliorated by moving slowly about (like FERRUM) but the great lassitude compels him to lie down. *532*

Chlorosis and pernicious anaemia would make one think of MANG, and also PIC AC and FERRUM. *724*

ARG NIT — Eructations of air accompanied by a mouthful of undigested food, like PHOS and FERRUM. Spitting it up; welling up in mouthfuls. *140*

AESC — "Eructations: sour, greasy, bitter." "Desire to vomit." "HEART-BURN AND GULPING UP OF FOOD AFTER EATING." It has a great DISTURBANCE OF DIGESTION, and we can see by these symptoms that we must class it with PHOS and FERR. As soon as the patient has swallowed the food, or a little while after, it becomes sour and he eructates it, until after a while he has emptied the stomach of its contents. Such is the state of PHOS, FERR, ARS, AESC and a few other medicines. *38*

SANG — A patient comes to you after exposure to cold; he cannot raise the arm; it hangs by his side; pain worse at night in bed, worse turning over (as he uses the shoulder muscle to turn over). It is probably in the deltoid, but you need not speculate on the tissues involved. SANG competes with FERRUM. All red faced highly flushed people who cannot raise the arm and have pain which is worse in the daytime, not night, and ameliorated by slow motion need FERRUM. SANG is not relieved by motion; it is aggravated by such motion as calls the arm into use. FERRUM has relief from slow motion, aggravated by rapid motion and the pain comes on in the daytime. While FERRUM has a uniformly red, plethoric face, SANG has a pale face. *902*

FERR PHOS — Rheumatic pain in right shoulder and upper arm, of a drawing, tearing character, aggravated by violent motion of arm, ameliorated by gentle motion (FERR), part sensitive to touch.......... ***536***

When it is a case of septicaemia SULPH goes to the very root of it.When the feet burn, when there is a hungry feeling in the stomach, the night aggravation with sinking and exhaustion, and when throughout the body there is a sensation of steam rising or hot flushes, one after another, you must give SULPH. Now, on the other hand, if in such a case, if there is a purplish appearance of the body, cold sweat all over, if there are remittent or intermittent chills, with thirst during the chill and at no other time, and the face is red during the chill, you must give FERRUM, as no other remedy looks just like that. ***972***

FERRUM PHOSPHORICUM

Every experienced physician must have met with many cases where for a time he felt unable to cope with the case because of his inability to reach the constitutional state that underlies this continual taking of cold. So he puzzles for a long time, and prescribes on the immediate attack and palliates it. For instance the immediate attack might look like BELL or BRY, FERRUM PHOS or ARS etc.; he treats that attack without taking into consideration the underlying constitutional state of the patient. It is quite a profitable business for one who has not much conscience and not much intelligence. But a conscientious physician feels worried and knows he is not doing what he ought to do by his patient, unless he reaches out for the remedy that touches the constitution. It is far more useful to keep people from taking colds than to cure cold. ***509***

FLUORIC ACID

AGAR — Leucorrhoea very profuse, dark, bloody, acrid, excoriating in parts. This remedy has been mentioned in relation to FL-AC. There are many points of relation. They are like each other in the leucorrhoea especially; copious and ACRID, so acrid that it keeps the parts raw and irritated around the genitals and the patient can't walk. In FL-AC there is, with the nervous symptoms, headache ameliorated by passing the urine, or headache if urination is not immediately attended to, with copious acrid excoriating leucorrhoea. ***47***

MERC — Eating away of the soft palate and the bone of the hard palate is often eaten away. Purulent formation in the Antrum of Highmore and fistulae from the mouth to the antrum. FL-AC and SIL are more frequently indicated in these fistulae, especially if the bone is involved. ***737***

PULS — Tumefaction about the penis. Foreskin dropsical (NIT-AC, FL-AC, CANN SAT). ***869***

PULS — Swelling of veins in the arms and hands. Varicose veins of the limbs like FL-AC. ***871***

Varicose veins of the thighs and legs have been cured by AESC (FL-AC). ***40***

GAMBOGIA

KALI-BICH — Diarrhoea after beer, like ALOE, CHINA, GAMBOGIA, LYC, MUR-AC and SULPH. ***621***

GELSEMIUM

Any little disturbance, a mental disturbance, a fright, or distress, or a grievance, will bring a young, sensitive woman home and to her bed, and she will go on with a spasm of the larynx. It is a laryngismus stridulus that can be heard all over the house. IGN stops it at once (GELS, MOSCHUS). ***595***

SQUIL — Quite similar to CANN IND or GELS in brain affections, but SQUIL has not many brain affections nor many febrile complaints. ***941***

You will find some deep seated brain troubles that will try your patience. Some cases go slowly and gradually into unconsciousness; rolling of the head for days; eyes lustreless; body emaciated, involuntary discharges of faeces or urine in the bed; tongue dry and parched, so shrivelled that it looks like leather, lips also; face withered and each day looks older; paralysis of one hand or one foot, or it seems that the whole muscular system is paralysed. Screaming out in pain, although not so shrilly as in APIS. A dose of ZINC will sometimes bring this patient back to life. In a few days after the remedy there will be a jerking and a quivering in the parts that were motionless, or its action will be shown in a copious sweat, much vomiting; sudden arousing that is alarming, for it looks like a threatened sinking, but this is the beginning of reaction. Now, for days and nights while this little one is coming back to consciousness, the restoration of sensation in the parts is accompanied with the tormenting formication, tingling, pricking, creeping and crawling. The mother and the father and the neighbours will want something done for it, but if you antidote, the case will return to where it was before. This suffering is but the awakening to life. It will go on in this way for a week or two and then will begin to show signs of falling back; it needs another dose of ZINC, which will again be followed by sweat, vomiting etc. You will see this in spinal meningitis. The early stage will be that of congestion and BELL may palliate, but with the onset of the symptoms enumerated above, ZINC is the only remedy that will cure. After the relief from GELS, BELL or BRY give ZINC. Rugged little fellows who hang on for weeks in this state, emaciating and unconscious............. ***1015***

SIL — Headache once a week (GELS, LYC, SANG, SULPH)................................. ***927***

EUP-PER — Painful soreness in the eyeballs, like BRY and GELS. The eyeballs are very sensitive to touch and sore to pressure; feels as if he had been struck a blow in the eye; sore, bruised pain in the eye. ***515***

SPONG — At times an adult takes cold and rawness of the larynx and trachea is the result. On going to bed she is taken with a spasmodic constriction of the larynx. Laryngismus stridulus is commonly found in women. IGN, GELS, LAUR and SPONG. IGN and GELS will cure 8 out of 10 cases. ***940***

When the (sexual) desire is so violent that it drives her to secret vice the remedies are GELS, GRATIOLA, ORIGANUM, NUX VOMICA, PHOS, PLATINA and ZINC. ***561***

KALI CARB — It is a severe labour, a prolonged labour; the uterus appears to be weak, and the pains are feeble; they are all in the back and do not go to the centre of operation as they should. Now this same kind of a pain may deceive you in taking another form. The pains begin in the back, appear to go to the uterus and then run up the back, which would turn you aside entirely from the KALI CARB pain into a pain that would indicate GELS.......... ***634***

GNAPHALIUM

RUTA — The severest forms of sciatica; pains commence in the back and go down the hips and thighs; tearing pains; comfortable during the day, but aggravated as soon as he lies down at night. GNAPHALIUM is a great sciatic remedy, and it also has this aggravation from lying down. *890*

GRAPHITES

ALUM — is not a medicine that would be selected for a cold settling in the throat, not a remedy for acute sore throat, but it is a deep acting anti-psoric and acts for months. Its greatest use is as a remedy for taking cold. In this respect it is like SIL, GRAPH and SULPH. *72*

ALUM — The skin indurates and ulcerates and becomes clumsy and unhealthy and constipation is produced, and so, after studying the remedy in that way, you are not surprised if it cures a fissure. If you look into the nature of NIT-AC, CAUST and GRAPH you will see why they have had a wonderful record for curing fissure. That is the way to study your Materia Medica; see what it does to the man himself, to his organs and tissues. *73*

A patient much debilitated with bronchial catarrh; susceptible to cold, to every change in weather, from change to damp weather, to every draft, to change of clothing; always taking new "cold". There is burning in the chest behind the sternum; thick, tough, ropy expectoration; spasmodic cough, and every cough ends in belching; eructations of gas, empty eructations. If to the burning in the chest, the severe pains in the larynx and trachea while talking and cough ending in belching you add heat in the palms and soles, SANG will patch him up and mitigate the troubles. Many such cases get SULPH, but to their destruction. There is a class of remedies that suits these phthisical patients better than SULPH, SIL and GRAPH; such remedies as PULS, SANG, SENECIO GRACILIS and COCCUS CACTI, which will palliate, mitigate his sufferings and may even build him up so that he could take a medium potency of a deep remedy. *900*

MANG — Irritability and low-spirited, like SULPH and GRAPH. It is similar to ARG MET, PHOS, GRAPH, and SULPH in its underlying tendency to tuberculosis. .. *723*

BAR-C — You will have patients to treat, where this slow development manifests itself in girls 18 to 25 years of age, who do the things they did when they were children, and say things as they said them when they were children. "Childish manner of doing things, and childish behaviour. Playing with dolls and saying foolish things." They have not come into womanhood. They are late in taking on the activities and uses of the woman. They lack the prudence of the woman. They have not become circumspect, and say things just as a boy or just as a little girl would say them. That is the dwarfishness of the mind. To appreciate that late development, and to see it in BARYTA CARB from all of its symptoms and peculiar features, leads to such remedies as GRAPH, SULPH and CALC, but nothing compared to this remedy. *221*

The CARBONS affect the veins more or less, relaxing and paralysing. *368*

PETR is not so closely related to SIL as it is to GRAPH and CARBO VEG, which are carbonaceous substances, and all carbonaceous products affect the back of the head.

"Pain from occiput over head to forehead and eyes, with transitory blindness; he gets stiff; loses consciousness." "Circumscribed pain in the occiput, aggravated on shaking the head." *818*

MANG — Dreadful flushes of heat like PSOR, LACH, SULPH and GRAPH, coming on in women who have been anaemic for some time. *725*

NAT-S — The next most important feature is in relation to the eyes. That is characteristic, and is equalled only by one remedy in chronic diseases where there is an aversion to life with photophobia, and that is GRAPH. You take these cases of chronic conjunctivitis, with granular lids, green pus, terrible photophobia, so much so that he can hardly open his eyes; the light of the room brings on headache, distress and many pains. Here NAT-S should be compared with GRAPH, because GRAPH has also an extreme aggravation from light in eye affections. *791*

Separation of the gums from the teeth. The teeth get loose. We hear about "the teeth rattling in his mouth". The CARBONS produce just such a state, a settling away and absorbing of the gums. They get spongy and bleed easily and hence looseness of the teeth with bleeding of the gums, which are very sensitive. *376*

BAR-C — "Spasm in the oesophagus. Difficulty in swallowing." The bolus of food goes down a little way, and then causes spasms, and he gags and chokes. This gagging and choking with a little food is a very strong feature in KALI CARB, GRAPH and MERC COR. This is also a strong feature of BARYTA CARB, but much stronger in MERC COR. *227*

PETR — He cannot eat without pain, but he has a gnawing hunger, which drives him to eat (LACH, GRAPH). *817*

This is chronic diarrhoea or constipation with stool covered with or followed by jelly-like mucus in SEPIA. Do not confound with GRAPH which has an enormous stool with much straining and sweating, and coated with and mixed with a substance looking like the cooked white of an egg, as if covered with albumen. *922*

ALOE — If there is an ulcerated spot or aphthous patch or inflamed surface thick jelly-like cakes of mucus may be peeled off, almost as thick as leather at times. At times the lower portion of the rectum is in this state and the patient will say that the lumpy stools are caked in jelly. The lumpy stools in GRAPH look as if embedded in coagulated white of egg. *61*

When an old man, who has been single for a long time, marries, his cramps will sometimes prevent him performing the act of coition. He has cramps in the calves and soles as soon as he begins the act. CUPR is especially useful in young men who have become PREMATURELY OLD FROM VICES, from strong drink, from late nights and various abuses, and these cramps are not unlikely to occur in such subjects. CUPR and GRAPH are the two remedies for cramps coming under these circumstances, but whereas CUPR is said to produce cramps that prevent the act, GRAPH is said to bring on cramps during the act. These two remedies, however, compare closely with each other, and hence if GRAPH corresponds to the constitution of the patient, it should be given, and the same in regard to CUPR. *489*

Until PHYT was known there was but one remedy for the old cicatrices in the mammary gland. Women who were confined years before, had abscesses of the breast which were poulticed and lanced, had a cicatrix left, and now in the present confinement they have trouble; inflammation in the old cicatrices; ulceration which eats off the lacteal glands or turns the ducts aside and twists them; high inflammation; throbbing and pain; milk bloody. GRAPH was the old routine remedy, but PHYT is a better remedy and suits the concomitants oftener. The symptoms usually found in an inflamed breast after confinement are: aching in the back and bone pains; fever and shivering. PHYT has these and falls into the very nature of the case. GRAPH has it only in a limited way. ***837***

PETR—Study closely the skin symptoms and compare with GRAPH and SULPH. ... ***819***

PETR — The eruptions on the surface and the state of induration are like GRAPH, but the oozing in PETR is thin and watery, and in GRAPH it is gluey, honey-like, sticky, viscid. You have indurations and cracks of the fingers, and rhagades in both remedies, but the horn-like warty growths, lifting up the quick of the nails, you will find only in GRAPH. ***819***

PHYT is somewhat like GRAPH in that it seeks out fissures in which to establish inflammation, induration and eruptions. Where the circulation is feeble it has the tendency to establish induration. ***838***

KALI SIL has cured the most stubborn cases of eczema where SULPH and GRAPH seemed indicated and failed. ***660***

Zona is a herpetic formation, great vesicular patches come out upon the body called "shingles", here we should compare THUJA, GRAPH, RHUS-T, KALI HYDR and MEZ. ***997***

DULC — Eruptions upon the scalp that look so much like crusta lactea that DULC has been found a very useful medicine. Extreme soreness, itching, and the itching is not relieved by scratching, and the scratching goes on until bleeding and rawness take place. Eruptions that come out upon the face, upon the forehead, all over the nose, but especially upon the cheeks, which become completely covered with these crusts; eczema of infants. Children only a few weeks old break out with these scalp eruptions, and DULC is one of the medicines that you will need to know. It is about as frequently indicated as any of the medicines. SEPIA, ARS, GRAPH, DULC, PETR, SULPH and CALC are about equally indicated, but of these, in this climate at least, I think SEP is probably more frequently indicated. ***507***

NIT-AC — Phagedenic blisters on the toes (GRAPH). ***801***

SIL — Corns (ANT-CRUD, GRAPH). Ingrowing toe-nails. ***934***

CARBON SULPH is a most useful remedy to restrain the growth of cancer (like GRAPH) and it has cured lupus. ***387***

SIL has also cured fistulous openings. Patients who have a tendency to phthisis are subject to abscesses about the region of the rectum that break inside or out and form complete or incomplete openings. These seem to take the place of what would otherwise come, and if healed by operation or other external means, the tendency is to end in chest trouble, either in the form of a fixed catarrh or tubercular infiltrations. SIL is one of the remedies that turns the constitution into order and in one to five years the opening ceases to be necessary and it will heal. Surgeons heal it up at once and for a time the patient is comfortable, but in a few years he breaks down. CAUST, BERB, CALC, CALC PHOS, GRAPH, SULPH etc. are suitable in such cases. SIL here follows THUJ well. ***932***

GRATIOLA

PHOS AC — If the diarrhoea slacks up the patient feels worse and on come symptoms of tuberculosis, weakness, prostration, brain-fag. Some patients say they are never comfortable unless they have diarrhoea. PODO is the very opposite. Take the same child; the stool is very copious and runs all over the floor, the mother wonders where it all comes from, but the stool is so OFFENSIVE, a horrible stench, and the patient looks as if dying; mouth and nose drawn, countenance hippocratic, almost unconscious. There is painless stool in both, but PHOS AC has not the great prostration. In PHOS AC the stool is whitish-grey, like dirty white paint; in PODO it is yellow. GRAT has a similar state of prostration, but the fluid is GREEN water; when seen it looks like light shining through a green glass; sometimes thicker, like green bile. *822*

GRINDELIA

SPONG — Cardiac affections accompanied with thick, green or yellow expectoration like pus and dyspnoea on falling asleep so that he must keep awake as long as he can, fear of sleep in advanced chest troubles. GRIND will palliate such a case and if the condition is only catarrhal and not tuberculous, it will cure. 940

HAMAMELIS

SARS — Eruptions appear in the spring. All the venous remedies are braced up by winter and go down in the spring, as LACH, SEC and HAMAM. *905*

SENECIO AUREUS — The whole urinary tract is painful and subject to bleeding. But bleeding especially in the absence of the menstrual flow is the feature of this remedy. Wherever there is an inflammatory spot or catarrhal condition of the mucous membrane, it will bleed in case the menstrual flow does not appear. We have other medicines having the symptoms of vicarious haemorrhage, such as HAMAMELIS, PHOS and BRY, but SENECIO has this condition strikingly, and is one of the newer remedies for such condition. *913*

HELLEBORUS NIGER

IGN has another thing-"Thinks she has neglected some duty." That is very much like PULS, HELL and HYOS. *596*

You will find some deep seated brain troubles that will try your patience. Some cases go slowly and gradually into unconsciousness; rolling of the head for days; eyes lustreless; body emaciated, involuntary discharges of faeces or urine in the bed; tongue dry and parched, so shrivelled that it looks like leather, lips also; face withered and each day looks older; paralysis of one hand or one foot, or it seems that the whole muscular system is paralysed. Screaming out in pain, although not so shrilly as in APIS. A dose of ZINC will sometimes bring this patient back to life. In a few days after the remedy there will be a jerking and quivering in the parts that were motionless, or its action will be shown in a copious sweat, much vomiting; sudden arousing that is alarming, for it looks like a threatened sinking, but this is the beginning of reaction. Now, for days and nights while this little one is coming back to consciousness the restoration of sensation in the parts is accompanied with tormenting formication, tingling, pricking, creeping and crawling. The mother and the father and the neighbours will want something done for it, but if you antidote, the case will return to where it was before. This suffering is but the awakening to life. It will go on in this way for a week or two and then will begin to show signs of falling back; it needs another dose of ZINC, which will again be followed by sweat, vomiting etc. You will see this in spinal meningitis. The early stage will be that of congestion and BELL may palliate, but with the onset of the symptoms enumerated above ZINC is the only remedy that will cure. The BELL case will have flushed face, hot head, rolling of the head, flashing eyes, throbbing carotids. The BRY case will be docile, purple, stupid, sleepy, ameliorated by quiet. The HELL cases will exhibit but little fever; cold extremities, tossing of the head, dilated pupils, unconsciousness, can hardly be roused; rolling head from side to side, but when the reflexes are abolished, ZINC comes in *1015*

HEPAR SULPHURICUM

KALMIA — In bed at night the pains become very severe and last all night. This night aggravation is especially true of the marked anti-syphilitic remedies. It is found under HEPAR and MERC; but in none of these do we find it as strikingly manifest as in the disease, or miasm, syphilis itself......... *668*

Syphilitic complaints are commonly worse at night and such anti-syphilitic remedies as MERCURIUS, STAPHISAGRIA, HEPAR, NIT-AC etc. are all worse at night. *186*

AURUM is full of nasal troubles, with foetid discharge. The bones of the nose necrose; syphilitic necrosis, the nose flattens down; the bones are discharged. You see these people walking about with flattened down nose and if you get near enough to them the stench will be observed. They are nearly all syphilitics. A few remedies have the power of curing this syphilitic nose condition; AURUM, MERCURY and HEPAR are three of them. I have cured this state a number of times with HEPAR. I once cured a man after the bones were completely softened, so that when the nose was handled it would bend right over; only a sort of cartilaginous structure held the nose in place. I gave that patient HEPAR. It cured him of syphilis after he had been filled in vain with MERCURY. *199*

There are some remedies that correspond to extreme irritation in very sensitive natures; like HEPAR where she faints with the pain; like NITRIC ACID who cannot bear the noise of vehicles going along the street, because it creates such violent sufferings; like COFFEA where footsteps aggravate all the complaints; he was so sensitive to pain that the noise of one entering the door when he was on the third floor aggravated his sufferings intensely, though no one else could hear it. In NUX VOMICA even the sound of footsteps increases the pain all over the body. BELL has in its nature all this sensitiveness to pain. It is a part of the general sensorium; the whole bodily state is intensified. The CHAM patient is oversensitive to pain; but we do not need to sympathise with the CHAM patient, he will fight it out himself. But you will pity the BELL patient, the PULS patient, the NIT-AC patient. *239*

SPIG — On the pain first beginning there is not so much hyperaesthesia, but as it goes on this increases and the eye becomes congested. I have seen the pains so severe that they produced perfect prostration, cold sweat, vomiting. The HEPAR patient is so sensitive to pain that he becomes unconscious, faints with the pain. *936*

The MAG CARB baby smells sour like the HEPAR baby. Wash it as you will and it smells sour; the perspiration is sour, the whole baby smells sour. *715*

NAT-P — The body smells sour (like HEPAR, SULPH, LYC)...................................... *773*

SULPH AC is often indicated in sour smelling babies like HEPAR, and it is as sensitive to touch and nearly as sensitive to cold... .... *976*

STRAM — High grade inflammation which it carries to the finish. Pus forms abscesses with excruciating pain (HEPAR, MERC, SIL, SULPH)..950

The mental state of the IODINE is that of anxiety, excitement, impulses, melancholy; he wants to do something, wants to hurry; he has impulses to kill. In this it is closely related to ARSENICUM and HEPAR. The ARS and HEPAR patients also have impulses to commit murder without being offended and without cause. The sensitiveness to heat will at once decide, for while IODINE is warm blooded, the ARS and HEPAR patients are always chilly...... *599*

The patient may not be known to be insane in anything else; he may be a good business man. Remedies also have this. These things are forerunners. It is recorded in HEPAR that a barber had an impulse to cut the throat of his patron with the razor while shaving him. The NUX VOM patient has an impulse to throw her child into the fire, or to kill her husband whom she dearly loves. The thought comes into her mind and increases until she becomes actually insane and beyond control and the impulse is carried into action. A NAT SULPH patient will say "Doctor, do you know how I have to resist killing myself. An impulse to do it comes into my mind." IODINE has the impulse to kill, not from anger, not from any sense of justice, but without any cause. An overwhelming anger is often a cause for violence, but the impulses are not of that sort in IODINE. While reading or thinking placidly at times a patient may have an impulse to do himself violence, and this finally grows until the end is a form of impulsive insanity................................. *599*

MEZ — Headache extending from the root of the nose to the forehead (MERC and HEPAR). Pain in the head causes faintness (HEPAR). *747*

PULS — Abscess in the middle ear; inflammation of the middle ear; copious thick, bloody discharge, then yellow-green. The case goes on night and day until rupture takes place. I have found this condition as an endemic, in which MERC, HEPAR and PULS were the most frequently indicated medicines. *861*

HEPAR competes with SILICA in syphilitic nasal catarrhs where the parts are phagedenic; HEPAR, MERC COR and ARS are the principal anti-syphilitics when there is phagedenic ulceration of the nose... *929*

PSOR — Horribly offensive discharge from the nose; gluey discharge from the nose; offensive like MERC, SIL, CALC-P, HEPAR. *853*

Most prescribers give HEPAR for every sticking or fishbone sensation in the throat; this is the old keynote, the old routine. NIT AC, ARG NIT, ALUM and NAT MUR all have it, but all differently. HEPAR : The tonsils are swollen, full, purple - quinsy. The patient is sensitive to the slightest draft, there is pain in the throat even on putting the hand out of bed; he sweats in the night with no relief; he is sensitive to every impression; feels everything ten times amplified. NIT AC: There are yellow patches in the throat; ragged, jagged ulcers in the throat, or it is inflamed and purple. The urine smells like horse's urine. ARG NIT: There is much hoarseness, the vocal cords being disturbed. The throat is swollen, patulous; the patient wants cold things, cold water, cold air. Adapted to those cases that have had ulceration of the os uteri with cauterisation. NAT MUR: There is extreme dryness of the mucous membranes, as if they would break; chronic dryness without ulceration. There is much catarrhal discharge like the white of an egg, with dryness of the mucous membranes when not covered by this mucus. The patient is extremely sensitive, sensitive to a change of weather. *771*

CARBO AN — The glands of the throat and axillae grow purple and indurated with no tendency to soften. Some of these medicines, after infiltrating a gland, will hurry up the inflammatory action, produce sloughing, rapid breaking down, with pus - like HEPAR, MERC and SULPH. But CARBO AN paralyses and infiltrates the little veins in the inflamed parts and there seems to be no tendency to suppuration........................368

BAR-C — "Inflammation of the tonsils." The inflammation is not so violent as that which comes on in BELL, it does not come on in a night, it does not go on rapidly to suppuration; but it is a very sore throat, has come on slowly and after many days of exposure and there is gradual growth and development, while that of BELL comes on with great rapidity. HEPAR is also rapid and goes on to suppuration. *227*

CAPS is useful in perplexing and troublesome chronic hoarseness. He has had a cold and remedies for the acute condition have been given, perhaps two or three remedies, ACON, BRY, HEP, PHOS, but all at once you wake up to his chronic constitutional state of hoarseness. He is rotund, chilly, red-faced, and the hoarseness disappears under CAPS. *367*

ALUMEN — The urine is very slow to start and when the patient stands to urinate the urine falls down perpendicularly, as in HEPAR. From this we see the sluggish action. *62*

KALMIA — A general weakness, prolonged weakness after confinement, or from the pain, as we find in HEPAR, but with the weakness these pains are threatening to leave their parts and go to the heart... *671*

BELL — The chest is so painful the child dreads the cough and screams. By the child's cry we know that it is going to have a coughing spell. Just like BRY, HEPAR and PHOS which have that feature more than any other remedies. *251*

CALC SULPH — Croupy cough, where there is much choking, when an experienced practitioner might well think of HEPAR - but it will be remembered that in HEPAR, uncovering a hand or throwing the covers off the chest will increase the croupy tendency and aggravate the croupy cough, and that the patient in HEPAR is very sensitive to a draft and to the air. In this patient (CALC SUL) uncovering is grateful. The patient throws off the covers and wants the air and seems to breathe better and croups less. It may seem strange that such a great difference should come between the sulphide and the sulphate of lime. *352*

The symptoms usually found in an inflamed breast after confinement are; aching in the back and bone pains; fever and shivering. PHYT has these and falls into the very nature of the case. GRAPH has it only in a limited way. If there is high fever; congestion to the head; throbbing carotids; much redness, and the redness radiates from the nipple, BELL is the remedy. When the entire gland is as heavy as a stone, and hard, and the patient is sensitive to motion and touch, BRY. MERC when the general symptoms agree. HEP and SIL after suppuration is inevitable, especially when the only comfort is obtained from heat. HEPAR when there is extreme pain and soreness, irritability and this relief from heat; it limits the suppuration and opens the part without pain. *838*

PSOR — It is not the sourness of HEPAR; in spite of washing the child smells so sour; like sour milk; the diaper, urine, faeces, and perspiration are sour. This is a strong general feature of HEPAR. The stool smells like spoiled eggs, so also the eructations and flatus. *855*

HYOSCYAMUS

IGN — At times she is taciturn; again she prattles and is loquacious, and talks to herself. She comes into a state in a little while where she delights to bring on her fits and to make a scare. The natural hysteric is born with that, and IGN will do her no good. But when this is brought on from conditions described, IGN is of the greatest benefit. It runs closely along by the side of HYOS. "A feeling of continuous fright, or apprehension that something is going to happen." *596*

IGN has another thing: "Thinks she has neglected some duty." That is very much like PULS, HELL and HYOS. Only AURUM believes that she has committed a great wrong. *596*

ANAC — Suitable in religious mania when the conflict between the external and internal will is kept up. It is analogous to HYOS. *104*

CANTH — Restlessness causing him to move constantly, a rage and delirium intermingled with amorous frenzy. This kind of mental conduct in CANTH is similar to what will take place in HYOS, PHOS and SEC, a violent delirious state intermingled with sexual ideas and talk. *362*

HYPERICUM

CIC was the old remedy for tetanus and spasms caused by splinters in the skin or under the nails, competing with BELL. At the present day we find the most frequently indicated remedies for injuries to nerves are LEDUM and HYPERICUM. *433*

When tetanus comes on from punctured wounds in the palms or soles or in other parts, think of HYPERICUM, or when you have a punctured wound to treat, give LEDUM at once and you will prevent tetanus. When the fingernails have been torn, or the nerves in sentient parts like the ends of the fingers have been torn and lacerated, HYPERICUM becomes the remedy. For the bruising of various parts, and when the patient feels as if bruised all over, no matter how extensively he is bruised, ARNICA is generally the remedy. It may be said, for punctured wounds study LEDUM; for lacerated wounds of sentient nerves study HYPERICUM; for bruises study ARNICA; for open lacerations and cuts study CALENDULA. *696*

IGNATIA

We notice the complaints of IGN how flitting and unexpected and intermittent everything is. *276*

AMBR GR — The symptoms are most erratic, as much so as in IGN and NAT MUR. Taken as a whole they can be reconciled but taken a few at a time they seem wonderfully inconsistent. You must get the whole remedy in order to comprehend it. *95*

Compare CIMIC with PULS, SEP, NAT MUR, LIL TIG, CAUL and IGN. *35*

GELS — There is a sense of weakness and goneness in the region of the heart, and this weakness and goneness often extends into the stomach, involving the whole lower part of the left side of the chest and across into the stomach creating a sensation of hunger, like IGN and SEPIA. There is a hysterical element in GELS and it has the same nervous hunger and gnawing. 545

NAT-C — Headache, chilliness and palpitation, better from eating (IGN, SEP, SULPH). *765*

CIC — Full of fear; fright will bring on convulsions, like OP, IGN and ACON. *434*

CAUL — She is hysterical, like IGN.. *398*

MOSCH — When they (hysterical girls) have been encouraged to resort to crafty cunning, to have every whim gratified from infancy to eighteen years of age they become fit subjects for MOSCH, ASAF, IGN and VALER. *750*

NUX-V — Full of hysterical manifestations. Europeans develop symptoms more often calling for NUX in their hysterical manifestations, while Americans oftener need IGN. *809*

THUJ — Pain localised in small spots. A nail driven in the head, side of the head and forehead, like IGN and ANAC............ *999*

SEPIA — Nausea violent; deathly sinking accompanied by an awful anxiety in the stomach. PHOS has more of the typical hunger which is relieved by eating. The IGN patient is always sighing; cannot get rid of "that feeling". OLEANDER has an all-gone empty feeling as if he would die; food does not relieve, is not digested, but passes undigested the next day. LYC has an all-gone feeling sometimes not better by eating, felt as markedly before as after eating, and after eating there comes a throbbing. KALI CARB has it also, without the amelioration from taking food; it is even intensified after eating, which is followed by a sensation of fullness and throbbing. In severe liver and heart affections the stomach is not able to keep up assimilation; palpitation, great weakness, liver congested, white stool. DIG comes in here with its deathly sinking not better by eating. In SEPIA this symptom is associated with loss of affections, the lump in the rectum, with the constipation, etc. *922*

At times an adult takes cold and rawness of the larynx and trachea is the result. On going to bed she is taken with a spasmodic constriction of the larynx. Laryngismus stridulus is commonly found in women, IGN, GELS, LAUR and SPONG. IGN and GELS will cure 8 out of 10 cases................. *940*

Copious colourless urine is one of SQUILLA's important symptoms and resembles IGN, but SQUIL is not a hysterical patient like IGN.. *941*

VALER — Inspirations grow more rapid and less deep until they cease; then she catches her breath by a sobbing effort, in spells (compare IGN, OX-AC). ***1009***

NUX-V — Chills are not better from any amount of covers; IGN chills are better uncovering. ***809***

INULA

INULA resembles NUX; has colic with urging to stool and to urinate. ***808***

IODUM

The LIL TIG patient suffocates in a crowded room, in the theatre, in church, like APIS, IOD, KALI IOD, LYC and PULS. ***701***

The PULS mental state in a man is that a woman would be to the detriment of his soul; it is a delusion, a fixed idea. IOD is full of fixed ideas. ANAC has a fixed idea that a devil is sitting on one shoulder talking into his ear, while an angel sits on the other shoulder talking into the other ear, and he halts between the two and says nothing.. .... ***893***

FL-AC — Often that "all-gone" sensation in the stomach. Is always eating and is relieved from eating, but like IOD it does not last long, for soon he becomes hungry again. Such medicines are very deep. We see that they go to the very root of assimilation and nutrition. ***542***

IOD is worse in a warm room; thick discharge from the nose which burns and excoriates and is yellowish-green; but there is one thing that differentiates it from all the others - the patient immediately begins to emaciate when the complaint comes on and is very hungry. KALI HYDR with the thick yellowish discharge, worse in a warm room, there is a great amount of rawness and burning in the nose; external nose very sore to pressure; sensitiveness in the root of the nose; whole face aches and patient is very restless; wants to walk in the open air which does not fatigue him. ARS IOD; anxiety, restlessness and weakness; frequent sneezing and copious watery nasal discharge that burns the lip. Burning, watery discharge from the eyes like ARS. ARS wants to be very warm; wants hot water applied to the eyes; the only relief is from sniffing hot water up the nose. ARS IOD is worse in a warm room and for days after sneezing the discharge thickens and becomes gluey, looking like THICK, YELLOW HONEY, this excoriates; much pain through the root of the nose and eyes; often rawness in the chest with dyspnoea. The remedies having the dyspnoea are ARSENIC, IODIDE OF ARSENIC, IODINE, KALI HYDR and SABADILLA; these are the ones I have found most frequently indicated in the asthmatic forms of hay fever. ***863***

NUX VOMICA has a free, easy breathing in the open air, but when he goes into the warm room his nose stuffs up, which also occurs at night, though the water drips on the pillow yet he stuffs up like PULS, BRY and the IODINE preparations, IODIDE OF ARSENIC and CYCLAMEN. ***864***

IPECACUANHA

That is one of the first things I observed, that outside of sycotics you will seldom find a cure for asthma. There is that peculiarity that runs through sycosis which gives you a hereditary disease, and asthma corresponds to that disease. Hence it is that SIL is one of the greatest cures for asthma; it does not cure every case, but when SIL corresponds to the symptoms you will be surprised how quickly it will eradicate it. While IPECAC, SPONG and ARS will correspond just as clearly to the supervening symptoms and to everything that you can find about the case, yet what will they do? They palliate; they repress the symptoms; but your asthma is no better off, your patient is not cured. ARS is one of the frequently indicated remedies for the relief of asthma; so also are BRY, IPECAC, SPONG and CARBO-VEG, but they do not cure; although they relieve surprisingly at times. *793*

In a case confused by remedies think of CALC, ARS, SULPH, SEP and IPECAC. Never give CHINA or NAT MUR for irregular symptoms and stages. *925*

Sometimes it is true it will appear to you that ACON is capable of coping with all there is in the disease. But there seems to be a lingering something that holds on, and such medicines as ARN and BELL and IP and BRY do have to come in to finish up the attack - or sometimes SULPH. Very commonly SIL. So we have to study the relations of medicines. *30*

ARN follows well after ACON and is complementary to ACON, IPECAC, and VERATRUM. *148*

The CADMIUM SULPH nausea is distressing. Nauseated all the way down to the abdomen, like IPECAC, ANT-T and ARS. *305*

CROTON TIG — Excessive nausea with vanishing of sight, vertigo, worse after drinking, with frequent discharges of yellow-green water from the bowels; excessive nausea, much water in the mouth. So we note the excessive nausea and not so great vomiting. The nausea is more like IPECAC, but in IPECAC we have nothing like the stools of CROTON TIG, we have only scanty little gushes, every minute a little gush, with tenesmus. Vomiting is the all-important symptom in the cholera infantum of IPECAC, and when the stomach is emptied there is overwhelming retching and exhaustion from it, and the stools are scanty; but in CROTON TIG the stools are copious, and while there is nausea the vomiting is seldom and scanty. *481*

The nausea of DIG is not like that of BRY and IPECAC. It is a singular nausea. The smell of food excites a deathly nausea, a sinking, a goneness, associated with cardiac troubles, with jaundice and liver troubles. The nausea is accompanied by a deathly feeling, as if he is sinking away. Sometimes the nausea is relieved by eating, but the sinking remains after eating, showing that it is something besides hunger. *501*

MERC, IPECAC and ACON are frequently indicated in epidemic dysentery that comes in HOT weather, and IPECAC, DULC and MERC are frequently indicated in the dysentery of COLD weather. You should go to the bedside of a case of dysentery with your repertory or go home and send medicine. Your first prescription should cure in epidemic dysentery, and if you work cautiously you will cure every case. *738*

In the uterine haemorrhage compare SABINA with IPECAC, which has a gush of bright red blood fully as copious as SABINA, but at the beginning of that gush, before it has kept on long enough to produce exhaustion, the face becomes pale, there is nausea and a feeling of faintness, syncope, out of proportion to the blood lost. *898*

APOC — "Shreds or pieces of membrane with the fluid blood. Menorrhagia, continuing or paroxysmal." That is a continuous flow until the patient is exhausted. That is like PHOS and IPECAC and SECALE....... *128*

CARBO VEG hardly ever has what may be called an active gushing flow, such as belongs to BELL, IPECAC, ACON, SEC and such remedies where the flow comes with violence; but it is a passive capillary oozing. The women suffer from this kind of bleeding; a little blood oozing all the time so the menstrual period is prolonged. *372*

Atony is everywhere present in the CARBO VEG constitution. The muscles are tired, the limbs are tired, the whole being is tired and relaxed. This is in contradistinction to the gushing found in BELL, IPECAC, SEC and HAMAMELIS, where the blood escapes in great gushes, followed quite naturally by a contraction of the uterus, for there is more or less tonicity in connexion with it. In CARBO VEG either in connexion with confinement or in an incidental haemorrhage, the uterus does not contract. Subinvolution from mere atony; no contraction; no tonicity; weakness and relaxation. *380*

Vomiting of pregnancy is not cured, although it may be temporarily relieved, by IPECAC as this is a medicine that corresponds merely to the nausea itself. In a large number of instances gagging and nausea are only second or third grade symptoms in the remedy that will cure. The condition really depends upon the constitutional state and the remedy that is to cure must be a constitutional remedy. SULPH, SEP and KALI CARB are among the remedies commonly indicated. Sometimes ARS is needed. Of course, if a pregnant woman has simply disordered her stomach and has vomited bile a few times the remedy might be IPECAC. When a pregnant woman has no constitutional symptoms at all, and upon examining the case you find nothing but the nausea, overwhelming deathly nausea, with continuous vomiting day and night, a single dose of SYMPHORICARPUS RACEMOSA will help. That is prescribing upon very limited information and should only be done in circumscribed or one-sided cases. It is not a long acting remedy, it is not a constitutional remedy and acts very much like IPECAC. *633*

NAT MUR is irregular enough in its nature to develop the chills into regularity. When it has come into better order, wait; either the whole case will subside, or another remedy will be clear. There are other remedies that can turn cases into order. Often cases spoiled by homoeopaths can be turned into order by SEP. Marked cases with congestion of the head, aching in the back and nausea are turned into order by IPECAC. The cure is permanent after homoeopathic prescribing; the chills do not return. *770*

You will cure more cases of intermittent fever with IPECAC and NUX VOM than with CHINA. *442*

JACARANDA CAROBA

MERC — Balanitis, offensive pus. In chronic balanitis when pus forms behind the glans and under the foreskin, gonorrhoeal or psoric, consult JACARANDA CAROBA. *739*

KALI ARSENICOSUM

KALI BICH — Sensitive to cold winds. CAUST, it will be remembered, is sensitive to cold dry winds. The KALIS generally are sensitive to cold, dry weather. *618*

Like the rest of the KALIS, KALI BICH has cured epilepsy. ***618***

GRAPH — From eruptions, catarrhal discharges, menstrual flow, ulcers, breath and perspiration there is marked offensiveness (like CARBO VEG, PSORINUM, KALI PHOS, KALI ARS). ***553***

ARG-M is a medicine of great use in horribly offensive leucorrhoea (KALI ARS, KALI PHOS). ***134***

CALC ARS — Excoriating yellow leucorrhoea, offensive bloody leucorrhoea. For offensive leucorrhoea it compares with KALI ARS and KALI PHOS. ***310***

KALI BICHROMICUM

In some of the old catarrhs no reaction seems to come after the most carefully chosen remedies, and all at once the doctor observes that the patient has a red face and it is cold and the end of the nose is red and cold, and the patient is fat and flabby and yet has not much endurance, never could learn at school, and if she exerts breaks out into a sweat and freezes in the cold air. He has a key to the patient and examines the patient by the key, that is by the drug, a bad practice and never to be resorted to except as a DERNIER RESORT and in stupid patients. When he gives CAPS to that patient it arouses her, it may not cure; but after it the SIL or KALI BICH or other remedy that was perhaps given before and did not act takes hold and cures. ***365***

CARBO VEG — Awful occipital headache, or headache over the eyes, or headache involving the whole head, with pounding like hammers. These states are like KALI BICH, KALI IOD and SEPIA. Many of these headaches are due to stopped catarrhal conditions. ***373***

As we go into the syphilitic affections that lead into the throat, we find ulcers of the soft palate which eat away the uvula, small ulcers which finally unite and destroy the soft palate and then commence to work on the osseous portion of the roof of the mouth. The odour that comes from the mouth when it is opened to show the throat is extremely offensive; very often like spoiled cheese. The medicines that are especially related, or especially useful in this form of ulceration in old syphilitics will be KALI BICH, LACH, MERC, MERC COR and HEPAR, but in those cases that have been mercurialised HEPAR and NIT AC should be thought of. ***575***

LAC-C is indicated especially in a glazed, shiny, red appearance of the throat, like KALI BICH. ***677***

LACH — The saliva is stringy and can be pulled out of the mouth in strings; white mucus or saliva. This is not an uncommon feature in diphtheria, in sore throat, in inflammation of the tongue and mouth and gums, and in inflammation of the salivary glands. When this mucus in thick, tough, yellow, stringy and ropy it is like KALI BICH.. ***690***

ALOE — There is much pain in the hepatic region, burning and heat etc. Mostly in the right hypochondrium you will find distension and fullness. It is pre-eminently a liver medicine. It is not as deep in its action as SULPH. You will often find that ALOE will serve as a palliative, when it will have to be followed by SULPH, SULPH AC, KALI BICH or SEPIA, the medicines that follow ALOE and are complementary to it, finishing its work. In persons who have a diarrhoea every time they drink beer you will most likely find that ALOE will agree with the symptoms but sometimes it will be KALI BICH, for these two remedies are very similar as to their stomach and bowel symptoms *59*

If you study together, side, by side ALOE, KALI BICH and SULPH, you will be astonished at their wonderful relation to the stomach and bowels. *58*

SEP — Chronic diarrhoea, stools jelly-like, lumpy. The acute diarrhoeas and dysenteries with jelly-like stools are more in keeping with KALI BICH and COLCH. This is chronic diarrhoea or in constipation with stool covered with or followed by jelly-like mucus in SEPIA. *922*

THUJA — Feeling as if the urine were constantly running along the urethra, like KALI BICH and PETROS. *1000*

SENEGA — The rattling in the chest is as marked as in ANT-T; the tenacious mucus is as copious, as gluey and stringy as in KALI BICH, so much is this the case that he can get it only part way up and with a spasmodic effort he swallows it, like SPONG and CAUST. *914*

This thick, tough mucus will lead most prescribers to give such medicines as KALI BICH, LACH and MERC COR, entirely overlooking the usefulness of SENEGA. *915*

LYC — The mucous discharge is almost as thick and tenacious as in KALI BICH. *709*

PULS; There is another class of remedies having the stuffing up of the nose not relieved by the discharge. There is a constant desire to blow the nose, yet he gets no relief. This makes me think of LACH, KALI BI, PSOR, NAJA and STICTA. *864*

KALI CARBONICUM

KALI BICH — Sensitive to cold winds. CAUST, it will be remembered, is sensitive to cold dry winds. The KALIS generally are sensitive to cold, dry weather. *618*

KALI BICH — Many of its symptoms are aggravated 2-3am. like KALI CARB... *618*

It is in the nature of AESC to have FLYING PAINS all over the body, like PULS and KALI CARB; flitting, sharp, shooting, tearing pains, flying from one part to another; they seem at times to be scarcely more than skin deep. Sometimes they fly along the course of the nerves. *37*

Like the rest of the KALIS, KALI BICH has cured epilepsy. *618*

MEZ — Sensation of goneness, fear, apprehension, faintness in the stomach, as if something would happen; every shock, pain and hearing bad news, cause this apprehensive, hungry, faint, weak, all-gone feeling in the pit of the stomach. It comes on when the doorbell rings, if the patient is expecting the postman, while waiting at the depot for the arrival of a friend, or the departure of the cars; on being introduced to someone, he experiences a thrill beginning in the stomach, is "frightened in the stomach". CALC, KALI-C, PHOS and MEZ have this. These "solar plexus" individuals often have a deep cracked tongue and are hard to cure. *748*

SIL and KALI CARB are the two principal remedies for the paroxysmal cough that comes on from scratching the auditory canal. I have seen them choke and gag and vomit when they needed KALI CARB after scratching the auditory canal. Spasmodic cough from scratching the auditory canal belongs principally to SIL and KALI CARB, but MANG has cured it. *724*

BAR-C — "Spasm in the oesophagus. Difficulty in swallowing." The bolus of food goes down a little way, and then causes spasms, and he gags and chokes. This gagging and choking with a little food is a very strong feature in KALI CARB, GRAPH and MERC COR. This is also a strong feature of BARYTA CARB, but much stronger in MERC COR. 227

OLEANDER has an all-gone empty feeling as if he would die; food does not relieve, is not digested, but passes undigested the next day. LYC has an all-gone feeling sometimes not better by eating, felt as markedly before as after eating, and after eating there comes a throbbing. KALI CARB has it also, without the amelioration from taking food; it is even intensified after eating, which is followed by a sensation of fullness and throbbing. 922

PULS — Most troublesome constipation with haemorrhoids; violent pains in the haemorrhoids, worse lying down, ameliorated from gentle motion, worse from the warmth of the bed, better moving about in the open air. The aggravation from lying down in extremely painful haemorrhoids is contrasted with AMM-C which has violently painful haemorrhoids relieved by lying flat on the back. In violently painful haemorrhoids with intense burning, think of ARS and KALI CARB. 867

SPONG — at times after great dyspnoea, white tough mucus forms in the air passages, difficult to expectorate; it comes up and often has to be swallowed (ARN, CAUST, LACH, KALI-C, KALI-S, NUX-MOSCH, SEP, STAPH). 939

SULPH AC — Ulceration of lungs (compare KALI CARB). 979

KALI HYDRIODICUM

Zona is a herpetic formation, great vesicular patches come out upon the body called "shingles", here we should compare THUJA, GRAPH, RHUS-T, KALI HYDR and MEZ. 997

KALI HYDR with the thick yellowish discharge, worse in a warm room, there is a great amount of rawness and burning in the nose; external nose very sore to pressure; sensitiveness in the root of the nose; whole face aches and patient is very restless; wants to walk in the open air which does not fatigue him. ARS IOD; anxiety, restlessness and weakness; frequent sneezing and copious watery nasal discharge that burns the lip. Burning, watery discharge from the eyes like ARS. ARS wants to be very warm; wants hot water applied to the eyes; the only relief is from sniffing hot water up the nose. ARS IOD is worse in a warm room and for days after sneezing the discharge thickens and becomes gluey, looking like THICK, YELLOW HONEY, this excoriates; much pain through the root of the nose and eyes; often rawness in the chest with dyspnoea. The remedies having the dyspnoea are ARSENIC, IODIDE OF ARSENIC, IODINE, KALI HYDR and SABADILLA; these are the ones I have found most frequently indicated in the asthmatic forms of hay fever. 863

KALI IODATUM

KALI BICH — Sensitive to cold winds. CAUST, it will be remembered, is sensitive to cold dry winds. The KALIS generally are sensitive to cold, dry weather. 618

MERC is not deep enough to cure the whole

constitution in psoric cases that are constantly taking cold. It cures the cold at once, but implants its own nature and the patient catches cold oftener. It should not be given often, not oftener than twice in a winter. KALI IOD is better for the same burning in the face, running coryza, and aggravation from heat and warmth of the bed, and it will cure the coryza in a night when apparently MERC is indicated. It is also an antidote to MERC. Don't give many doses of MERC in psoric cases; look for a deeper medicine. ***736***

IOD also has oedema of the hands and feet, and carries this tendency with it into the IODIDE OF POTASSIUM, which has oedematous swellings like those we find in kidney affections. It is capable of putting a stop to cases of Bright's disease in the early stage. ***601***

Like the rest of the KALIS, KALI BICH has cured epilepsy. ***618***

IOD — While attempting to keep still, he is overwhelmed with impulses, impulses to tear things, to kill himself, to commit murder, to do violence. He cannot keep still and so he walks night and day. This remedy carries the same feature into the IODIDE OF POTASSIUM, so that it makes the IODIDE OF POTASSIUM patient walk. But there is this difference; the KALI IOD patient can walk long distances without fatigue, and the walking only seems to wear off his anxiety, whereas in IODINE there is great exhaustion; he becomes extremely exhausted from walking and sweats copiously even from slight exertion. ***598***

The LIL TIG patient suffocates in a crowded room, in the theatre, in church, like APIS, IOD, KALI IOD, LYC and PULS. ***701***

CARBO VEG — Awful occipital headache, or headache over the eyes, or headache involving the whole head, with pounding like hammers. These states are like KALI BICH, KALI IOD and SEPIA. Many of these headaches are due to stopped catarrhal conditions. ***373***

MEZ — Violent headaches and brain affections; pains rending, tearing; boring; head painful to touch; syphilitic affection of the brain; headaches through the sides of the head as if in the bone; feels as if the head would be crushed (closely related to MERC and KALI IOD). ***747***

A marked feature of the KALI BICH throat is its oedematous uvula. This symptom is also found in APIS, KALI-I, LACH, MUR-AC, NIT-AC, PHOS, SULPH-AC and TAB. ***620***

When you get an old gouty subject who has big toe joints and finger joints, and they are sore and inflamed every now and then, you might think that KALI CARB covers the case very suitably; he is disturbed in just such weather, he is pallid and sickly, his complaints come on at 2 or 3 o'clock in the morning, he has shooting pains. But these gouty patients are often incurable, and if so, to undertake to cure them would be a dreadful calamity, because the aggravations would last so long. If you give KALI CARB to one of these incurable patients in very high potency it will make your patient worse, and the aggravation will be serious and prolonged, but the 30th may be of great service. KALI IOD, when it is indicated in the gouty state, acts as a soothing and palliative remedy, but KALI CARB seems to be a dreadful medicine to handle, it is a sharp and two-edged sword. ***636***

KALI MURIATICUM

KALI BICH — Sensitive to cold winds. CAUST, it will be remembered, is sensitive to cold dry winds. The KALIS generally are sensitive to cold, dry weather. *618*

Like the rest of the KALIS, KALI BICH has cured epilepsy. *618*

KALI NITRICUM

KALI BICH — Sensitive to cold winds. CAUST, it will be remembered, is sensitive to cold dry winds. The KALIS generally are sensitive to cold, dry weather. *618*

Like the rest of the KALIS, KALI BICH has cured epilepsy. *618*

ARG NIT — Here is a striking feature. "Patient cannot lie on the RIGHT side because it brings on so much palpitation." We have plenty of remedies with palpitation worse from lying on the left side, but remedies with palpitation worse lying on the right side are rare (ALUMN, BAD, KALM, KALI NIT, LIL TIG, PLAT, SPONG). This is uncommon, strange, rare and peculiar. *138*

KALI PHOSPHORICUM

KALI BICH — Sensitive to cold winds. CAUST, it will be remembered, is sensitive to cold dry winds. The KALIS generally are sensitive to cold, dry weather. *618*

GRAPH — From eruptions, catarrhal discharges, menstrual flow, ulcers, breath and perspiration there is marked offensiveness (like CARBO VEG, PSORINUM, KALI PHOS, KALI ARS). *553*

Like the rest of the KALIS, KALI BICH has cured epilepsy. *618*

CALC ARS — Excoriating yellow leucorrhoea, offensive bloody leucorrhoea. For offensive leucorrhoea it compares with KALI ARS and KALI PHOS. *310*

HEPAR — Copious leucorrhoea with the same offensive, cheesy smell. The leucorrhoea is so copious that she is compelled to wear a napkin and the napkins, I have been told by women who have been cured by HEPAR, are so offensive that they must be taken away and washed at once because the odour permeates the rooms. This horribly offensive odour that is so permeating is often cured by KALI PHOS. It has really one of the most penetrating odours, so much so that when a woman suffers from this leucorrhoea the odour can be detected when she enters the room. *574*

ARG-M is a medicine of great use in horribly offensive leucorrhoea (KALI ARS, KALI PHOS). *134*

KALI SULPHURICUM

KALI BICH — Sensitive to cold winds. CAUST, it will be remembered, is sensitive to cold dry winds. The KALIS generally are sensitive to cold, dry weather. *618*

ANT TART — In children that have frequent attacks of bronchitis, from cold wet weather, from cold rainstorms in the autumn, in the spring and in coloudy weather. No sooner do they get over one cold than another cold comes on. The acute stage is never violent with them, but they keep having these passive rattling colds. Recurrent rattling in the chest. Chilly, and pale. Those florid children that do not look sick when they have a cold, are more or less vigorous, have a rattling in the chest, but do not come down with weakness and are not prostrated by it, but keep on rattling, they call for KALI SULPH. *111*

Like the rest of the KALIS, KALI BICH has cured epilepsy. *618*

SPONG — at times, after great dyspnoea, white tough mucus forms in the air passages, difficult to expectorate; it comes up and often has to be swallowed (ARN, CAUST, LACH, KALI-C, KALI-S, NUX-MOSCH, SEP, STAPH). *939*

AURUM MUR is one of the most useful remedies for catarrh of the nose in patients who are sensitive to the warm room. It classes with PULSATILLA and KALI SULPHURICUM, as both of these are better in the open air. *202*

KALI SILICATUM

KALI BICH — Sensitive to cold winds. CAUST, it will be remembered, is sensitive to cold dry winds. The KALIS generally are sensitive to cold, dry weather. *618*

The relationship between TUB and CALC is very close. They are interchangeable; that is, the one may be indicated for a while, and then the other. They are both deep acting remedies - also SIL is closely related to TUB, on the same plane of action, going deep into the life in a similar way; CALC, TUB, SIL and the SILICATES. *1003*

Like the rest of the KALIS, KALI BICH has cured epilepsy. *618*

KALMIA

STANNUM — The pain sometimes begins at sunrise, increases until noon and gradually diminishes, and ceases with sunset. On the other hand, it may begin at any time, as often at 10am. and increasing for 10 or 20 minutes, then gradually decrease until gone. A few other remedies have these sun headaches. KALM has a similar headache, not so regularly increasing and diminishing, but especially worse at noon. *942*

ARG NIT — Here is a striking feature. "Patient cannot lie on the RIGHT side because it brings on so much palpitation." We have plenty of remedies with palpitation worse from lying on the left side, but remedies with palpitation worse lying on the right side are rare (ALUMN, BAD, KALM, KALI NIT, LIL TIG, PLAT, SPONG). This is uncommon, strange, rare and peculiar. *138*

ABROT — A suddenly suppressed rheumatism of any joint followed by violent cardiac symptoms; it is much like LEDUM, AURUM and KALMIA. *17*

In acute endocarditis the principal remedies are SPONG, ABROT, SEP, and KALM. NAJA in valvular diseases. *941*

SPONGIA — Hypertrophy of the heart (KALM, NAJA, SEP). *939*

KREOSOTUM

LACH — From the wounds there is much bleeding. SMALL WOUNDS BLEED much, like PHOS and KREOSOTE. *683*

In BRY there is a keynote which really applies to a dozen or more remedies, "He wants something and he knows not what." It is a very important symptom of BRY. It is a symptom that calls for BRY only when the rest of the symptoms agree. You go to a child who is being carried in the arms of the nurse and wants one toy after another; you get the toy he wants and he does not want it and throws it right back at you. When that case is looked into thoroughly it may be covered by KREOSOTE.................................. *278*

Until ALETRIS FARINOSA was known KREOS was the most promising remedy for copious frothy eructations with vomiting; ALET-F must take the place of KREOS in the vomiting of pregnant women, when the symptoms agree. *54*

STAPH — Meibomian tumours (CON, THUJA), in irritable children (KREOS). *946*

LAC CANINUM

GUAIACUM — The rheumatic joints are more painful from warmth (LAC-C, LED, PULS). *562*

LAC FELINUM

I remember a patient who had been travelling about from oculist to oculist, who had many visual troubles, and no glasses would suit. She had one sharp, stinging pain over the left eye day and night and she could only sleep when worn out. LAC FEL cured. Constant fine stinging pain over left eye was brought out by the provers of cat's milk........... *937*

LACHESIS

A haemorrhagic patient should have a dose of MILL or LACH before having teeth extracted. *749*

Nowadays we frequently find the dry hacking cough in the hands of doctors who have given too much LACH. LACH is commonly given to oversensitive women; and it produces many of those conditions; it sometimes cures great troubles but leaves behind for weeks a dry, hacking cough that stops her from sleeping. Sometimes it comes on after the first sleep, which is commonly around 11 o'clock; a dry, hacking cough from lying down. BELL will cure this old effect of LACH, the nervous state, the excitability and the cough. BELL will be suitable as an antidote to LACH, that is for its acute symptoms. CALC is an antidote for the more chronic effects of LACH. *256*

AMM-C — A congestive headache comes on in wet weather and from weather changes. Sensation as if the brain would come out through the forehead and eyes. "Pulsating, beating in the forehead as if it would burst." The headache is worse from stepping, especially the headaches that come at the menstrual period. Headache worse in the morning. This medicine in such headaches, with the symptoms I have described, shows its antidotal relationship to LACH, because LACH produces all this state of prostration. In the old textbooks you will notice this expression "Inimical to LACH." This means that when LACH has been given in high potency and has acted curatively, AMM-C is unlikely to act curatively after it and is sometimes capable of disturbing the case, confusing it and mixing up the symptoms. But when LACH has been given in too low potency and the patient has been poisoned with the crude medicine, this remedy then becomes an antidote, used in a high potency, because of the similarity of its action. It will overcome many of the poisonous symptoms of the case. *99*

LAC-C — An oversensitive state prevails, a general hyperaesthesia of the skin and all parts. It makes women violently hysterical and causes all sorts of strange and apparently impossible symptoms. For example, a woman lay in bed for days with the fingers abducted and would go wild if they would touch each other. The fingers were not aggravated from hard pressure but she would scream if they touched. This state is difficult to cure outside of LAC-C and LACH. LACH has produced a similar condition. The sensitiveness of the abdomen so that the sheet cannot be permitted to touch the skin belongs to both. Another strange state is a peculiar vertigo, a condition, when walking, in which she seems to be floating in mid-air, or when lying as if she were not on the bed. Other remedies have this. The sensation as if floating or not touching the bed, or sinking down, belongs to LACH. The sensation of gliding when walking is strong under ASARUM EUROPEUM. *675*

The KALI CARB patient is oversensitive to all the surrounding things, oversensitive to touch; shivering from the simplest and lightest touch, even when hard pressure is agreeable. Violently ticklish in the soles of the feet; I have often examined the feet when a patient would shiver and draw up the feet and scream out "Dont tickle my feet!"; I had probably touched it so lightly that I did not know I had touched it at all. In LACH also gentle touch is painful, while hard pressure is agreeable, but here it is not so much the ticklishness. In LACH the abdomen is so sensitive that the touch of the sheet is painful. I have seen LACH patients using a hoop to keep a light sheet from touching the abdomen. You may know then that you are in the realm of LACH, and that it is like those persons who are unable to bear the slightest touch upon the neck and suffer from uneasiness on wearing a collar. All that however is different from this KALI CARB state of ticklishness. *629*

The hardness and purple colour are what are peculiarly SEPIA. SEPIA stands on a par with LACH for this purple aspect....... *919*

ASAF — In old syphilitics with this kind of venous face, subject to bleeding, ulcers turn black or become purple. In this there is a similarity to LACHESIS. *184*

DIG — Constant desire to take a deep breath. When he goes to sleep the breath seems to fade away, then he wakes up with a gasp. LACH, PHOS, CARBO VEG and some other remedies have that; remedies that affect the cerebellum particularly, producing a congestion of the cerebellum. *500*

In cardiac and asthmatic troubles SPONG resembles LACH in the rousing up from sleep in suffocation; after sleep the dyspnoea is worse. The PHOS dyspnoea is often increased after sleeping, with suffocation. LACH has it in a marked degree; in phthisis when the patient is about to die, there is sweat on going to sleep; dyspnoea on going to sleep and on waking. LACH palliates and must be repeated. 940

GRAPH — He suffocates when falling asleep (LACH). *558*

CARBO VEG — The patient coughs until the chest is sore, as if he had been beaten all over the chest. All night he has paroxysms of coughing. He sleeps into a paroxysm of coughing, like LACH. He rouses up from sleep with coughing, gagging, sweat and suffocation. *384*

SEPIA — The cough is a violent one. Cough during first sleep (LACH. In irritable children CHAM). *919*

SQUIL — Dry cough at 11pm.,worse from cold water and cold air (RUMEX). BELL has cough at 11pm.,worse from uncovering, red face, congestion in head. LACH has cough soon after going to sleep, which may be 11pm. *942*

We often study remedies by contrast. SABAD travels from left to right, and at once a good practitioner associates it with LACH. The soreness, pain and inflammatory conditions of the throat commence on the left side and spread to the right in both SABAD and LACH. But warm things aggravate the pain in LACH; they cause a spasmodic condition with a sensation of choking and therefore he wants cold things, which relieve; they are swallowed more easily and ameliorate the pain in the throat. SABAD on the other hand is relieved by heat, either inside or outside. *892*

Like LACH, BROMIUM in many instances picks out the left side of the body. *273*

SARS — Eruptions appear in the spring. All the venous remedies are braced up by winter and go down in the spring, as LACH, SEC and HAMAM. *905*

ARS is also like the condition that has been brought about from the absorption of animal poisons. It goes to the very root of the evil, as it is similar to the symptoms brought on from a dissecting wound. ARS and LACH are medicines that will go to the cause at once and antidote the poison, establishing harmony and turning things into order. *159*

Old debauchees, enfeebled by wine and women, with weak heart, lungs, brain and bladder, emaciated and shrivelled. Prematurely old, a man of 40 looks to be 80, feet swollen, totters about on a staff. NUX will palliate in the early periods of breakdown, but the time comes when he is weak in body and mind and must have such remedies as SARS, LACH, SEC etc. *905*

Women needing SULPH are full of HOT FLASHES, such as they are likely to have at the climacteric period, and here it competes with LACH and SEP. *972*

MANG — Dreadful flushes of heat like PSOR, LACH, SULPH and GRAPH, coming on in women who have been anaemic for some time. *725*

At times you will see a woman having little shiverings followed by flashes of heat and red splotches in the face, and then she fans vigorously; cannot fan fast enough, and she wants the doors and windows open. Such is SULPH as well as LACH and many others. *957*

SARS is suitable in low forms of chronic disease, especially in complex states resulting from mixed miasm; especially in cases of sycosis and syphilis; cases made complex by MERCURY, sycosis, syphilis and psora. Weakness stamps itself upon the whole economy, as in MERC, LACH and other remedies. The tissues become flabby, refuse to heal when injured, ulcerate from slight causes. After an injury an open sore remains and is indolent or becomes phagedenic and spreads like ARS, LACH and MERC COR. Weakness all over the body; a paralytic feeling. *904*

It is important to compare the symptoms of

NAJA with those of the other snakes. The patient is disturbed by closeness of the collar, < after sleep. There are exhaustion and trembling, trembling of the muscles. Its direction is somewhat like LACH, from left to right, i.e., the ovarian pains, the diphtheria, the joint affections go from left to right. NAJA like LACH is < in damp weather. On inflamed surfaces NAJA produces greyish exudations. It does not partake so extensively of this character as do LACH and CROT. There is only a shadow of the septic in NAJA, but it is extensive in LACH and extremely marked in CROT. NAJA is not as subject to haemorrhage as either LACH or CROT. *755*

NAJA has more nervous, LACH more septic symptoms. NAJA, marked agitation without sepsis, LACH, all the nervousness with a tendency to haemorrhage and sepsis; black blood, like charred straw; dark clotted blood. NAJA has surging of the blood upwards, like LACH - a distressing symptom. There is marked dyspnoea, cardiac or otherwise.. .... *755*

SEPIA — The sensation of a lump in the throat (like LACH), but the latter is better from swallowing. The same in worm troubles indicates CINA. Uneasiness fo the collar and corsets like LACH. Worse in the first sleep like LACH. *921*

LEDUM comes up well after the study of LACH, for we find in the pathogenesis many features similar to those in LACH. It has the mottled aspect and the same puffed and bloated appearance of the face. It is antidotal to LACH, to the poison of insects, to the poison of APIS and to animal poisons. *695*

CROT-H — The low form of delirium, muttering, talking to himself is a peculiar form of loquacity. It differs somewhat from LACH. Both have loquacity. The LACH loquacity is so rapid that if anyone in the room commences to tell something the patient will take it up and finish the story, although he has never heard anything about it, so active is his mind. No one is permitted to finish a story in the presence of a LACH patient. One will commence to tell something. He will say, "Oh yes, I understand it!" and he will go off on another line and will finish up with something completely different. CROT-H does that too, but CROT-H will take it up and will mumble and stumble over his words in a clumsy manner. It is a low passive state like intoxication; in LACH it is wild excitement. *475*

COCC-C — Apprehensiveness, especially at 2 to 4am. This state may alternate with loquacity and liveliness, like LACH. ... *455*

It is a strange thing to see a bright little girl of 8 or 9 years old taking on sadness, melancholy and commencing to talk of the future world and the angels and that she wants to die and go there, and she is sad and wants to read the Bible all day. That is a strange thing; and yet CALC has cured that. ARS has cured that state, and also LACH. *319*

SPONG — Wakens at night in great fear, and it is some time before he can rationalise his surroundings, (AESC, LYC, SAMB, LACH, PHOS, CARBO VEG). *938*

SIL — Flushes in the face during the day (SULPH, SEP, LACH). *934*

AGAR — Red nose, as if frostbitten. It is as good as LEDUM and LACH for the red tipped nose in old drunkards. *44*

HYOS — "Twitching of the muscles of the face when attempting to put out the tongue."

It trembles like it does in LACH, catches onto the teeth from its great dryness, and the jaw hangs down, relaxed; the mouth wide open. *585*

CAUST — The symptom of thirst with aversion to drinking is very much like LACH. The two run very close together in the paralytic condition of the throat... *402*

AMM-C — In diphtheria when the nose is stopped, the child starts from sleep gasping for breath. Here again we observe its relation to LACH and the ophidia, for soon after the patient drops to sleep he wakes up suffocating. *100*

As we go into the syphilitic affections that lead into the throat, we find ulcers of the soft palate which eat away the uvula, small ulcers which finally unite and destroy the soft palate and then commence to work on the osseous portion of the roof of the mouth. The odour that comes from the mouth when it is opened to show the throat is extremely offensive; very often like spoiled cheese. The medicines that are especially related, or especially useful in this form of ulceration in old syphilitics will be KALI BICH, LACH, MERC, MERC COR and HEPAR. *575*

A marked feature of the KALI BICH throat is its oedematous uvula. This symptom is also found in APIS, KALI-I, LACH, MUR-AC, NIT-AC, PHOS, SULPH-AC and TAB. *620*

MERC has chronic throat troubles and syphilitic ulcers and patches. The inflammation extends upwards and downwards, red and pale patches, the red looking as if they would ulcerate or suppurate. The red spots become quite purple, but the more purple they are the more they are like LACH. *738*

PETR — He cannot eat without pain, but he has a gnawing hunger which drives him to eat (LACH, GRAPH). *817*

LAC-C — Severe pain in the region of the right ovary, ameliorated by the flow of bright red blood, is again somewhat like LACH. These pains take alternate sides. *677*

LAC-C — Horrible sights are presented to the mental vision, not always snakes, and she fears the objects will take form and present themselves to her eyes. This is analogous to LACH, which has the feeling that the atmosphere is full of hovering spiritis, although he never sees them. In LAC-C she cannot bear to be alone. In LACH the patient wants to be alone to indulge the strange fancies, and when alone she feels as if she were floating out of the window and over the grassy plains, but a sound will bring her back to the world again. This is on the borderland of insanity or delirium. *676*

SENEGA — "Copious accumulation of tough mucus in air-tubes, which causes the greatest, often ineffectual, efforts at coughing and hawking for its expulsion." This thick, tough, mucus will lead most prescribers to give such medicines as KALI BICH, LACH and MERC COR, entirely overlooking the usefulness of SENEGA. *915*

SPONG — at times, after great dyspnoea, white tough mucus forms in the air passages, difficult to expectorate; it comes up and often has to be swallowed (ARN, CAUST, LACH, KALI-C, KALI-S, NUX-MOSCH, SEP, STAPH). *939*

PULS — A general feature of the skin is itching and burning, but a more marked PULS state is a LACH appearance of the skin. It is mottled, erysipelatous; spotted, purplish in spots; veins engorged; capillaries tumid; a vasomotor paralysis of the capillaries or veins producing a mottled appearance. *858*

Carbuncles that come upon the neck and upon the back begin with a pustule, and then several come, and they are surrounded by little pustules and papules and there is pitting upon pressure. For these carbuncles you will need to study particularly ARS, ANTHR, LACH, SEC and CROT-H. They are the medicines that have in their nature malignancy and manifestation. *477*

CROT-H — There is some reason to think that this will be more or less a heart remedy from the great cardiac weakness it produces. But the other snake poisons like NAJA, LACH and ELAPS have had more clinical application than this one *477*

NAJA — These are symptoms in connexion with hay fever : The rawness in the throat and larynx; dreadful aching in the throat extending to the larynx, which swallowing does not relieve. The LACH state is expressed more by a lump in the throat; grasping of the throat with a sense of choking. *756*

There is another class of remedies having the stuffing up of the nose not relieved by the discharge. There is a constant desire to blow the nose, yet he gets no relief. This makes me think of LACH, KALI BI, PSOR, NAJA and STICTA. *864*

CROT-H — In PUERPERAL FEVER there is a continued oozing of black, offensive blood that will not coagulate; bleeding from every orifice of the body as well as from the uterus. Imagine a woman who is pregnant suffering from typhoid fever. She aborts and a low zymotic state comes on with the symptoms that I have described and with all the appearances as if she would bleed to death after the abortion. The blood will not coagulate and the flow continues. Or in a woman during a typhoid fever menstruation comes on. It is not a true menstrual flow, that is, it does not resemble the ordinary flow, because it is copious, dark and liquid, a continuous oozing with all the grave symptoms described, and especially the besotted countenance, the comatose state, the appearance as if she were intoxicated, lying as one dead. When aroused every muscle trembles; if the tongue is protruded it trembles, and there is inability to articulate. CROT-H may save her life. Would it be possible to think of graver states of sickness than such as are produced by the ophidia? When a physician sees these states coming on he immediately thinks of a class of remedies that can cover such a state, remedies like BAPT, ARS, SEC and the OPHIDIA, and sometimes ARN, PHOS and PYR. *477*

AIL — "Eruption plentiful with a bluish tint Typhoid scarlatira." "Eruption is slow to make its appearance, remains livid." "Body and limbs covered with an irregular patchy eruption of a very livid colour." Here you see but one type of scarlet fever. This low type of fever sometimes needs SULPH or PHOS or BELL or BAPT or LACH. *52*

You now think of the remedies that are typical of all zymotic states; the prostration, the aggravation after sleep, general stupor and delirium, and almost at a glance you see LACH, the type of such forms of disease. Its picture comes into your mind speedily. . *53*

ARN is one of the sheet anchors in certain seasons, in the malarial valleys of the West, for intermittent fever. In congestive chills, in those dreadful attacks with prostration, stupor, mottled skin, with congestion that comes on suddenly, with anxiety. The doctors know these fevers, they dread them and can only cope with them by using such remedies as ARN and LACH and other deep acting medicines. *143*

Post-diphtheritic paralysis is a serious condition and only a few remedies can cure it. CAUST is one of them. LACH and COCC are also important. *401*

LATRODECTUS MACTANS

OX-AC — Stitching, tearing pains behind the sternum going to shoulders and arms; worse on left side, with blueness of nails and lips; cold sweat; paralysis of lower limbs; spasmodic respiration (compare LACTRODEDTUS MACTANS). *815*

LAUROCERASUS

At times an adult takes cold and rawness of the larynx and trachea is the result. On going to bed she is taken with a spasmodic constriction of the larynx. Laryngismus stridulus is commonly found in women, IGN, GELS, LAUR and SPONG. IGN and GELS will cure 8 out of 10 cases. *940*

LEDUM PALUSTRE

HYPERICUM—Lingeringsore bruised places on bones, in joints and upon cartilages. But LEDUM comes in very often as a preventive medicine. It is a preventive medicine when an accident hapens to the ends of the fingers, if a patient steps on a nail or tack or sticks a splinter under a finger nail or into the foot. If a horse picks up a nail, pull it out and give him a dose of LEDUM; there will never be trouble, he will not have lock-jaw. These punctured wounds, rat bites, cat bites, etc. are all made safe by LEDUM, i.e., LEDUM prevents the shooting pains that naturally come and the nerves will never be involved. We will have no trouble if we can give it at once. Again if the pain is a dull aching in the part that was injured, in the wound, LEDUM is still the remdy; if it shoots from the wound up the nerve of the arm it is more like HYPERICUM. A sensitive nervous woman steps on the tack during the day, and she feels all the day where the tack went in, lies down in bed and it aches so violently she cannot keep it still. LEDUM will prevent any further trouble, but if that goes on until the morning the pains will be shooting up the leg, calling for HYPERICUM. I mentioned the use of LEDUM when a horse picks up a nail. Now if a nail goes through the thin part of the hoof and strikes the coffin bone that horse is a almost sure to die with tetanus; the veterinarians know nothing for it though they poultice it and put on liniments etc., that horse will die with tetanus; but if a dose of LEDUM is a given before the tetanus comes on it will save the animal from tetanus; after the jerking comes on LEDUM will not do but HYPERICUM must be given. HYPERICUM belongs to lacerated wounds and when there is laceration of parts that are full of small nerves, sentient nerves, give it at once. Do not waste time with ARNICA because there is soreness, for the soreness is of much less importance than the danger from nerves in lacerated wounds. In punctured wounds give LEDUM at once. Whatever sequences come on, of course, have to be met in accordance with the state and symptoms of the case, ... *590*

AGAR — Red nose, as if frostbitten. It is as good as LEDUM and LACH for the red tipped nose in old drunkards. *44*

KALMIA — "Wandering rheumatic pains in the region of the heart". "When articular rheumatism has been treated externally and cardiac symptoms ensue". Rheumatism that goes from the lower to the upper limbs. Not uncommonly you will meet such things. These "rubbers" that go around the streets with a strong liniment and considerable magnetism frequently cause a rheumatism to leave the knee joint and, when it does that, the heart is likely to be the organ that suffers. Then, KALMIA, AURUM, BRYONIA, RHUS-TOX, LEDUM, CALC, ABROTANUM and sometimes CACTUS are remedies that prove suitable for such cardiac affections. *670*

ZINC — Aching in the dorsal, lumbar and sacral regions, better from walking and worse rising from a seat. (In RHUS the aching is in the sacral region and better when walking and coming on while sitting. CALC, RHUS, PHOS, SULPH and SEP have this in the highest degree. ZINC occupies a lower grade in the aggravation when rising from a seat, as do PETR and LEDUM.) *1014*

GUAIACUM—The rheumatic joints are more painful from warmth (LAC-C, LED, PULS). *562*

BERB — Finally the gouty deposits become prominent in the fingers and after the gout has determined itself then we have sore fingers; but these correspond more closely to LEDUM, SULPH, AESC and LYC where the disease has become marked and located in the joints. *261*

LILIUM TIGRINUM

Compare CIMIC with PULS, SEP, NAT MUR, LIL TIG, CAUL and IGN. 35

ARG NIT — Here is a striking feature: "Patient cannot lie on the RIGHT side because it brings on so much palpitation." We have plenty of remedies with palpitation worse from lying on the left side, but remedies with palpitation worse lying on the right side are rare (ALUMN, BAD, KALM, KALI NIT, LIL TIG, PLAT, SPONG). This is uncommon, strange, rare and peculiar. *138*

LITHIUM CARBONICUM

KALMIA — CALC, LITH CARB, LYC, NAT MUR and PULS are the remedies that are closely related and should be compared. *671*

LYCOPODIUM

NAT-P — The body smells sour (like HEPAR, SULPH, LYC). *773*

When patients are under constitutional remedies, they need caution about certain kinds of food that are known to disagree with their constitutional remedy. A BRYONIA patient is often made sick from eating sauerkraut, from vegetable salads, chicken salad, etc. so that you need not be surprised, after administering a dose of BRY for a constitutional state, to have your patient come in and say that she has been made very ill from eating some one of these things. It is well to caution persons who are under the influence of PULS to avoid the use of fat foods, because very often they will upset the action of the remedy. It is well to say to patients who are under LYC, "See that you do not eat oysters while taking this medicine." *286*

Persons who are subject to BRY conditions suffer in church, at the opera, in close warm rooms, like LYC. Girls that faint every time they go to church are relieved by IGN. . *280*

The LIL TIG patient suffocates in a crowded room, in the theatre, in church, like APIS, IOD, KALI IOD, LYC and PULS. *701*

MAG CARB is especially useful if the history has been a tubercular one. Losing flesh and craving meat in those who are tubercular, or in those that are from tubercular parents. Patients suffering from a dry cough. There are persons who have simply this tendency who go along year after year in this withered state with the little hacking cough, not rousing up into much. Finally some favourable circumstance arises and the tuberculosis comes on rapidly after it has remained in a sluggish state for a long time. There are a few remedies more likely to be associated with that condition than any others - ARS, CALC, LYC, MAG CARB and TUB. They fit into this lingering state, this prelude to active phthisis. They sometimes set a patient thriving, but mind you, these cases are hard cases to manage. They are difficult to find remedies for. Their trouble is so latent, the symptoms do not come out and sometimes you will have to read between the lines. They are the one sided cases spoken of by Hahnemann. ***716***

LYC is stupid, the dread of undertaking anything is from a general knowledge of inability. In SIL it is imaginary. ***926***

TAR-H — Restlessness of the limbs in the evening, in bed before going to sleep, like ARS and LYC.................................... ***990***

SPONG — Wakens at night in great fear, and it is some time before he can rationalise his surroundings (AESC, LYC, SAMB, LACH, PHOS, CARBO VEG). ***938***

He wakes up confused and wonders where he is. You will see that in children especially - they wake up in the morning in a bewildered state, such as you will find in ALUM, AESC, LYC. ***69***

SIL — Headache once a week (GELS, LYC, SANG, SULPH)................................. ***927***

PHOS — Fan-like motion of the nose, like LYC.. ***828***

PYR — Fan-like motion of the alae nasi (LYC). ***872***

SULPH AC — Weak chest and great dyspnoea. Rapid movement of the wings of the nose like LYC. Rapid movement up and down of the larynx during the dyspnoea. ***979***

LACH — The dyspnoea and the distress about the throat are increased by taking something warm. Now, in the sore throat of LYC warmth often benefits, but it is also true that in some cases of LYC sore throat they want cold drinks and cold feels good to the throat. ***691***

AURUM IOD has cured goitre. It has cured enlarged thyroid with fast pulse and protruding eyes. The goitre is right sided, like LYC.. ***192***

CYCLAMEN — Satiety after the first mouthful (LYC) and then he loathes food...... ***496***

KALI SULPH — Fulness after eating EVER SO LITTLE (LYC). ***664***

RHOD — Feels full after a little food (LYC). ***877***

SEPIA — Nausea violent; deathly sinking accompanied by an awful anxiety in the stomach. LYC has an all-gone feeling sometimes not better by eating, felt as markedly before as after eating, and after eating there comes a throbbing........... ***922***

CARBO VEG — The idea is that the patient gets relief from belching, from eructation, but under LYC and CHINA it seems that no relief comes. They belch copiously and yet seem just as full of wind as ever, and sometimes even seem to be worse....... ***378***

KALI IOD has all the flatulence and belching of CARBO VEG and LYC. ***640***

The relaxed condition in weakly infant boys, that so much disposes to inguinal hernia, is often overcome by NIT AC, and the hernia cured (LYC, NUX VOM). *799*

If you watch a chronic SANG patient you will notice that the stomach will be disordered for a week; spitting up bile; much flatulence; sour, hot eructations; then all at once this will disappear, and a diarrhoea which fairly floods him comes on suddenly; a bilious, gushing stool. NAT SULPH, SANG, PULS and LYC cure this alternation of diarrhoea and constipation. *903*

KALI-BICH — diarrhoea after beer, like ALOE, CHINA, GAMBOGIA, LYC, MUR-AC and SULPH. *621*

ALOE — Diarrhoea from eating oysters out of season. You might be disposed to give LYC because in the textbooks poisoning from oysters is laid down under LYC. I do not know that you would be justified in saying poisoning from oysters in season is LYC and out of season is ALOE, but there is a tremendous poisoning effect about oysters in the hot weather and in the breeding season that is not found at any other time. A great many people bloat up, become nauseated, purge tremendously, vomit everything for several days after eating oysters. Now, when that group of symptoms is present LYC will cure and will remove the tendency to get sick from oysters. But if you notice those who get sick have a cholera-like trouble from eating oysters in the hot season you will find that is where ALOE is the remedy. *58*

LEDUM has red sand in the urine as marked as LYC. *698*

SIL — Slow recovery after pneumonia (LYC, SULPH, PHOS, SIL, CALC). Flushes, rattling in the chest. Flushes in the face during the day (SULPH, SEP, LACH), rattling in the chest like ANT TART, flushes like SULPH and LYC. *934*

KALI CARB — There is sensitiveness of the body to weather changes, to cold air and to wet, a continuous dry, hacking cough, with gagging, the aggravation from three to five in the morning, and the patient has flying neauralgic pains. These symptoms gradually increase and the patinet dates them back to his pneumonia. He says, "Doctor, I have never been well since I had pneumonia." The catarrhal state has settled in his chest and there is a chronic tendency to take cold. These cases are threatening to go into phthisis and will hardly get better without KALI CARB. In this tendency for catarrhal states to locate in the chest KALI CARB should be thought of as well as PHOS, LYC and SULPH. *627*

BERB — Finally the gouty deposits become prominent in the fingers, and after the gout has determined itself then we have sore fingers; but these correspond more closely to LEDUM, SULPH, AESC and LYC where the disease has become marked and located in the joints. *261*

When it is a case of septicaemia SULPH goes to the very root of it.When the feet burn, when there is a hungry feeling in the stomach, the night aggravation with sinking and exhaustion, and when throughout the body there is a sensation of steam rising or hot flushes one after another, you must give SULPH. Now, on the other hand, if in such a case, with the hot sweat and other general features, you have one rigor following another in rapid succession, and no end to them, you cannot get out of the case without LYC, which goes as deeply into the case as SULPH. *973*

RUMEX is one of the most valuable palliatives in advanced phthisis; it will often carry a case through another winter. With RUMEX, PULSATILLA, SENEGA, ARS and NUX VOM you can patch up the last years of a phthisical patient. You will remove the sore bruised aching all over the body of a consumptive by ARN, and it will suit the cough and gagging and retching and make him sleep. Later PYR may be needed for the aching in the bones and distressing cough. You patch him up year after year. Sometimes ARS is the remedy and it has to be more frequently repeated; sometimes it is LYC, PULS, PYR or ARN. These medicines help him along, and they have often to be changed, but finally the breakdown occurs, and these medicines are no longer suitable. An awful dyspnoea gradually creeps on the patient; there is craving for air; the breathing space is becoming diminished. Dropsy comes on in the extremities. The heart gives out; there is emaciation; the hippocratic countenance is seen; there is cold sweat, blue face, sinking. Even now we can palliate with TARENT-C. Sometimes it has to be repeated. It will relieve for days and give a euthanasia, not a stupefaction as produced by morphine, benumbing the senses, but an actual comforting. *888*

LYSSIN

HYOS — Another thing running through the remedy in insanity and in the delirium of fevers is a fear of water, fear of running water. Of course, hydrophobia, which is named because of that symptom being a striking feature, has fear of water, but some remedies also have that fear of water. "Anxiety on hearing running water. A fear of water." That runs through BELL, HYOS, CANTH and, of course, the nosode HYDROPHOBINUM (LYSSIN). STRAM has the fear of anything that might look like water, shining objects, fire, looking glass. Fear of things that have in any manner whatsoever the resemblance to fluids, and hence the sound of fluids. HYDROPHOBINUM (LYSSIN) has cured "involuntary urination on hearing running water. Involuntary discharge from the bowels on hearing running water." It has cured a chronic diarrhoea when that symptom was present. *583*

MAGNESIA CARBONICA

Like MAG CARB, MAG MUR has inablility to digest milk. Milk causes pain and it is passed undigested - lienteric stools...... *718*

MAG PHOS — If well proved we would probably have many liver symptoms, because both MAGNES and PHOS have liver symptoms. *721*

MAG MUR : Constipation of infants, as in MAG CARB. Chalky stools like MAG CARB. *719*

MAGNESIA MURIATICA

MAG PHOS — If well proved we would probably have many liver symptoms, because both MAGNES and PHOS have liver symptoms. *721*

SIL — Headache worse from cold air. PSOR wears a fur cap even in summer. MAG MUR is better from wrapping up the head, but still wants to be in the air. *927*

CARD MAR — Dragging pain in right hypochondrium when lying on left side; like ARN, MAG-M, NAT-S and PTEL........ *397*

MAGNESIA PHOSPHORICA

COLOC — The faceache is especially important, because COLOC is one of the most frequently indicated remedies for neuralgia of this region. There are three remedies which are indicated in faceache more often than any others, BELL, MAG PHOS and COLOC. The BELL pains are as violent as any, and are accompanied by red face, flashing eyes, hot head and great sensitiveness of the part to touch. In COLOC the pains come in waves, are better from heat, from pressure, worse if anything during rest, and are brought on by excitement or vexation. They are generally on the left side; while those of BELL are on the right, and are caused by cold. MAG PHOS has tearing pains that shoot like lightning along the nerves and are relieved by heat and pressure. *466*

BRY is worse from motion and not better from heat - NUX is both and is more suited to portal congestion, the neuralgias etc.; is worse from slightest pressure (COLOC is better from the slightest pressure - MAG P is better from pressure and heat). *808*

MALANDRINUM

The dreadful EFFECTS OF VACCINATION are often cured by SULPH. In this it competes with THUJA and MALANDRINUM. *960*

MEDORRHINUM

I do not use TUB merely because it is a nosode or with the idea that generally prevails of using nosodes; that is, a product of the disease for the disease and for the results of the disease. This I fear is too much the prevailing thought in using nosodes. In certain places it prevails and is taught that anything relating to syphilis must be treated with SYPH; that anything relating to gonorrhoea must be treated with MED, anything psoric must be treated with PSOR, and anything that relates to tuberculosis must be treated with TUB. That will go out of use some day; it is mere isopathy and it is an unsound doctrine. It is not the better idea of Homoeopathy. *1001*

There are probably several varieties of urethral discharges, but there is one that is sycotic, and when that has been suppressed, it has produced a miasm with soreness in the bottom of the feet, in the knees and particularly through the back and loins and sciatic nerves, in the knees and ankle joints. Sometimes it affects the upper extremities, but particularly the lower. Most violent aggravation when keeping still, like RHUS, great aching that increases so long as he keeps still, he is very often compelled to keep the bed and then he constantly moves and turns. An antisycotic must be selected. While this group of symptoms would be cured by RHUS when the case is not sycotic, when these symptoms come from suppressed gonorrhoea MED or THUJA will cure. *997*

CALC PHOS — Gonorrhoeal rheumatism when of long standing, and worse in every change to cold weather (MED). *336*

SIL — Rheumatism of the soles of the feet. Cannot walk (ANT-CRUD, MED, RUTA). 934

MERCURIUS

As SULPH is to Psora, so is MERC to syphilis and THUJA to sycosis. *960*

ARG-NIT — The baby had MERCURIAL STOOLS, sure enough, they were grass green. Well, CHAM has grass green stools, and ARS and MERC and lots of remedies have grass green stools. Routinist that I was in those days I could not get anything but MERC out of it, and although the baby had gotten MERC, ARS and CHAM, there was no relief, there was no relief until I found that the mother had been eating candy. The baby did not get well until it got ARG-NIT and the mother stopped eating sugar. 140

Where catarrhal discharge has been thick and yellow and then stops suddenly from a cold and a coryza comes on, BELL is worthless. Always bear in mind that you select for suppressed catarrh a medicine that is within the sphere of the symptoms that have been suppressed. Hence the medicine for thick greenish-yellow discharges might be MERC, SULPH or PULS; then you are within the range of medicines capable of restoring the flow and at the same time beginning a curative effect on the state of the tissue, leaving the patient in a much better state. *243*

These condylomata could not come without having some constitutional basis, these warts have a cause, and that cause seems to be less able to make the patient sick if he has the warts, he feels better when he has the warts. Strange to say, when these warts have been suppressed we get symptoms of NIT AC, THUJA, MERC and STAPH. *997*

SARS is suitable in low forms of chronic disease, especially in complex states resulting from mixed miasm; especially in cases of sycosis and syphilis; cases made complex by mercury, sycosis, syphilis and psora. Weakness stamps itself on the whole economy, as in MERC, LACH and other remedies. The tissues become flabby, refuse to heal when injured, ulcerate from slight causes. After an injury an open sore remains and is indolent or becomes phagedenic and spreads like ARS, LACH and MERC COR. Weakness all over the body; a paralytic feeling. *904*

NAT-S — In chronic gonorrhoea, with greenish or yellowish-green discharge. Instead of gonorrhoea running off into a white, gleety discharge, it keeps up a yellowish, thick, greenish discharge. It competes here with THUJA and MERC, both of which are antisycotics. *793*

Syphilitic complaints are commonly worse at night and such anti-syphilitic remedies as MERCURIUS, STAPHISAGRIA, HEPAR, NIT-AC etc. are all worse at night. .. *186*

STAPH — Nightly bone pains ASAF, MERC, SIL. *948*

AURUM is full of nasal troubles, with foetid discharge. The bones of the nose necrose; syphilitic necrosis, the nose flattens down; the bones are discharged. You see these people walking about with flattened down nose and if you get near enough to them the stench will be observed. They are nearly all syphilitics. A few remedies have the power of curing this syphilitic nose condition; AURUM, MERC and HEPAR are three of them. I have cured this state a number of times with HEPAR. *199*

KALMIA — In bed at night the pains become very severe and last all night. This night aggravation is especially true of the marked anti-syphilitic remedies. It is found under HEPAR and MERC; but in none of these do we find it as strikingly manifest as in the disease, or miasm, syphilis itself. *668*

MEZ — Worse from the warmth of the bed (hence related to MERC and syphilis). *748*

HEPAR is also a complement and antidote to potentised mercury. When MERC has been administered and has done all it can do as a curative remedy, or when it has acted improperly and has somewhat mixed up the case and it is necessary to follow it with the natural complement or antidote and prepare for another series, HEPAR is to be thought of as one of the natural followers of MERC. It is very well known that MERC is not followed well by SIL. SIL does not do useful work when MERC is still acting or has been acting. This is the time that HEPAR becomes an intercurrent remedy. SIL follows well after HEPAR and HEPAR follows well after MERC and thus HEPAR becomes an intercurrent in that series............. *574*

KALI-IOD — It is a deep acting medicine and closely related to MERC. It has ulcerations and catarrhal states and glandular affections like MERC. It is similar in its action to MERC and is an antidote to it.. .... *637*

RUTA is related to and is an antidote to MERC. *892*

A certain class of physicians used to call PODO "vegetable mercury". PHYT ought to be called "vegetable mercury" because it is so full of symptoms analogous to MERC. *839*

VERAT — You would naturally suppose that heat would be comforting; so it is at times to the abdomen and other parts when there is coldness, but it aggravates the pains (MERC). *1012*

STRAM — High grade inflammation which it carries to the finish. Pus forms abscesses with excruciating pain (HEPAR, MERC, SIL, SULPH). *950*

PODO — The body is offensive; offensive sweat; compare SEP, MERC, ALOE, SULPH, MUREX, NUX-V. *851*

CARBO AN — The glands of the throat and axillae grow purple and indurated with no tendency to soften. Some of these medicines, after infiltrating a gland, will hurry up the inflammatory action, produce sloughing, rapid breaking down, with pus - like HEPAR, MERC and SULPH. But CARBO AN paralyses and infiltrates the little veins in the inflamed parts and there seems to be no tendency to suppuration...................... *368*

BROM — The process of inflammation is slow; not that violent, rapid kind like we find in BELL and MERC. *271*

MEZ — Violent headaches and brain affections; pains rending, tearing; boring; head painful to touch; syphilitic affection of the brain; headaches through the sides of the head as if in the bone; feels as if the head would be crushed (closely related to MERC and KALI IOD). Headache extending from the root of the nose to the forehead (MERC and HEPAR).. *747*

NUX-V — The coryza and some head symptoms are worse from the warmth of the bed like MERC, yet worse uncovering; worse from eating and from motion; head is worse from heat. *809*

I have seen syphilitic iritis of the most severe character cured with STAPH, HEPAR, MERC, NIT-AC, KALI IOD and many other remedies. The inflammatory process stops at once, there are no adhesions, no deformity and no troubles remaining behind. *638*

Abscess in the middle ear; inflammation of the middle ear; copious thick, bloody discharge, then yellow-green. The case goes on night and day until rupture takes place. I have found this condition as an endemic, in which MERC, HEPAR and PULS were the most frequently indicated medicines... ***861***

KALI BICH — With the catarrhal conditions there is much suffering from the malar bones, like MERC. ***619***

PSOR — Horribly offensive discharge from the nose; gluey discharge from the nose; offensive like MERC, SIL, CALC-P, HEPAR. ***853***

CULEX — Periodical attacks of salivation for months; at night the pillow is wet and the daytime the saliva accumulates and causes constant swallowing. If you prescribe a remedy on one symptom, this patient will probably be given MERC. ***484***

CROT-H — Ulcers in the mouth. Ulcers after MERC in those who are passing forth saliva on the pillow at night. ***476***

BAPT — Canker sores in the mouth. "Putrid ulceration of the whole buccal cavity." Now, with all this trouble saliva pours into the mouth, is thick and ropy and runs all over the pillow; like we find in MERCURY. ***212***

As we go into the syphilitic affections that lead into the throat, we find ulcers of the soft palate which eat away the uvula, small ulcers which finally unite and destroy the soft palate and then commence to work on the osseous portion of the roof of the mouth. The odour that comes from that mouth when it is opened to show the throat is extremely offensive; very often like spoiled cheese. The medicines that are especially related, or especially useful in this form of ulceration in old syphilitics, will be KALI BICH, LACH, MERC, MERC COR and HEPAR, but in those cases that have been mercurialised HEPAR and NIT AC should be thought of. 575

SULPH — As in MERC he must sit long at stool because of a feeling as if he could not finish. Such is the typical MERC state - a slimy stool with the sensation as if he could not finish. SULPH often cures this state after MERC fails. It is the natural follower of MERC when the latter has been misunderstood and given. In dysentery when this tenesmus is of the most violent character, when the stool is pure blood, when it is attended also with much urging to urinate, MERC COR gives the quickest relief. If the tenesmus is less violent and there is not much straining to urinate, or if it is altogether absent, MERC SOL is the more natural remedy. These medicines run very close to SULPH in dysentery but are more commonly indicated than SULPH. In SULPH patients of course SULPH will be the suitable remedy in dysentery. ***969***

CULEX — After stool he has the sensation that he has not finished, so he sits and strains until blood comes (MERC). ***485***

NUX-V — In diarrhoea and dysentery there is straining without relief, but as soon as he passes a little stool there is relief. In dysentery MERC has the constant urging; MERC COR tenesmus with great desire to urinate. ***805***

After stool KALI BICH has tenesmus, like MERC. ***621***

AGAR — Sensation as if the rectum would burst, even after stool (MERC, SULPH). ***45***

PULS — A striking feature is, when the menstrual flow is present there is milk in the breasts. In girls at puberty - milk in the breasts; a premature establishment of milk. In non-pregnant women, milk in the breasts (CYCL, MERC)..................................... ***870***

PHYT — Almost any excitement centres in the mammary gland; fear or an accident;

lumps form, pains, heat, swelling, tumefaction; even violent inflammation and suppuration. No other remedy in the Materia Medica centres so in the mammary gland. MERC is similar; when the patient takes cold the glands become sore. *837*

The symptoms usually found in an inflamed breast after confinement are: aching in the back and bone pains; fever and shivering. PHYT has these and falls into the very nature of the case. MERC when the general symptoms agree. *837*

BENZ-AC — Another feature that seems almost like metastasis. Take an individual who is going around with more or less rheumatic aches in the joints; he takes cold and all this ceases, but the next day he comes down with inflammation of the tongue or sore throat, or INFLAMMATION OF THE STOMACH; so that he vomits everything he eats. The gout goes to different parts and in this instance it goes to the stomach; and then BENZ-AC, ANT-C or SANGUINARIA is likely to be useful. When it goes to the throat or is followed by swelling of the tongue MERC and BENZOIC ACID should be thought of. *258*

PHYT — DIPHTHERIA. In certain epidemics; great tumefaction of the throat; swelling of the glands of the neck, parotid and submaxillary; aching in the bones; foetor from the mouth, with heavily coated tongue; great aching in the back; nose bleed; soreness of the muscles. Analogous to MERC; they are closely related in diphtheria. At times in diphtheria we can only obtain the foetor, loaded tongue, exudation, swollen glands and stiff neck. This looks like MERC or one of the MERCURIES. The PROTOIODIDE is RIGHT-SIDED and stays there or may go to the left side. The BINIODIDE goes from LEFT to RIGHT. The MERC CYANIDE has a thick green membranous cast extending from the nose to the throat. In PHYT we have many features of MERC. *837*

MERCURIUS CORROSIVUS

SARS — After an injury an open sore remains and is indolent or becomes phagedenic and spreads like ARS, LACH and MERC COR. *904*

ARS and MERC COR are the two principal medicines for spreading ulcers that eat in every direction, very offensive. *163*

NIT-AC — SPREADING ULCERS - The ulcers discharge a brown, bloody water, offensive. Phagedenic ulcers (ARS, AUR-M-N, CAUST, MERC-C). *800*

HEPAR, MERC COR and ARS are the principal anti-syphilitics when there is phagedenic ulceration of the nose. *929*

As we go into the syphilitic affections that lead into the throat, we find ulcers of the soft palate which eat away the uvula, small ulcers which finally unite and destroy the soft palate and then commence to work on the osseous portion of the roof of the mouth. The odour that comes from the mouth when it is opened to show the throat is extremely offensive; very often like spoiled cheese. The medicines that are especially related, or especially useful in this form of ulceration in old syphilitics will be KALI BICH, LACH, MERC, MERC COR and HEPAR, but in those cases that have been mercurialised HEPAR and NIT AC should be thought of. *575*

BAR-C — "Spasm in the oesophagus. Difficulty in swallowing." The bolus of food goes down a little way, and then causes spasms, and he gags and chokes. This gagging and choking with a little food is a very strong feature in KALI CARB, GRAPH and MERC COR. This is also a strong feature of BARYTA CARB, but much stronger in MERC COR. *227*

CANTH — It is rare that one suffering from gonorrhoea has this violent inflammation, with burning and tenesmus of the bladder and rectum, but in such a case this remedy is indicated. The intensity and rapidity are features of CANTH. It brings on pain and excitement found in no other remedy. Next to it comes MERC COR. *364*

SENEGA — "Copious accumulation of tough mucus in air-tubes, which causes the greatest, often ineffectual, efforts at coughing and hawking for its expulsion." This thick, tough, ropy mucus will lead most routine prescribers to give such medicines as KALI BICH, LACH and MERC COR, entirely overlooking the usefulness of SENEGA. *915*

MERC and SULPH will sit and strain, and all the salts of MERC have the same state. MERC) COR has a more violent attack, with violent urging to stool and to urinate, and intense suffering, with burning in the parts and the passage of pure blood............. *738*

In dysentery when the tenesmus is of the most violent character, when the stool is pure blood, when it is attended also with much urging to urinate, MERC COR gives the quickest relief. If the tenesmus is less violent and there is not much straining to urinate, or if it is altogether absent MERC SOL is the more natural remedy. These medicines run very close to SULPH in dysentery but are more commonly indicated than SULPH. *969*

LIL TIG has also a dysentery that you will hardly be able to distinguish from MERC COR, so marked is the tenesmus, mucus and blood. The stool is merely mucus mingled with blood and the tenesmus is as great and the burning in the anus as marked as in MERC COR. LIL TIG is especially suited to those attacks of dysentery that come on as an occasional chronic manifestation in nervous patients such as I have described. Now do not think that because this patient is nervous, that she is weak or liliputian or lean; for it is especially suitable for those with full veins; apparently plethoric, full bodied, fleshy, rotund women who are very nervous, and especially at the change of life. Recurrent dysenteric attacks with every cold in those who suffer from pelvic and abdominal relaxation, mental irritability as described, palpitation and fluttering of the heart, with nervous constitutions. You do not see MERC COR in such a picture. If it were a dysentery alone I would not be able to tell which it was... *702*

MERCURIUS IODATUS FLAVUS

MERC is one of the best palliatives in cancer of the uterus and mammae. It will restrain and sometimes cure epithelioma. I knew one case cured by the PROTO-IODIDE, an ulcerated, indurated lump in the breast, as large as a goose egg, with knots in the axilla, blueness of the part, and no hope. The 100th attenuation, given as often as the pains were very severe, took it away and she remained well. *740*

MEZEREUM

In ALUM at the beginning there in no eruption, but he scratches until the skin is off and then come the crusts. You must here prescribe not for the eruption, but for the itching of the skin without the eruption. Now in MEZEREUM, ARSENICUM, DOLICHOS and ALUMINA the skin itches and he scratches until it bleeds, and then he gets relief. Of course, after this there is an apparent eruption, because crusts form. *71*

Zona is a herpetic formation, great vesicular patches come out upon the body called "shingles", here we should compare THUJA, GRAPH, RHUS-T, KALI HYDR and MEZ. *997*

RUTA — Eruptions on the skin with itching, which changes place after scratching like MEZ. *892*

MILLEFOLIUM

In the uterine haemorrhage compare SABINA with IPECAC, which has a gush of bright red blood fully as copious as SABINA, but at the beginning of that gush, before it has kept on long enough to produce exhaustion, the face becomes pale, there is nausea and a feeling of faintness, syncope, out of all proportion to the amount of blood lost. MILLEFOLIUM produces a gushing flow, but it has a continuous dribbling day after day, a continuous flow of bright red blood. *898*

MOSCHUS

IGN — Any little disturbance, a mental disturbance, a fright, or distress, or a grievance, will bring a young, sensitive woman home and to her bed, and she will go on with a spasm of the larynx. It is a laryngismus stridulus that can be heard all over the house. IGN stops it at once (GELS, MOSCHUS). *595*

MURIATIC ACID

LYC — We also see that the jaw drops as in OPIUM and MURIATIC ACID. *710*

A marked feature of the KALI BICH throat is its oedematous uvula. This symptom is also found in APIS, KALI-I, MUR-AC, NIT-AC, PHOS, SULPH-AC and TAB. *620*

PODO — Prolapse of rectum and anus during vomiting (MUR AC). *850*

KALI-BICH — Diarrhoea after beer, like ALOE, CHINA, GAMBOGIA, LYC, MUR-AC and SULPH. *621*

MUREX

PODO — There body is offensive; offensive sweat; compare SEP, MERC, ALOE, SULPH, MUREX, NUX-V. *851*

PODO — Prolapsus of the uterus; prominent are MUREX, SEP, NAT MUR. SEP is better sitting or lying; worse walking. Aversion to coition; hot flushes; constipation with sense of lump in the rectum, or better by stool. MUREX has the following: The only relief is to press on the vulva; not better lying down; she then has pains in the back and hips compelling her to walk; yet this aggravates. Strong sexual desire. Pain in the right ovary, which crosses entire body to left breast. Pain shooting up in the uterus. *851*

The close relation between SEPIA and MUREX is worth considering. The muscular relaxation, dragging down in the abdomen and pelvis, aggravated from exertion and walking, ameliorated by sitting with the limbs crossed and ameliorated by pressure on the genitalia would be like both remedies; but add to this the copious menstrual flow and violent sexual desire and MUREX must be considered and SEPIA eliminated. Both have extremely empty feeling in the stomach. SEPIA has diminished sexual desire and often aversion. MUREX has great soreness and congestion of the uterus, and she is constantly reminded of the uterus. MUREX has acute pain in the right side of the uterus which crosses the body diagonally upward to the left side of the chest, or left breast. It cures violent dysmenorrhoea. It has been useful in cancer of the uterus. Watery, greenish, thick, bloody leucorrhoea, causing itching. *924*

NAJA

In acute endocarditis the principal remedies are SPONG, ABROT, SEP, and KALM. NAJA in valvular diseases. *941*

SPONGIA — Hypertrophy of the heart (KALM, NAJA, SEP). 939

There is another class of remedies having the stuffing up of the nose not relieved by the discharge. There is a constant desire to blow the nose, yet he gets no relief. This makes me think of LACH, KALI BI, PSOR, NAJA and STICTA. PSORINUM has the copious, watery, bland discharge from the nose, it may be excoriating, it has both. The stuffing up of the nose generally takes place in the open air; he is relieved in a warm, close room and by lying down. NUX VOMICA has a free, easy breathing in the open air, but when he goes into the warm room his nose stuffs up, which also occurs at night, though the water drips on the pillow yet he stuffs up like PULS, BRY and the IODINE preparations, IODIDE OF ARSENIC and CYCLAMEN. *863*

NATRUM ARSENICOSUM

If you compare BORAX with other NATRUMS you will find an astonishing likeness in nervous excitability. Aggravation from noise, oversensitive to noise and overexcitement of the nerves run through all the SODIUM family. They are wonderfully intense people. *267*

NAT-S — The satiety of life, aversion to life; the great sadness, the great despondency coupled with the irritability and dread of music - music makes her weep, makes her sad, makes her melancholy - this symptom runs through the NATRUMS, which it receives from the NATRUM side of its family. *789*

NAT-C — When asleep the child jumps, cries, springs up and grasps the mother; a nervous, cold baby, easily startled like the BORAX baby. So are the NATRUM babies in general. *765*

NAT-C — Music causes a tendency to suicide, melancholy, weeping and trepidation; playing the piano is so exhausting that she must lie down; music causes great sadness which increases to a religious insanity. This is true of all the SODIUMS. .... *.763*

BORAX — Like all the salts of SODIUM the nose suffers from chronic inflammation of the mucous membrane, a catarrhal state, with copious discharge, and crusts in the nose; stoppage of the nose. The whole NATRUM family has these dry crusts in the nose, and copious discharge from the nose. 267

NAT-C — All the NATRUMS take away the desire to go to stool; no ability to bear down; stool large and hard, great effort to pass it. *765*

NATRUM CARBONICUM

Take a robust looking fellow, who declares himself fairly well, out to lunch with you. You have noticed for some time that his nose is all the time peeling off; at once there is a star. He never talks about his health. Pretty soon the door slams and he jumps. That is the second point. Then he tells you how much he eats, how well it affects him, how good he feels after eating, and you have noticed yourself that he eats a good deal. You have not said one word about his health to him. You have not asked him to tell you any symptoms. Finally you shove the pitcher of milk over to him and he says "Oh, I can't drink milk; if I take milk it gives me diarrhoea; I never think of taking it." Who could not prescribe for that fellow without taking him into the office? Who could think of anything except NAT CARB for such a case? Sometimes you can find out the whole story by getting a stubborn patient to go and dine with you. *42*

If you compare BORAX with other NATRUMS you will find an astonishing likeness in the nervous excitability. Aggravation from noise, oversensitive to noise and overexcitement of the nerves run through all the SODIUM family. They are wonderfully intense people. *267*

NAT-S — The satiety of life, aversion to life; the great sadness, the great despondency coupled with the irritability and dread of music - music makes her weep, makes her sad, makes her melancholy - this symptom runs through the NATRUMS, which it receives from the NATRUM side of its family. *789*

BORAX — There is another feature like NAT MUR and NAT CARB - in both male and female it takes away sexual desire - it benumbs the patient and hence the mind and sexual organs are in a state of indifference. *268*

Both NAT CARB and NAT MUR have the general nervous tension of NATRUM, but one is a chilly patient, the other warm blooded. *767*

BORAX — Like all the salts of SODIUM the nose suffers from chronic inflammation of the mucous membrane, a catarrhal state, with copious discharge, and crusts in the nose; stoppage of the nose. The whole NATRUM family has these dry crusts in the nose, and copious discharges from the nose. *267*

NAT-C and SIL are both useful when the mother's milk causes diarrhoea and vomiting. The routinist is likely to give such medicines as AETHUSA, entirely forgetting SIL. The latter, as well as NAT-C, has sour vomiting and sour curds in the stool. "Aversion to the mother's milk and vomiting." "Diarrhoea from milk". Put these two together. *931*

NAT-S — Vesicular eruptions around the mouth and chin and various parts of the body; little, fine water blisters, very much like NAT-M and very much also like NAT-C. So you see it runs into the NATRUMS. *794*

NAT-P — Weakness of the ankles in children (NAT-C). ***778***

NATRUM MURIATICUM

AGAR — Children are late learning to talk and walk, thus combining the features of two remedies, NAT MUR which has the symptom "late learning to talk" and CALC CARB which has the symptom "late learning to walk". ***42***

"Late walking" is CALC. "Late learning to walk" is BARYTA CARB. BARYTA CARB competes also with BORAX and NAT MUR. All three of these medicines have a peculiar kind of tardiness in the development of the brain, so that they are late learning to do things; late in developing. ***221***

CALC — Defective formation of bone. A keynote has grown "Late learning to walk" because the legs are so weak. It is not late learning to walk, but late walking. It knows how to walk, but it can't walk. NAT MUR has brain trouble, in which the child is late learning to do things. ***315***

Where the child is losing flesh, slow learning to do things, slow learning to walk, or the legs are not strong enough to support the body, or it is behind in mental development CALC PHOS is one to be examined, (like BARYTA CARB, BORAX, PHOS AC, NAT-M, CALC-C). ***334***

BAR-C — The infant looks like a little old person, like the state we find in NAT MUR and CALC. ***226***

ARS — Then threre are dreadful occipital headaches, so severe that the patient feels stunned or dazed. They come on after midnight, from excitement, from exertion, they come on from becoming heated in walking, which produces determination of blood to the head. NAT MUR is a medicine analogous to ARS in its periodicity and in many of its complaints. It has congestive headaches from walking and becoming heated; especially from walking in the sun. ***156***

IOD — As in NAT MUR and ABROT, he emaciates while he has at the same time an enormous appetite. The nutrition is so disturbed that there is no making of flesh, and hence the emaciation. ...., ***601***

ABROT — The emaciation begins IN THE LOWER LIMBS AND GRADUALLY SPREADS UPWARD so the face is last affected; that is the opposite of LYC, NAT MUR and PSOR. ***17***

If you compare BORAX with other NATRUMS you will find an astonishing likeness in the nervous excitability; NAT-C and NAT-M. Aggravation from noise, oversensitive to noise and overexcitement of the nerves run through all the SODIUM family. They are wonderfully intense people. ***267***

Compare CIMIC with PULS, SEP, NAT MUR, LIL TIG, CAUL and IGN. ***35***

AMBR GR — The symptoms are most erratic, as much so as in IGN and NAT MUR. Taken as a whole they can be reconciled but taken a few at a time they seem wonderfully inconsistent. You must get the whole remedy in order to comprehend it. ***95***

SEPIA — A peculiar feature is amelioration from hard pressure. The patient commonly puts a book low down on the chair and presses the back against it. SEPIA does not seem to get the amelioration from lying on the back as NAT MUR does. ***924***

There is another feature which is like NAT MUR and NAT CARB in BORAX - in both male and female it takes away sexual desire - it benumbs the patient and hence the mind and sexual organs are in a state of indifference. *268*

NAT-C — A nervous, cold baby, easily startled like the BORAX baby. So are the NATRUM babies in general. Accumulation of mucus in the throat and posterior nares, generally yellow in colour, while with NAT-M it is white; the latter spits up copious, thick, white mouthfuls. *765*

PHOS AC — Falling out of the hair is a striking feature; falling of the hair from the genitals, whiskers, eyebrows, head. It is closely related to NAT MUR and SEL in falling out of the hair. SEL has falling out of the hair from the head, eyebrows and lashes, beard and genitals, from all over the body. NAT MUR causes the hair to become very thin; during confinement the hair falls from the genitals. *823*

LYC — While the abdomen is distended he is so nervous that he cannot endure any noise. The noise of the crackling of paper, ringing of bells or slamming of doors goes right through him and causes fainting, like ANT-CRUD, BORAX and NAT-MUR. . *704*

NAT-C — Music causes a tendency to suicide, melancholy, weeping and trepidation; playing the piano is so exhausting that she must lie down; music causes great sadness which increases to religious insanity. This is true of all the SODIUMS, but especially so of NAT-C; aggravation from the slam of a door, a pistol shot, which causes a headache and complaints in general, aggravated from music. *763*

NAT-S — The satiety of life, aversion to life; the great sadness, the great despondancy coupled with the irritability and dread of music - music makes her weep, makes her sad, makes her melancholy - this symptom runs through the NATRUMS, which it receives from the NATRUM side of its family; NAT-C, NAT-M and NAT-S all have it. *789*

AMBRA GRISEA — But while concentration of the mind is difficult he is compelled to sit and DWELL UPON THE MOST DISAGREEABLE THINGS that force themselves upon him and he cannot get rid of them. It is somewhat analogous to NAT MUR, but the peculiar feature of NAT MUR is that she delights to dwell upon past unpleasant occurences and lies awake at night thinking about them. AMBR GR is forced to dwell upon such things. *92*

One thing running through AMBRA GRISEA is that the PRESENCE OF OTHER PERSONS AGGRAVATES THE SYMPTOMS; also the MARKED AGGRAVATION FROM CONVERSATION. A woman, when attended by a nurse, is unable to have a stool without sending the nurse into another room. In spite of much straining she can do nothing unless alone. It is said that in NAT MUR the patient cannot urinate in the presence of other persons. The urine will not start when anyone is around. That is a sort of general feature of AMBR GR. *92*

A woman loses her child or her husband. A sensitive, delicate woman, and she suffers from this grief. She has headaches, trembles, is excited, weeps, is sleepless, unable to control herself. In spite of her best endeavours her grief has simply torn her to pieces. She is unable to control her emotions and her excitement. IGNATIA will quiet her and tide her over the present moment. In all of these instances where all of these conditions brought on from such troubles keep coming back, where your patient dwells upon them, dwells upon the cause, and the state keeps recurring, NAT MUR will finish up the case. It will nerve her up and help her to bear her sufferings. Especially useful in constitutions that have been overwrought at school, in science, music, art. Of course it is natural for very sensitive girls to go into the arts, such as music, painting etc. A daughter comes back from Paris after a number of years close application to her music. She is unable to do anything. She flies all to pieces. Every noise disturbs her. She cannot sleep at night. Excitable, trembles, jerks, cramps in the muscles, weeps from excitement and from every disturbing word. IGN will tone her up wonderfully. Sometimes it will complete the whole case. But especially in these oversensitive girls is NAT MUR very commonly the chronic. It is the natural chronic of IGN. When the troubles keep coming back and IGN comes to a place when it will not hold any longer. Another place where IGN and NAT MUR run close together. A sensitive, overtired girl, after she has been working in music and in art and in school has tired herself out, is unable to control her affections. Her affections rest on someone who she would despise. That would be a singular thing, one may not be able to understand it. A sensitive girl, though she would not let anyone but her mother know of it, falls in love with a married man. She lies awake nights, sobs. She says, "Mother, why do I do that. I cannot keep that man out of my mind." At other times, a man entirely out of her station, that she is too sensible to have anything to do with, she just thinks about him. IGN, if it is very recent, will balance up that girl's mind. If not, NAT MUR comes in as a follower................*593*

HELL - It is an apathetic state; she appears sad and melancholy, whereas perhaps she does little thinking. Any attempt at consolation, so long as the patient is able to think, only aggravates the trouble. Like NAT MUR, the complaints are aggravated by consolation, but the complaints of NATRUM MUR are not at all like these. If the HELLEBORE patient is able to meditate upon his symptoms, they seem to grow better. 567

CIC — Memory a blank for hours or days with or without convulsions. Convulsions generally take the place of the ecstatic or cataleptic condition. NAT MUR is somewhat similar to the mental condition of this remedy, as the NAT MUR patient goes about doing all her household work and other functions and next day knows nothing about it. NUX MOSCH is another remedy that has such a complete blank when going about doing things, a complete abstraction of mind. ***434***

STANNUM — The pain sometimes begins with sunrise, increases until noon and gradually diminishes, and ceases with sunset. On the other hand, it may begin at any time, as often at 10am. and increasing for 10 or 20 minutes, then gradually decrease until gone. A few other remedies have these sun headaches. KALM has a similar headache, not so regularly increasing and diminishing, but especially worse at noon. CACT has a sun headache. NAT MUR has never been known to cause it, but has cured it, especially when beginning at 10am., and worse from 2 to 3pm. SANG has headache coming and going with the sun. ***942***

Some SULPH headaches that I have known present a peculiar appearance before the eyes; a rhomboidal figure, obliquely placed, with saw teeth on the upper side and the body filled with spots. Sometimes this figure is seen toward one side of the object looked at, sometimes toward the other, but it is seen equally distinctly by both eyes at the same time. These saw teeth are flashes of light and the base of the figure grows increasingly dark until you get all the colours of the rainbow. Whenever he disorders his stomach he has this peculiar vision. Sometimes it comes on in the morning after eating and sometimes at noon after eating. It comes also in the evening when he is hungry and delays his eating. These zig-zags come very often with that hungry all-gone feeling in the stomach. We have the same state of affairs, similar appearance of zig-zags and flickerings in both NAT MUR and PSOR before the headache. They are warning of headache. These zig-zags, flickerings, sparks, stars and irregular shapes appear before the eyes periodically and may last an hour or so. In the head there is much throbbing. ***963***

BAR-C — A sensation of weight in the brow with headaches as if the forehead was pressing down over the eyes. Like CARBO VEG, CARBO AN and NATR MUR. ... ***225***

PSOR — Increased growth of hair on the face; a fuzz (NAT-M, SULPH, CALC). ***856***

RUTA — Pain in the eye, above and through the eye when he attempts to use the vision, that is, aggravation from overexertion of the vision. From looking at fine print, fine sewing. This overexertion of vision brings about redness, pain and inability to concentrate the vision on one point. Headache follows. Here ARG NIT resembles RUTA. ARG NIT and NAT MUR are the two remedies most frequently used, but ONOSMODIUM is a very frequently indicated remedy for headaches from eyestrain. ***890***

BORAX — Like all the salts of SODIUM the nose suffers from chronic inflammation of the mucous membrane, a catarrhal state, with copious discharge, and crusts in the nose; stoppage of the nose. The whole NATRUM family has these dry crusts in the nose, and copious discharges from the nose. NATRUM MUR predominantly produces WHITE discharge, and so does BORAX; NATR SULPH produces YELLOW discharge from the nose, even yellowish-green. BORAX is laid down as producing greenish discharge; its characteristic discharge, which is a general of the remedy, is a white discharge. The face of the infant is pale and clay coloured. "Children have small vesicles around the mouth and on the forehead." NATR MUR produces herpetic eruptions around the mouth in all its febrile states, and when the patient takes cold. BORAX is sometimes forgotten, and NAT. MUR is thought of because it is better known. ***267***

BAPT — He can swallow fluids but he cannot swallow solids. Every particle of solid food gags; but he can swallow liquids. NATR MUR and quite a number of other remedies have spasms of the oesophagus coming on with nervous complaints. ***213***

All the NATRUMS take away the desire to go to stool; no ability to bear down; stool large and hard, great effort to pass it. ***765***

Great straining at stool belongs to many remedies but especially to ALUMINA, ALUMEN, CHINA, NAT MUR, NUX VOM, NUX MOSCH, and SIL. ***932***

KALI CARB runs very close to NAT MUR in many of its old, long standing bladder troubles. In old cases of gleet and long standing cases of urinary troubles that follow gonorrhoea these two medicines are useful, both suitable in the scanty, white, gleety discharge that remains. In both, the urination is painful. In NAT MUR the burning is AFTER URINATION. Where there is scanty gleety discharge and the burning is very marked and only AFTER urination, and the patient is extremely nervous and fidgety, NAT MUR will cure. If the burning is DURING and AFTER URINATION and you have the broken down constitution we have described then the remedy may be KALI CARB. *631*

PODO — Prolapsus of the uterus; prominent are MUREX, SEP, NAT MUR. *851*

PULS — Most troublesome cases of prolapsus. It competes with SEP, BELL, NAT MUR, NUX-V and SEC; all of these are remedies with great relaxation, bearing down; some have even cured procidentia. *870*

NAT-C — Crusty eruptions on the skin that have not been vesicular; but most NAT-C and NAT-M eruptions are of the vesicular form. *763*

PETR — Herpetic eruptions about the mouth (NAT-M), about the genitals, lips, face and the patches become crusty and ooze much. *817*

NAT-S — Also vesicular eruptions around the mouth and chin and various parts of the body; little, fine water blisters, very much like NAT-M and very much also like NAT-C. So you see it runs into all the NATRUMS. *794*

ANAC; —Warts on the palms like NAT MUR. *105*

PULS — When the hay fever comes on, all the other symptoms are better, she feels nothing except the hay fever, however all the symptoms interweave with each other. The NAT MUR symptoms will be worse in the morning and until toward noon, while in PULS they are worse in the evening, the nose filling up with thick, yellowish-green, ropy mucus, and when the nose has been cleared, a dry, burning, smarting feeling remains; if the room is warm at night she cannot sleep. NAT MUR is a little like that in the smarting and inability to sleep at night in a warm room. In NAT MUR too the discharge may continue day and night. *863*

In cold cases of suppressed malaria, SEPIA brings back the chill, but its most useful sphere is after a bad selection of the remedy and the case becomes confused. Where a remedy has been selected for only a part of the case and changed it a little but the patient gets no better. It will be seen that the fever, chill, and sweat are just as erratic as can be. NAT MUR is one of the greatest malarial remedies, but it is full of order like CHINA, SEPIA is full fo disorder. In a case confused by remedies think of CALC, ARS, SULPH, SEP and IPECAC. Never give CHINA or NAT MUR for irregular symptoms and stages. *925*

When EUP PER has been apparently indicated by intermittents, and it has not proved of sufficient depth to root out the intermittent, there are two remedies, either of which is likely to follow it, and these are NAT MUR and SEP. These two remedies are very closely related to EUP PER, and take up the work where it leaves off, when the symptoms agree. *513*

It is not an uncommon thing for a malarial fever that has lingered a long time to be attended with swelling of the lower limbs. EUP-PER very strongly competes with NAT MUR, CHINA and ARS in such lingering malaria. *516*

NATRUM PHOSPHORICUM

If you compare BORAX with other NATRUMS you will find an astonishing likeness in nervous excitability. Aggravation from noise, oversensitive to noise and overexcitement of the nerves run through all the SODIUM family. They are wonderfully intense people. 267

NAT-C — A nervous, cold baby, easily startled like the BORAX baby. So are the NATRUM babies in general. ***765***

NAT-C — Music causes a tendency to suicide, melancholy, weeping and trepidation; playing the piano is so exhausting that she must lie down; music causes great sadness which increases to a religious insanity. This is true of all the SODIUMS. ***763***

BORAX — Like all the salts of SODIUM the nose suffers from chronic inflammation of the mucous membrane, a catarrhal state, with copious discharge, and crusts in the nose; stoppage of the nose. The whole NATRUM family has these dry crusts in the nose, and copious discharges from the nose. ***267***

NAT-C — All the NATRUMS take away the desire to go to stool; no ability to bear down; stool large and hard, great effort to pass it. ***765***

NATRUM SULPHURICUM

If you compare BORAX with other NATRUMS you will find an astonishing likeness in the nervous excitability. Aggravation from noise, oversensitive to noise and overexcitement of the nerves run through all the SODIUM family. They are wonderfully intense people. ***267***

NAT-C — A nervous, cold baby, easily startled like the BORAX baby. So are the NATRUM babies in general. ***765***

NAT-C — Music causes a tendency to suicide, melancholy, weeping and trepidation; playing the piano is so exhausting that she must lie down; music causes great sadness which increases to a religious insanity. This is true of all the SODIUMS. ***763***

A NAT SULPH patient will say, "Doctor, you do not know how I have to resist killing myself. An impulse to do it comes into my mind." IODINE has the impulse to kill, not from anger, not from any sense of justice, but without any cause. ***599***

NUX-V — Driven by impulses to commit acts that verge upon insanity - the destruction of others. NAT-SUL has a strong impulse to destroy himself. ARG NIT also, particularly by jumping from a height, but he avoids placing himself in such a position. ***804***

BORAX — Like all the salts of SODIUM the nose suffers from chronic inflammation of the mucous membrane, a catarrhal state, with copious discharge, and crusts in the nose; stoppage of the nose. The whole NATRUM family has these dry crusts in the nose, and copious discharges from the nose. NATRUM MUR predominantly produces WHITE discharge, and so does BORAX; NATR SULPH produces YELLOW discharge from the nose, even yellowish-green. BORAX is laid down as producing greenish dicharge; its characteristic discharge, which is a general of the remedy, is a white discharge. ***267***

CARD MAR — Dragging pain in right hypochondrium when lying on left side; like ARN, MAG-M, NAT-S and PTEL. ***397***

NAT-C — The most troublesome constipation; stool hard, dark, smooth and crumbling. All the NATRUMS take away the desire to go to stool; no ability to bear down; stool large and hard, great effort to pass it. ***765***

ALOE is useful also in old chronic sufferers from this trouble, those who suffer from constipation, who go many days without a stool, but feel every little while, or several times in the day that they must go to stool, and then only a little wind passes. NAT SULPH will very commonly overcome that state. *60*

ABROT — The diarrhoea is his great relief like NAT SULPH and ZINCUM. *17*

NAT MUR and NAT SULPH were used by the homoeopaths to clear up chronic diarrhoea, the old army diarrhoea. *769*

If you watch a chronic SANG patient you will notice that the stomach will be disordered for a week; spitting up bile; much flatulence; sour, hot eructations; then all at once this will disappear, and a diarrhoea which fairly floods him comes on suddenly; a bilious, liquid, gushing stool. NAT SULPH, SANG, PULS and LYC cure this alternation of diarrhoea and constipation. *903*

SEPIA — Spasmodic dry cough in the evening until midnight; holds the chest during cough (BRY, NAT SULPH, PHOS). *919*

MED — Asthma in children of sycotic parents (NAT SULPH). *730*

SIL — Especially the asthma of old sycotics, or in the children of sycotic parents. It competes with NAT SULPH in such cases. The patient is pale, waxy, anaemic, with great prostration and thirst. *934*

NATRUM SILICATUM

SIL is closely related to TUB, on the same plane of action, going deep into the life in a similar way; CALC, TUB, SIL and the SILICATES. *1003*

If you compare BORAX with other NATRUMS you will find an astonishing likeness in nervous excitability. Aggravation from noise, oversensitive to noise and overexcitement of the nerves run through all the SODIUM family. They are wonderfully intense people. *267*

NAT-C — A nervous, cold baby, easily startled like the BORAX baby. So are the NATRUM babies in general. *765*

NAT-C — Music causes a tendency to suicide, melancholy, weeping and trepidation; playing the piano is so exhausting that she must lie down; music causes great sadness which increases to a religious insanity. This is true of all the SODIUMS, ... *763*

BORAX — Like all the salts of SODIUM the nose suffers from chronic inflammation of the mucous membrane, a catarrhal state, with copious discharge, and crusts in the nose; stoppage of the nose. The whole NATRUM family has these dry crusts in the nose, and copious discharges from the nose. 267

NAT-C — The most troublesome constipation; stool hard, dark, smooth and crumbling. All the NATRUMS take away the desire to go to stool; no ability to bear down; stool large and hard, great effort to pass it. 765

NITRIC ACID

As you might suppose, ALUM has fissures; you would naturally expect this when you consider what kind of mucous membranes and tissues this patient manufactures. He suffers greatly from constipation, he does much straining, the mucous membrane is thickened and swollen and hence we have a fissure. If you look into the nature of NIT-AC, CAUST and GRAPH you will see why they have had a wonderful record for curing fissure. That is the way to study your Materia Medica; see what it does to the man himself, to his organs and tissues......... *73*

Sometimes a patient comes to you with erratic symptoms and you may study for hours over these symptoms and see very little order in them, you will realise that the leading features have been left out and that something is lacking. Someone has applied nitric acid or calomel or something else and driven these figwarts away. These condylomata could not come without having some constitutional basis, these warts have a cause, and that cause seems to be less able to make the patient sick if he has the warts, he feels better when he has the warts. Strange to say, when these warts have been suppressed we get symptoms of NIT AC, THUJA, MERC and STAPH. *997*

Syphilitic complaints are commonly worse at night and such anti-syphilitic remedies as MERCURIUS, STAPHISAGRIA, HEPAR, NIT-AC etc. are all worse at night.... *186*

In this relationship to syphilis and mercury HEPAR is closely allied to STAPH, ASAF, NIT-AC, SIL etc. *575*

There are some remedies that correspond to extreme irritation in very sensitive natures; like HEPAR where she faints with the pain; like NITRIC ACID who cannot bear the noise of vehicles going along the street, because it creates such violent sufferings; like COFFEA where footsteps aggravate all the complaints; he was so sensitive to pain that the noise of one entering the door when he was on the third floor aggravated his sufferings intensely, though no one else could hear it. In NUX VOMICA even the noise of footsteps increases the pain all over the body. BELL has in its nature all this sensitiveness to pain. It is a part of the general sensorium; the whole bodily state is intensified. The CHAM patient is oversensitive to pain but we do not need to sympathise with the CHAM patient, he will fight it out himself. But you will pity the BELL patient, the PULS patient, the NIT-AC patient. *239*

NUX-V — Impulses are strongly marked at times. The woman has impulses to destroy her husband or to throw her children into the fire; the impulse is intermingled with violent temper, cannot be contradicted or opposed; if a chair is in the way he kicks it over; if, while undressing, a part of his clothing should catch on a button he would pull it off because he is so mad at it (like NIT AC). *804*

GLON — The weight of the hat is a very common aggravation in headaches in school-children. The little ones work all day in a hot stuffy room and feel better in the open air, but the weight of the hat seems an encumbrance as in NIT-AC and CALC PHOS. *550*

I have seen syphilitic iritis of the most severe character cured with STAPH, HEPAR, NIT-AC, MERC and KALI IOD and many other remedies. The inflammatory process stops at once, there are no adhesions, no deformity and no troubles remaining behind. *638*

In those syphilitic cases that have been mercurialised HEPAR and NIT AC should be thought of. NIT AC is very closely related to HEPAR; it is just as chilly; it has the sensation of sticks in the throat and in inflamed parts. It has fine ulcers in the throat, upon the tonsils and in the larynx. NIT AC competes with HEPAR. You think of the two together. Both have sensation of a fish bone or stick in the throat...... *575*

-Most prescribers give HEPAR for every sticking or fishbone sensation in the throat; this is the old keynote, the old routine. NIT AC, ARG NIT, ALUM and NAT MUR all have it, but all differently. HEPAR: The tonsils are swollen, full, purple - quinsy. The patient is sensitive to the slightest draft, there is pain in the throat even on putting the hand out of bed; he sweats in the night with no relief; he is sensitive to every impression; feels everything ten times amplified. NIT AC: There are yellow patches in the throat; ragged, jagged ulcers in the throat, or it is inflamed and purple. The urine smells like horse's urine. ***771***

ARG-NIT — "Sticks" in the throat like fishbones. NIT-AC, HEPAR and ARG-NIT are the most striking remedies for the fish-bone sensation. ***139***

A marked feature of the KALI BICH throat is its oedematous uvula. This symptom is also found in APIS, KALI-I, LACH, MUR-AC, NIT-AC, PHOS, SULPH-AC and TAB. ***620***

CYCL — Desires lemonade (NIT AC, BELL, SAB). ***496***

THUJ — Cauliflower excrescences upon the cervix uteri, about the anus (like NIT-AC), about the labia majora and mucous membranes generally. ***997***

BENZOIC ACID — Sudden stoppage or slacking up of the quantity of urine; it becomes scanty, high coloured and pungent, smelling like that of a horse (NIT AC)..... .... ***258***

NAT-C — Urine offensive like that of a horse, from a vegetable or milk diet. This is not so marked as in NIT-AC, but resembles it. ***763***

In strictures and constrictions of an inflammatory character in the urethra there is a tendency to ulcerate and with this the sensation of a stick is felt. ARG NIT, NIT AC and HEPAR run close together for this kind of inflammation and will cure the inflammatory stricture before it becomes a complete and permanent fibrinous structure. ***576***

PULS — Tumefaction about the penis. Foreskin dropsical (NIT-AC, FL-AC, CANN SAT). ***869***

When the case is of sycotic origin, small or large white gelatinous polypi form in the larynx and they are sore, causing loss of voice or cracked voice; when they cause choking or uneasiness HEPAR is one of the remedies. HEPAR, CALC, ARG NIT and NIT AC and sometimes THUJA are the remedies related to such conditions.... ***575***

NUX MOSCHATA

SABAD — A sleepiness comes on from thinking, meditating, reading. While meditating in a chair he falls asleep, like NUX MOSCH and PHOS AC. ***893***

CIC — Memory a blank for hours or days with or without convulsions. Convulsions generally take the place of the ecstatic or cataleptic condition. NAT MUR is somewhat similar to the mental condition of this remedy, as the NAT MUR patient goes about doing all her household work and other functions and next day knows nothing about it. NUX MOSCH is another remedy that has such a complete blank when going about doing things, a complete abstraction of mind. ***434***

BRY — With this dry brown tongue, however, he loses his taste for water and does not want it; dry mouth and thirstless like NUX MOSCH. *285*

Great straining at stool belongs to many remedies but especially to ALUMINA, ALUMEN, CHINA, NAT MUR, NUX VOM, NUX MOSCH, and SIL. *932*

SPONG — at times, after great dyspnoea, white tough mucus forms in the air passages, difficult to expectorate; it comes up and often has to be swallowed (ARN, CAUST, LACH, KALI-C, KALI-S, NUX-MOSCH, SEP, STAPH). *939*

NUX VOMICA

PODO — The body is offensive; offensive sweat; compare SEP, MERC, ALOE, SULPH, MUREX, NUX-V. *851*

There are some remedies that correspond to extreme irritation in very sensitive natures; In NUX VOMICA, even the noise of footsteps increases the pain all over the body. BELL has in its nature all this sensitiveness to pain. It is a part of the general sensorium; the whole bodily state is intensified. .. *239*

In many medicines reaction is slowed down, but in BELL it is intensified. So it is in NUX VOMICA and ZINCUM. When the case is very acute, but sometimes also when the case is somewhat chronic, this sensibility is marked. *239*

In RUMEX the nerves are sensitive to the open air; a nervous sensitiveness to open air as marked as in NUX. *888*

The ZINC patient is nervous and extremely sensitive, excitable, trembling, quivering, twitching of muscles, tearing pains along the course of nerves, tingling, excited on the least provocation; oversensitiveness in one part and lacking in feeling in another. This extreme sensitiveness is like NUX, which is inimical. The overworked and excitable persons belong to NUX and ZINC. NUX is sensitive to the higher potencies....... *1013*

CHAM — Excessive sensibility of the nerves, so excessive that only a few remedies equal it, such as COFF, NUX-V and OP...... *415*

COFF — All the nervous disturbances possible are found in this medicine, and they are all aggravated by noise. Even the opening of the door or the ringing of the doorbell produces great suffering. Such patients are so sensitive that they hear sounds which those in a state of health cannot hear. Perhaps no other medicine in the Materia Medica approximates this sensitiveness of hearing where it is accompanied with pain, unless it be NUX VOM. Those practitioners who do not know this generally resort to NUX VOM for pains aggravated from voices in another room, or from the sound of children. *456*

COFF — Such persons sometimes become sensitive to coffee and they drink it in great quantities; the face becomes red; headaches come on, and other symptoms of COFFEA. Stopping the coffee brings out quite a proving, and you have to study CHAM and NUX VOM for an antidote. In all these remedies you get opposite effects. *458*

In dipsomania the sinners who have been drinking a great many drinks in a day sometimes get to that state in which they must get up during the night for a drink or they will not be able to get up in the morning. In the morning the first three or four drinks will be thrown up, but the next one will stay down; they must take a number until one sticks. They have got to that state in which they must keep on taking it. If they sleep too long the first few drinks will come up, and so they must get up in the night or the whisky will not stay down in the morning until they have taken a number of drinks. You will see this in lawyers who do a great amount of work on stimulants. NUX, ARS and CAPS will do something for them if they will co-operate with you. *367*

Old debauchees, enfeebled by wine and women, with weak heart, lungs, brain and bladder, emaciated and shrivelled. Prematurely old, a man of 40 looks to be 80, feet swollen, totters about on a staff. NUX will palliate in the early periods of breakdown, but the time comes when he is weak in body and mind and must have such remedies as SARS, LACH, SEC etc. *905*

SANG — Headache from stomach disturbances, overeating, rich food, drinking wine. Almost as useful as NUX in old drinkers. *902*

If you have administered ACON in too many doses or given it too strong and your patient is slow in recovering from the attack, or your patient has taken ACON himself unwisely, then COFFEA or NUX will often put the patient in a better condition. *31*

GRATIOLA is a great remedy for nervous prostration; marked lassitude, with mental and bodily weakness. It is closely related to COFFEA and NUX VOMICA and especially useful for the weakness of will and neuralgic pains in coffee drinkers. *560*

COFF — So full of ideas that she lies awake nights making plans, thinking of a thousand things; utterly unable to banish the thoughts that flood the mind; hears the clocks on distant steeples, as do OP, CHINA and NUX VOM. Hears the dogs barking. So great is the brain activity, the mental excitement, that she hears noises that are purely imaginary. *457*

IODINE — The MENTAL STATE of this patient is that of excitement anxiety, impulses, melancholy; he wants to do something, wants to hurry; he has impulses to kill. The NUX VOM patient has an impulse to throw her child into the fire, or to kill her husband whom she dearly loves. The thought comes into her mind and increases until she becomes actually insane and beyond control and the impulse is carried into action. *599*

When the desire is so violent that it drives her to secret vice the remedies are GELS, GRATIOLA, ORIGANUM, NUX VOMICA, PHOS, PLATINA and ZINC. *561*

CIC — Between the convulsions the patient is mild, gentle, placid and yielding, which distinguishes it from NUX VOM and STRYCHNINE convulsions. The NUX convulsions are all over the body and are worse from touch and draft, blueness and purple colour of the body, but between the convulsions the patient is very irritable. Of course when they go out of one convulsion into another you cannot see this, but when out of the convulsion, the NUX patient is very irritable. *434*

SULPH — Persistent neuralgias in those that live in a malarial climate, when the short acting remedies given for the neuralgia, such as BELL and NUX-V, have only for a short time mitigated the suffering. If upon studying the whole case you find he turns out to be a SULPH patient, SULPH will permanently cure the neuralgia. *966*

The AGAR patient has spells in which a little muscle of the face or a few fibres of a muscle will quiver for a few minutes and stop, and then in another part of the face the same thing, an eyelid will quiver, and then another set of fibres, sometimes so bad as to nearly drive him crazy. Such is an AGAR state as well as NUX VOM. *45*

The relaxed condition in weakly infant boys, that so much disposes to inguinal hernia, is often overcome by NIT AC, and the hernia cured (LYC, NUX VOM). *799*

Great straining at stool belongs to many remedies, but especially to ALUMINA, ALUMEN, CHINA, NAT MUR, NUX VOM, NUX MOSCH, and SIL. *932*

SEPIA has the ineffectual urging like NUX VOM. She may go on for days with no urging and then the effort is as if she were in labour. *923*

NIT-AC — constant fruitless urging (NUX-V). *799*

PULS has (like NUX) frequent urging to stool without any stool, or frequent urging with only a scanty stool; goes many times before can pass a stool, NUX or PULS. Frequent unsuccessful urging in a chronic case is looked upon as a keynote to NUX, but many remedies have it. PULS is one. *866*

CYCL — Irritable prostate gland, with stitching pains; urging to stool and urine (NUX). *497*

PHOS AC — Later there is sexual impotence; aversion to coition; loss of sexual desire; no erections; penis becomes relaxed in the middle of an embrace and he cannot finish the act (NUX-V). *820*

PULS — Most troublesome cases of prolapsus. It competes with SEP, BELL, NAT MUR, NUX-V and SEC; all of these are remedies with great relaxation, bearing down; some have even cured procidentia. *870*

ARUM — The sneezing is like an ordinary coryza, with repeated chills over the body and aching in the bones as if the bones would break, like NUX, EUPATOR, ARN, RHUS, BRY and ARS that have aching all over during "cold". *180*

The DULC coryza is worse going out in the open air and better from motion. The NUX VOM coryza is better in the open air. The patient feels much aching distress in the nose. The NUX VOM patient ordinarily wants warmth and warm air and a warm room, but with the coryza he is the very opposite; he wants motion in the open air, he looks for cool air, for it relieves the distressing sensation. In the warm room there is a tickling sensation in the nose, and the nose will drip, night and day. The NUX VOM coryza is worse in the house and worse in the night, and worse in the warm bed, so that the discharge will run all over the pillow. In DULC it is more fluent in the house, in the warmth, and less fluent in the cold air, in a cold room. With the DULC coryza, if the patient should go into a cold room pain will commence in the nasal bones and he will begin to sneeze, and water will be discharged from the nose. That very state would relieve a NUX-V patient. ALL-C is made worse in a warm room; like NUX-V, is better in cold, open air. *508*

EUP PER — The subject is extremely sensitive to the cold air, as much so as in NUX VOM. NUX has aching in the bones as if they would break; he wants the room hot, and wants to be covered with clothing, which relieves; often the slightest lifting of the covers increases the chilliness, which is true also of EUP PER, so they run close together. In NUX we have the dreadful irritability of temper; in EUP PER we have overwhelming sadness. The NUX patient is not likely to say much about dying; he is too irritable to go into the next world; not so with EUP PER, he is full of sadness........... *515*

NUX VOMICA has a free, easy breathing in the open air, but when he goes into the warm room his nose stuffs up, which also occurs at night, though the water drips on the pillow yet he stuffs up like PULS, BRY and the IODINE preparations, IODIDE OF ARSENIC and CYCLAMEN. *863*

SABAD — HAY FEVER; when there is spasmodic sneezing, fluent coryza; nostrils stuffed up; inspirations through nose laboured; snoring; itching in the nose; profuse bleeding from the nose; bright red blood comes from the posterior nares and is expectorated; very sensitive to the smell of garlic; coryza with severe frontal pains and redness of the eyelids; violent sneezing; copious watery discharge from the nose. When the itching extends to the larynx and trachea, with great irritability and sensitive to cold: NUX VOM............................. *894*

RUMEX is one of the most valuable palliatives in advanced phthisis; it will often carry a case through another winter. With RUMEX, PULSATILLA, SENEGA, ARS and NUX VOM you can patch up the last years of a phthisical patient. You will see ACETIC ACID recommended for the diarrhoea in phthisis. You had better let such conditions alone, unless they are very marked. If the diarrhoea is very exhausting use some simple medicine like this one (RUMEX), to slack it up. But the phthisical patient is better off with a little diarrhoea, a loose morning stool. It is the same with the night sweats; if he does not have them he will have something more violent....................... *888*

MERC has a well defined dysenteric condition. Slimy, bloody stools with much straining, he feels as if he could never finish, even when no more is passing, a "NEVER GET DONE" FEELING. This is the very opposite of NUX and RHUS in DYSENTERY. These are relieved if a little stool is passed, but MERC and SULPH will sit and strain, and all the salts of MERC have the same state. *738*

OLEANDRUM

SEPIA — all-gone, hungry, empty feeling in the stomach sometimes not relieved by eating. At times a grawing pain, a sinking, a grawing hunger which is not always relieved by eating. OLEANDER has an all-gone empty feeling as if he would die; food does not relieve, is not digested, but passes undigested the next day...................... *921*

In PSOR we find the haste of SULPH, the flatulence of OLEAN and ALOE, and difficulty of expelling a soft stool like ALUM, CHINA and NUX-M. *855*

ONOSMODIUM

RUTA — This overexertion of vision brings about redness, pain and inability to concentrate the vision on one point. Headache follows. Here ARG NIT resembles RUTA. ARG NIT and NAT MUR are the two remedies most frequently used, but ONOSMODIUM is a very frequently indicated remedy for headaches from eyestrain. *890*

PIC AC — The eye symptoms are due to loss of tone in the eye muscles of such as are suffering from brain-fag. Looking, reading fine print and exertion of vision will bring on the headache and eye symptoms (ONOSMODIUM). ***840***

CALC — A wonderful remedy for eyestrain (ONOSMODIUM). ***323***

OPIUM

Excessive nervous irritability stands out perhaps as one of the most prominent features of BELL in contrast with medicines like OP that deprive the patient of all sensitivity. The more congestion there is in BELL the more excitability. The more congestion there is in OP the less excitability. And yet they are very similar in many respects; very similar in aspect; in the appearance of eyes and face; in the pathological states. If I were to prescribe on the pathological state, the congestion of the brain, the appearance, without taking in the intensity of the one or the other I would not be able to distinguish between OP and BELL. They often antidote each other.... .... ***238***

CHAM — Excessive sensibility of the nerves, so excessive that only a few remedies equal it, such as COFF, NUX-V and OP. Of course, without hearing a lecture on OPIUM you naturally think of OPIUM as capable of producing stupor. Those of you who have seen the awful state of mind and distress that follow the administration of the crude opium will understand what I mean by the CHAM sensitivity. ***415***

PSOR — It is not the dry heat of BELL, yet it is as intense. It is a steam. He is covered with a boiling sweat in fevers. Head and body hot, and hot air or steam beneath the covers, (OPIUM has this, but it is in a violent congestion to the head, an apoplectic condition). ***856***

NUX-V — Sharp fever and sweat, or a hot sweat like OP (but OP in a hot sweat wants the covers off, while NUX cannot raise the covers). ***807***

When coffee furnishes a crutch it is a sure sign that drinking it must be stopped. So it is with tea or any beverage. Such persons sometimes become sensitive to coffee and they drink it in great quantities; the face becomes red; headaches come on, and other symptoms of COFFEA. Stopping the coffee brings out quite a proving, and you have to study CHAM and NUX VOM for an antidote. In all these remedies you get opposite effects. Now OP will illustrate that. The first effect of OP is to constipate. Let several doses be given, and as the effects of the OP wear off he may have diarrhoea. OP eaters can seldom stop because a diarrhoea comes on. If you should ever have an OP case and diarrhoea comes on PULS will nearly always control it. But there are individuals who reverse that. Often small doses of OP will bring on dysentery, and if it is increased, bloody dysentery and inflammation of the bowels come on. Of course, one is action, the other the reaction. ***458***

ACON — "Vertigo that comes on from fear, from sudden fear, and the fear of the fright remains." There is a remnant of that fear left, but it will lead you on more strongly towards OPIUM. ***21***

ARN — It is also seen in persons who have gone through a railroad accident, of through some shock, who are sore and bruised from injury. They rouse up in the night with a fear of sudden death, with an expression of terror; the horrors they really went through are repeated. This is similar to OP, only the OP fear remains, even in the daytime. ARN dreams of it. ***143***

CIC — Full of fear; fright will bring on convulsions, like OP, IGN and ACON. 434

COFF — So full of ideas that she lies awake nights making plans, thinking of a thousand things; utterly unable to banish the thoughts that flood the mind; hears the clocks on distant steeples, as do OP, CHINA and NUX VOM. ***457***

NUX-M — The sleepiness and the dazed state are two things combined, and when combined are difficult to cover by a remedy. This state is somewhat like OP. ***802***

KALI MUR — Pain in the occiput, like a weight, holds the head fast to the pillow (like OP). ***642***

LYC — We also see that the jaw drops as in OPIUM and MURIATIC ACID. This occurs in a state marked by great exhaustion and indicates a fatal tendency. ***709***

GLON — In threatened apoplexy, and when apoplexy has taken place, if the violent pressure keeps on, think of this remedy. The clot may not be at first in the place to take life, it may be outside of the lifeline, but if the congestion continues that blood clot will increase. Such medicines as GLONOINE and OPIUM relieve the blood pressure when the symptoms agree. They equalise the circulation and the patient may not die. A paralytic condition in one arm or leg may go on for a while, and at the end of many weeks or months the motion may be regained, and the patient may recover; whereas if the suitable remedy had not been administered to reduce that blood pressure the continued congestion would certainly have ended in death in a few days. The stertorous breathing, the coma, the history, and the general appearance of an apoplectic patient are found in GLON, but the intense heat that comes on in many cases of apoplexy along with the shiny skin and coldness of the extremities are the guiding features. OPIUM is the most frequently indicated medicine, but it must not be administered in large doses. The highest potencies are the best, and one single dose is enough. ***550***

PLUMB — Apoplexy. Stupor, when OP is sufficiently similar to remove the cerebral congestion which always surrounds the apoplectic clot, PLUMB may follow. PLUMB, PHOS and ALUM are three sheet anchors. They conform to the symptoms often when the first state has been like OP. ***847***

SULPH — Then we have SEPTICAEMIC CONDITIONS, with purulent lochia or suppression of the lochia. You may go to a case in which, on the third day, there has been a chill, the lochia has been suppressed, the woman has a high temperature and is covered from head to foot in sweat. As you put your hand under the covers you feel steam come up from the body so that you want to take your hand away; it is so hot. She is dazed and is sensitive over the whole abdomen. You know now the meaning of suppression of the lochia; you have a PUERPERAL FEVER on hand. STUDY CLOSELY FOR SULPHUR instead of hunting around among ACON, BRY, BELL, OP etc. With these you will make a total failure in most instances, but SULPH fits into just such a state and has cured many cases of puerperal fever. ***972***

ORIGANUM

When the (sexual) desire is so violent that it drives her to secret vice the remedies are GELS, GRATIOLA, ORIGANUM, NUX VOMICA, PHOS, PLATINA and ZINC. *561*

OXALIC ACID

VALER — Inspirations grow less deep and more rapid until they cease; then she catches her breath by a sobbing effort, in spells (compare IGN, OX-AC)..................... *1009*

Oysters seem to poison the LYC patient just as onions are a poison to the THUJA patient. The OXALIC ACID patient cannot eat strawberries. *704*

PAEONY

PULS — Most troublesome constipation with haemorrhoids; violent pains in the haemorrhoids, worse lying down, ameliorated from gentle motion, worse from the warmth of the bed, better moving about in the open air. She becomes so nervous in a room while at rest that the pains seem intensified and she must move about. "Haemorrhoids; painful, protruding, blind, with itching and stitches in anus." The aggravation from lying down in extremely painful haemorrhoids is contrasted with AMM-C which has violently painful haemorrhoids relieved by lying flat on the back. In violently painful haemorrhoids with intense burning, think of ARS and KALI CARB. In those with sticking, tearing pains, study AESC. Looking over a number of years I have been forced to use in these cases a remedy not yet fully proven. In painful haemorrhoids in a broken down constitution, where the whole disease seems to culminate in the haemorrhoids; bleeding, protruding; a mere touch almost causes a convulsion; it causes her to scream out at the top of her voice; it is so painful that she feels that death would be a relief; she lies in bed holding the nates far apart with her hands; after every stool she has 3 or 4 hours of intense suffering. In these cases look up the PAEONY. The haemorrhoids it cures look like the flowers of the plant, they are so inflamed, so red and bleeding; oozing; tender to touch; patient is so worn out with the pain. It has many times relieved the pain and cured these enormous haemorrhoidal tumours. I have cured them after they have been operated on, and all sorts of violence done to them, without relief. Do not go to this drug if you can find a remedy that covers ALL THE PATIENT. Many patients will not confess to any other symptoms, and some of these will suffer so much from the haemorrhoids alone that you will really need this remedy. *867*

When piles are so painful that she breaks out in sweat, becomes anxious, and pulsates all over, on the slightest touch or at stool, NIT AC has been useful. (Compare PAEONIA and STAPH.) *799*

PARIS QUADRIFOLIA

With this inflammatory condition there is a sensation very commonly present in the CROTON TIG eye cases, as if the eye were drawn backwards by a string, or as if the optic nerves were dragging the eyes backwards into the head. This drawing in the back of the eyes as with a string is also peculiar to PARIS QUADRIFOLIA, but the conditions are different in PARIS Q. In headaches from overuse of the eyes in engravers or those doing fine needlework, with much neuralgia in the head, due probably to the overuse of the eyes, when the pains in the eyes are not attended with inflammation but are more of the type of dull aches and pains that you might call only rheumatic or neuralgic, with this sensation as if the eyes were drawn back into the brain; in these neuralgic cases use PARIS Q. But in the inflammatory conditions such as I have described, with the same drawing back as with a string, CROTON TIG is the remedy. ***480***

PETROLIUM

"Imagines someone is walking beside her." In the proving of SIL that was observed very strongly. It has been observed in PETR and CALC. ***317***

BRY — Sometimes he has several stools in the morning that will satisfy for the whole 24 hours, or only one or two in the afternoon and 5 or 6 in the morning, during the night no stools at all, because when he keeps quiet in bed and comfortable he has not much urging to stool; every motion or keeping on the feet increases the urging to stool. Some would think of it as a diarrhoea only in the daytime and would associate it with PETR, but with PETR, no matter how much he moves about at night, he will not have a stool, but will have all of the stools in the daytime. ***289***

In old gleety discharge where there is a continued itching, tingling in the urethra and the last drop will remain, discharging for a long time. There are two remedies better for this than many others, PETR and AGAR. ***46***

STAPH — Crawling etc. in the female external genitals, COFF, PLAT, PETROL, APIS, TARENT HISP. ***947***

ZINC — Aching in the dorsal, lumbar and sacral regions, better from walking and worse rising from a seat. (In RHUS the aching is in the sacral region and better when walking and coming on while sitting. CALC, RHUS, PHOS, SULPH and SEP have this in the highest degree. ZINC occupies a lower grade in the aggravation when rising from a seat, as do PETR and LEDUM.) ***1014***

DULC — Eruptions that come out upon the face, upon the forehead, all over the nose, but especially upon the cheeks, which become completely covered with crusts; eczema of infants. Children only a few weeks old break out with scalp eruptions, and DULC is one of the medicines that you will need to know. It is about as frequently indicated as any of the medicines. SEPIA, ARS, GRAPH, DULC, PETR, SULPH and CALC are about equally indicated, but of these, in this climate at least, I think SEP is probably more frequently indicated. ***507***

CROTON TIG is a remedy for vesicular and pustular eruptions upon the genital organs. It is closely related to PETR, which has fine red vesicular and granular elevations, intermingled with fine red rash upon the genitals, itching intensely, worse at times by scratching until burning comes on and then bleeding, which relieves. ***482***

PETROSELINUM

THUJA — Feeling as if the urine were constantly running along the urethra, like KALI BICH and PETROS................. ***1000***

PHOSPHORIC ACID

Where the child is losing flesh, slow learning to do things, slow learning to walk, or the legs are not strong enough to support the body, or it is behind in mental development, CALC PHOS is one to be examined, (like BARYTA CARB, BORAX, PHOS AC, NAT-M, CALC-C)................................ ***334***

FERR PHOS — The general physical anxiety is more like PHOS AC. ***531***

SABAD — "Mental exertion aggravates the headache and produces sleep." A sleepiness comes on from thinking, meditating, reading. While meditating in a chair he falls asleep, like NUX MOSCH and PHOS AC. ***893***

COCC — The mind appears like approaching imbecility, and as you look upon the true COCC case you wonder if the patient has not been growing insane for a year or two, because the mind seems almost a blank. He looks into space and slowly turning the eyes toward the questioner answers with difficulty. It occurs in nervous prostration, in typhoid fever. It is so nearly like PHOS AC that the two remedies must be individualised. ***450***

Purging is sometimes present in ARS, but generally he does not have much purging such as we find in PODO, PHOS AC. ***162***

SQUILLA has a loose morning cough and a dry evening cough (ALUM, CARBO-VEG, PHOS-AC, SEP, STRAM, PULS). ***941***

NUX-M — Useful in the coma of typhoid and intermittent fever. When aroused she remembers nothing; looks dazed; looks about and wants to know who the people are around and what they are doing. It is a state in which the patients answer questions slowly after a long interval, and then look confused again. They give an answer that has no relation to the question asked, or answer correctly. We find such a state in typhoid, in hysteria, after shock, after fear, blighted affections, or the loss of a friend. NUX-M is more suitable after shock ending in this kind of trouble than in typhoid. It is also useful in typhoid, but where there is great weakness, sliding down in bed, and nervous trembling, PHOS AC is a better remedy. NUX-M does not relate so completely to the general image of a typhoid as does PHOS AC. ***802***

When treating a low form of continued fever with extreme prostration, ARS, MUR-AC and PHOS-AC force themselves upon the mind. With ARS there has been the anxious restlessness; with PHOS-AC there has been the mental prostration and then the muscular weakness; and with MUR-AC the muscular weakness comes first, and there has been history of restlessness and the mind has been stronger than could be expected. With this great muscular exhaustion, with jaw hanging down and the patient sliding down in bed and soon the involuntary stool and urine, MUR-AC is forced upon the mind. Paralytic weakness is what it must be called. Soon the tongue is paralysed, as well as the sphincters of the bladder and rectum. It seems to be eminently fitted for the lowest forms of zymotic fever when the above symptoms are present. He finally becomes unconscious.

There has been some restlessness, but nothing like ARS and RHUS TOX. He refuses to talk because it frets him to do so. PHOS-AC is slow answering questions because of exhaustion of mind which makes him unable to think. *752*

CALADIUM is suitable in low, murmuring, exhaustive cases of typhoid fever that are running a very sluggish course, not a very active delirium; but muttering; a low form of semi-consciousness, very often coma or stupefaction like PHOS AC, a dazed mind.... .... *307*

PHOSPHORUS

When a periodic sick headache is interrupted by SANG, if a deeper acting drug, an anti-psoric is not given, the headache will return or something worse will come on, as SANG does not go deep into the nature of the case. I remember a case in which the patient missed his SANG headache and an epithelioma developed which was cured by PHOS. I am convinced that if PHOS had been given at the end of the attack the cancer would not have developed, as PHOS was his constitutional remedy. *900*

There are instances where rubbing is of benefit, but not in rheumatism. In paralysed muscles it is a beneficial exercise, for then rubbing can take the place of exercise of the patient himself, of the muscles. But rubbing is not admissible if it is used to reduce pain. The more agreeable it is, the worse for the patient. In a PHOS patient you would be astonished what wonderful relief they can get from rubbing. There is no person more inclined to be weak in the vitality, in the internal economy, than the PHOS patient. He is an excitable, weakly patient - feels better by rubbing and craves it, but if he has rheumatism in the knees and the knee is rubbed the rheumatism may go to the heart. The PHOS patient loves to be rubbed, because rubbing relieves the symptoms; he loves to be magnetised. *670*

If to the burning in the chest, the severe pains in the larynx and trachea while talking and cough ending in belching you add heat in the palms and soles, SANG will patch him up and mitigate the troubles. Many such cases get SULPH, but to their destruction. There is a class of remedies that suits these phthisical patients better than SULPH, SIL and GRAPH; such remedies as PULS, SANG, SENECIO GRACILIS and COCCUS CACTI, which will palliate, mitigate his sufferings and may even build him up so that he could take a medium potency of a deep remedy. But the deeper remedies ought to be avoided if the vital force is low, if the body is too much damaged to be repaired. Hahnemann warned against the use of PHOS in such cases of deficient vitality. SANG is a surface remedy; it does excellent palliation. *900*

PETR — Very sensitive to change in weather, like PHOS and RHOD; aggravated before a thunderstorm. *819*

MANG is similar to ARG MET, PHOS, GRAPH, and SULPH in its underlying tendency to tuberculosis. *723*

LACH — SMALL WOUNDS BLEED MUCH, like PHOS and KREOSOTE. A prick of a pin WILL ooze great drops of blood. *683*

BAR-C has some of the paralytic conditions analogous to the complaints of old apoplectics, and it has been very useful in re-establishing the supply and flow of nerve force along the nerves. It parallels PHOS and is an excellent remedy for old paralytic conditions that have come on from a rupture of a blood vessel, and therefore pressure upon the nerve supply. *224*

We know that PHOS will burn and it intensifies the tendency to ulcerate, makes the ulcer go deeper, while ARG NIT sets it healing. *137*

When the flashes (of heat) begin in the chest about the heart it is more like SULPH, but when in the back or in the stomach it is more like PHOS. *957*

There is great exhaustion in RUTA. The legs give out on rising from a chair, the patient totters and makes several efforts on rising from a seat. Routinists give PHOS and CON for this. RUTA and PHOS both have violent unquenchable thirst for ice-cold water. Compare PHOS and CON because of the weakness through the hips and thighs. *890*

RHOD — Fear of thunder in nervous persons (PHOS). *877*

CANTH — Restlessness causing him to move constantly, a rage and delirium intermingled with amorous frenzy. This kind of mental conduct in CANTH is similar to what will take place in HYOS, PHOS and SEC, a violent delirious state intermingled with sexual ideas and talk. *362*

GRATIOLA is one of our best remedies for nymphomania. When the desire is so violent that it drives her to secret vice the remedies are GELS, GRATIOLA, ORIGANUM, NUX VOMICA, PHOS, PLATINA and ZINC. *561*

MED — Sees faces that peer at her from behind the furniture (PHOS). *728*

SPONG — Wakens at night in great fear, and it is some time before he can rationalise his surroundings (AESC, LYC, SAMB, LACH, PHOS, CARBO VEG). *938*

DIG — Constant desire to take a deep breath. When he goes to sleep the breath seems to fade away, then he wakes up with a gasp. LACH, PHOS, CARBO VEG and some other remedies have that; remedies that affect the cerebellum particularly, producing a congestion of the cerebellum. *500*

You will find some deep seated brain troubles that will try your patience. Some cases go slowly and gradually into unconsciousness; rolling of the head for days; eyes lustreless; body emaciated, involuntary discharges of faeces or urine in the bed; tongue dry and parched, so shrivelled that it looks like leather, lips also; face withered and each day looks older; paralysis of one hand or one foot, or it seems that the whole muscular system is paralysed. Screaming out in pain, although not so shrilly as in APIS. A dose of ZINC will sometimes bring this patient back to life. In a few days after the remedy there will be a jerking and quivering in the parts that were motionless, or its action will be shown in a copious sweat, much vomiting; sudden arousing that is alarming, for it looks like a threatened sinking, but this is the beginning of reaction. Now, for days and nights while this little one is coming back to consciousness, the restoration of sensation in the parts is accompanied with the tormenting formication, tingling, prickling, creeping and crawling. The mother and the father and the neighbours will want something done for it, but if you antidote the case will return to where it was before. This suffering is but the awakening to life. It will go on in this way for a week or two and then will begin to show signs of falling back; it needs another dose of ZINC, which will again be followed by sweat, vomiting etc. You will see this in spinal meningitis. Rugged little fellows who hang on for weeks in this state, emaciating and unconscious. You must take the mother aside and inform her what will happen if the child returns to consciousness. If you do not you may be turned out of the house. A person advanced in years cannot stand such an ordeal, but it is astonishing how the little ones can endure the prolonged congestion and inflammation. After scarlet fever and badly treated meningitis; tubercular meningitis. I have carried these severe forms of brain disease through on PHOS which has a picture somewhat like that of ZINC. There is no record of recovery from tubercular meningitis, but a homoeopath can cure some of these cases, though it may take two or three months to go down and come up out of it, with two or three relapses...... ***1015***

There are SEPIA headaches that particularly affect the occiput, worse in the morning; great pain through the eyes and temples; relieved by sweat, worse on beginning to move; throbbing felt on stooping, worse on going upstairs. The PHOS headache is relieved by sleep, but continued rapid motion aggravates. Cannot endure it............ ***920***

LYC and especially PHOS and PSOR have headaches with great hunger. At or about the beginning of the attack there is a faint all-gone hungry feeling which eating does not satisfy. Such is the nature of PHOS and PSOR when the appetite and the headache are associated....................................... ***706***

With the headache and many complaints SANG has a faintness; like a hunger, yet not for food. A sinking, faint, "all gone" empty feeling. It is like PHOS with its "hungry headache". PSORINUM leads all others in "hungry headaches" but PSOR wants to eat and cannot get enough. SANG has a hunger, but not for food; aversion at the thought and smell of food. PSOR can eat a wolf meal and so can PHOS. It is a false hunger with the headache in SANG. 903

AURUM MUR — Caries of the lower jaw like PHOSPHORUS and exostosis of right cheek bone. ***203***

MEZ — Sensation of goneness, fear, apprehension, faintness in the stomach, as if something would happen; every shock, pain and hearing bad news, cause this apprehensive, hungry, faint, weak, all-gone feeling in the pit of the stomach. It comes on when the doorbell rings, if the patient is expecting the postman, while waiting at the depot for the arrival of a friend, or the departure of the cars; on being introduced to someone, he experiences a thrill beginning in the stomach, is "frightened in the stomach". CALC, KALI-C, PHOS and MEZ have this. These "solar plexus" individuals often have a deep-cracked tongue and are hard to cure. ***748***

A marked feature of the KALI BICH throat is its oedematous uvula. This symptom is also found in APIS, KALI-I, LACH, MUR-AC, NIT-AC, PHOS, SULPH-AC and TAB. ***620***

SEPIA — Nausea violent; deathly sinking accompanied by an awful anxiety in the stomach. PHOS has more of the typical hunger which is relieved by eating. ... ***922***

ARG NIT — Eructations of air accompanied by a mouthful of undigested food, like PHOS and FERRUM. Spitting it up; welling up in mouthfuls. ***140***

FERRUM — Sometimes there are eructations of food by the mouthful like PHOS. PHOS was the remedy with all the old masters for spitting up of food by the mouthful until the stomach was empty. ***529***

CUPR — The stool is gushig, copious, and is accompanied by dreadful exhaustion PHOS is also to be thought of in relation to CUPR. It also has cramps in the bowels, exhaustive diarrhoea, sinking as if dying, but commonly with heat of the skin, with burning internally, with gurgling of all the fluids taken into the stomach; as soon as they come to the stomach they commence to gurgle, and gurgle all the way through the bowel, A drink of water seems to flow through the bowel with a gurgle. Now this gurgle in CUPRUM commences at the throat; he swallows with a gurgle; gurgling in the oesophagus when swallowing. *491*

APIS — The anus protrudes with stool and seems to remain open, an open anus like PHOS and PULS. *121*

GRAPH — Long narrow stools like PHOS. *557*

MAG CARB — "Stools green, like scum on a frog pond; sour, frothy; with white floating lumps like tallow, bloody, mucous." Floating like lumps of tallow is more characteristic of PHOS, and many times DULC has cured it. *715*

KALI CARB — Constant irritation calling his attention to the genitals, brought on from abuse, from vice, from excesses. PHOS is a medicine that is abused in this sphere. Many physicians look upon it as one of the great remedies for the weakness of the genital organs. In PHOS the genital indications are extreme excitement, too active erections, a disorderly strength of the genital organs. Beware of giving it in impotency or in weakness, as this is often associated with very feeble constitutions and PHOS not only fails to cure, but seems to add to the weakness. It is a weakness that you will learn is a vital weakness. PHOS will set patients to running down more rapidly who are suffering from a vital weakness, who are always tired, simply weak, always prostrated and want to go to bed. *633*

LYC — One of the most prominent remedies in impotency. Persons of feeble vitality, overwrought persons, overtired persons, with feeble genital organs seldom need PHOS, but LYC is a typical remedy where the young man has abused himself with secret vices and has become tired in his spine, brain and genital organs. If this patient makes up his mind that he will live a somewhat decent life and marries, he finds that he is impotent sexually, that he is not able to obtain erections, or that the erections are too feeble or too short, and that he is not a man. *712*

BELL — The chest is so painful, the child dreads the cough and screams. By the child's cry we know that it is going to have a coughing spell. Just like BRY, HEPAR and PHOS which have that feature more than any other remedies. *251*

When the uterus is continually oozing, but every little while the flow increases to a gush and with every little gush of bright red blood the woman thinks she is going to faint, or if there is gasping, and the quantity of the flow is not sufficient to account for such prostration, nausea, syncope, pallor, IPECAC is the remedy. When with the gushing of bright red blood there is an overwhelming fear of death, ACONITE. If your patient, while going through the confinement, has had a hot head, an uncontrollable thirst for ice cold water, and after the confinement everything has gone on in an orderly way, and the placenta has been delivered, and although you have no reason to expect such haemorrhage, it comes on, PHOS will nearly always be the remedy. *607*

SENECIO AUREUS — The whole urinary tract is painful and subject to bleeding. But bleeding especially in the absence of the menstrual flow is the feature of this remedy. Wherever there is an inflammatory spot or catarrhal condition of the mucous membrane, it will bleed in case the menstrual flow does not appear. We have other medicines having the symptoms of vicarious haemorrhage, such as HAMAMELIS, PHOS and BRY, but SENECIO has this condition strikingly, and is one of the newer remedies for such condition. *913*

APOC — "Shreds, or pieces of membrane with the fluid blood. Menorrhagia, continuing or paroxysmal." That is, a continuous flow until the patient is exhausted. That is like PHOS and IPECAC and SECALE. *128*

In old, troublesome lingering haemorrhages, starting up fresh on the slightest provocation, SABINA will stop the gush, the acute stage, but it does not hold, the haemorrhage recurs, and then an antipsoric is needed. PHOS is somewhat like SABINA. It has a copious bright red flow which may or may not contain clots. The striking features are outside the flow. There is pinched countenance, extremely dry tongue and mouth, violent unquenchable thirst craving ice-cold water. The haemorrhage is bright red, in a gush or continuous oozing. *899*

SENEGA — "Dry cough with aphonia; worse in cold air and from walking." is like PHOS and RUMEX. These two remedies cause a cough which commences when he goes out into the air. SENEGA has another feature like PHOS, in that the cough is so violent that it makes him shake from head to foot; it brings on a tremulous feeling all over the body.. *915*

SEPIA — Spasmodic dry cough in the evening until midnight; holds the chest during cough (BRY, NAT SULPH, PHOS). *919*

EUP PER has a dry, hacking, teasing cough, that seems to rack the whole frame, as if it would break him up, it is so sore, and he is so much disturbed by motion. A great amount of tribulation is found in the respiratory tract, in the bronchial tubes. We find a cough in capillary bronchitis that shakes the whole frame, analogous to BRY and PHOS. *515*

BRY — Great soreness in the trachea; rawness and tightness in the trachea, even suffocation, like PHOS. *291*

CALC — The expectoration is sweetish very often, like PHOS and STANNUM...... *328*

In cardiac and asthmatic troubles SPONG resembles LACH in the rousing up from sleep in suffocation; after sleep the dyspnoea is worse. The PHOS dyspnoea is often increased after sleeping, with suffocation. *940*

SULPH — The NOSE, the INNER CHEST and LUNGS furnish us with localities for much trouble. The patient has had pneumonia and it has gone on to the period of infiltration; you have taken the case in this advanced stage after BRY has overcome the threatening features, and now when the patient should rally he does not rally; he perspires all over, is tired and has a strange and singular consciousness that "there is something wrong in there, a load in there;" difficult breathing; flashes of heat yet not much fever; sometimes coldness alternating with flashes of heat. I have often heard them say, "There is a great load in there, doctor, I cannot get rid of it." Upon close examination you find there is hepatisation and now comes the time for such remedies as PHOS, LYC and SULPH, and SULPH leads them all. When BRY has been sufficient for the earlier symptoms or when ACON has cleared them up, there has been too much for these remedies to relieve, then hepatisation comes on. If this is confined to only a small area it will keep up quite a chronic course, but SULPH will clear it up. If however it is a double pneumonia, or the hepatisation involves a considerable portion of the lung and the remedy given has not been sufficient and the case is advancing toward a fatal issue, it may be that all at once at two or three o'clock in the morning he begins to sink; his nose is pinched; his lips are drawn, he takes on a hippocratic countenance, is covered with cold sweat, he is too feeble in every part of his body to move, he only moves his head a little in a restless manner. Unless you are called at once and give him a dose of ARS he will die. You give the ARS and you have done well, but ARS has no ability to remove the results of inflammation. But though it cannot CURE that hepatised lung it acts as a vital stimulant; it warms up the patient and makes him feel he is going to get better; but, mark this, in 24 hours he will die unless you follow the ARS with the proper remedy. You must not wait upon your remedy too long in these cases. Just as soon as he rallies, and the reaction is at its highest pitch, give him the antidote and natural follower of ARS, which is SULPH, and in 24 hours that patient will say, "I am getting better." As sure as you exist today, it will do just that thing. There are times that you will see clearly that PHOS is the medicine to follow ARS with. If such a patient rallying under ARS goes into a fever, if a hot fever comes on with burning thirst and he cannot get enough ice cold water, you must follow it with PHOS and it will do in that case what SULPH will do in the other. *974*

We would think of ALUM when singers break down in the voice from paralysis or from overwork of the voice. The voice lets down and becomes feeble and when taking cold there starts up a peculiar kind of tickling. ALUM is very useful in these cases. There is a kind of hoarseness that you may discover to be a little different from the paralytic hoarseness of ALUM and ARG MET. This hoarseness of which I speak belongs to this same class of people; on first beginning to use the voice it seems that they must get rid of some mucus by clearing the throat until the voice can get to work. The vocal cords, on beginning to work, are covered with mucus, and on getting rid of it they can do very good work, so long as they keep at it. That is PHOS. In such cases the use of the voice becomes painful. The vocal cords are painful after motion and the larynx is painful to touch. Sometimes this is so marked that it is like stabbing with a knife on trying to use the voice. *76*

Now in ARUM as in PHOS the voice is ameliorated from clearing the vocal cords of a little mucus. *182*

MANG — Constant accumulation of mucus, more forms as soon as he clears it. Hemming all the time and annoying everybody. ARG MET, SIL, SULPH, PHOS and MANG all do that. Each hem brings up a mouthful of mucus. *726*

CAPS — is useful in perplexing and troublesome chronic hoarseness. He has had a cold and remedies for the acute condition have been given, perhaps two or three remedies, ACON, BRY, HEP, PHOS, but all at once you wake up to his chronic constitutional state of hoarseness. He is rotund, chilly, red-faced, and the hoarseness disappears under CAPS. It is the same with the cough. After making several blunders you wake up and see that it is a CAPS case and that you have never yet gotten at the root of the trouble. This shows the importance of getting at the things general first. If there is much acute suffering of course you must give an acute remedy, but if the patient has delayed recovery and convalescence is slow the next remedy should be the remedy for the patient. Sometimes it is SULPH, PHOS, LYC and sometimes it is CAPS. If the patient has a good constitutional state he will get over the cold on the acute remedy, but the old gouty, rheumatic, flabby patients need a constitutional remedy. *367*

PHOS has this hoarseness, but especially

aphonia relieved by hemming up a little mucus from the vocal cords. The CAUST hoarseness is due to a weakness of the vocal cords. PHOS has an inflammatory state and the continual accumulation of mucus impedes speech. RUMEX has the accumulation of tough, gelatinous, gluey mucus and he continually scrapes the larynx............ *886*

The CALC voice is that of PAINLESS HOARSENESS. The vocal cords are tired and cannot endure strain; almost a paralytic weakness. Sometimes a copious flow of mucus from the larynx. Much irritation in the larynx, but weakness. Not that burning and rawness that we find in BELL and PHOS, but painless hoarseness. In PHOS it is painful, in BELL it is very painful. *327*

SPONG — The larynx is sensitive to touch in croup etc. like PHOS. *940*

ZINC — Aching in the dorsal, lumbar and sacral regions, better from walking and worse rising from a seat. (In RHUS the aching is in the sacral region and better when walking and coming on while sitting. CALC, RHUS, PHOS, SULPH and SEP have this in the highest degree. ZINC occupies a lower grade in the aggravation when rising from a seat, as do PETR and LEDUM.) *1014*

MERC — Paralysis of the lower limbs, and twitching, jerking and quivering of the paralysed parts. ARG NIT, PHOS, SEC, STRAM and MERC have twitching of the muscles of the paralysed parts. *741*

MANG — Red, sore spots here and there on the scalp (like PHOS), as if erysipelas would develop. *723*

SENEGA has sometimes cured pleuro-pneumonia when there was the extreme exhaustion of PHOSPHORUS and ARSENICUM. In such cases SENEGA has caused reaction; it has such weakness. *916*

In the exudative stage of pneumonia, the stage of hepatisation, LYC may save the life of the patient. It is closely related in the period of hepatisation to PHOS and SULPH. *709*

SIL especially suits the later stages of pneumonia and the old, chronic complaints following pneumonia. Slow recovery after pneumonia (LYC, SULPH, PHOS, SIL, CALC). *934*

PLUMB — Apoplexy. Stupor, when OP is sufficiently similar to remove the cerebral congestion which always surrounds the apoplectic clot, PLUMB may follow. PLUMB, PHOS and ALUM are three sheet anchors. They conform to the symptoms often when the first state has been like OP. *847*

"Doctor, I have never been well since I had pneumonia." The catarrhal state has settled in his chest and there is a chronic tendency to take cold. These cases are threatening to go into phthisis and will hardly get better without KALI CARB. In this tendancy for catarrhal states to locate in the chest KALI CARB should be thought of as well as PHOS, LYC and SULPH. *627*

CADMIUM SULPH — After an apoplectic attack when the patient recovers, but weakness of one arm and leg remains, it competes with PHOS. *305*

AIL — "Eruption plentiful, of a bluish tint. Typhoid scarlatina." "Eruption is slow to make its appearance, remains livid." "Body and limbs covered with an irregular patchy eruption of a very livid colour." Here you see but one type of scarlet fever. This low type of fever sometimes needs SULPH or PHOS or BELL or BAPT or LACH. That you may be able to distinguish one from another and keep the picture of each remedy clearly in mind requires a prolonged study of the Materia Medica. It is an easy matter to compare remedies for yourself after you have first studied each one separately. You can then bring out many comparisons and especially in this case at the bedside. If you go to the bedside with a good knowledge of the generals of Materia Medica you will be surprised at the number of symptom pictures which will come into your mind, called up by the signs of the sickness. When you go to the bedside of scarlet fever you should not call to mind the names of these medicines which you may have heard recommended for scarlet fever; let the appearance of the patient bring to mind such remedies as appear like the patient, regardless of whether they have been associated with scarlet fever or not. When you see the rash perhaps you will say that looks like an ACON rash, but there is such scanty zymosis in the nature of ACON that it is no longer thought of. BELL is not suitable, for in that remedy the rash is shiny or smooth, the typical Sydenham rash. On the other hand you will say PULS has a measly rash, and often associated with a low form of fever, but not so low as the typhoid type, so PULS goes out of your mind. You now think of the remedies that are typical of all zymotic states; the prostration, the aggravation after sleep, general stupor and delirium, and almost at a glance you see LACH, the type of such forms of disease. Its picture comes into your mind speedily. You see another case of scarlet fever where there is a scanty rash, the child before you keeps picking the skin from the lips and nose, lies in a state of pallor and exhaustion, no rash to speak of, urine nearly suppressed; almost in a moment you think of ARUM TRIPH. It is the aspect of things which will call the remedy to mind. In another case you will have all the purple appearance I have spoken of in AIL; horrible foetor, a good deal of sore throat, and the child cannot get water cold enough, wants a stream of water running down the throat all the time; you may safely trust to PHOS. In these low types of sickness there is always something to tell the story, if you will only listen, study and wait long enough. *52*

BELL — The temperature I described among the generals as being so marked, so intense that you will carry it with you for hours after you have touched a BELL case. It differs wholly from the APIS case, which has a rough rash. BELL smooth and shining. APIS wants to be cool, wants to be uncovered, BELL wants to be warm, wants a warm room; APIS has no thirst to speak of; in BELL it is the exception to have no thirst, generally thirsty for water, a little and often. The intense dryness of the mucous membranes and skin. Coldness of the extremities with hot head. In ARUM TRIPHYLLUM there is a constant picking of the mouth, with suppressed or scanty urine; pale surface, only here and there a little rash; the itching of the fingers, toes, nose and lips will lead you to prescribe ARUM. You remember the BAPT case, with that mental state where he is feeling all over the bed "to get the pieces together". On the other hand where there is no rash to speak of, now and then a patch enough to make a diagnosis, or the diagnosis is made from someone else having the disease in the family, the child is swallowing ice water, but vomiting it up when it gets warm in the stomach, who would not give PHOS? So it is at the bedside we pick out the distinguishing things and see that these remedies are not at all alike. *254*

In PUERPERAL FEVER there is a continued oozing of black, offensive blood that will not coagulate; bleeding from every orifice of the body as well as from the uterus. Imagine a woman who is pregnant suffering from typhoid fever. She aborts and a low zymotic state comes on with the symptoms that I have described and with all the appearances as if she would bleed to death after the abortion. The blood will not coagulate and the flow continues. Or in a woman during a typhoid fever menstruation comes on. It is not a true menstrual flow, that is, it does not resemble the ordinary flow, because it is copious, dark and liquid, a continuous oozing with all the grave symptoms described, and especially the besotted countenance, the comatose state, the appearance as if she were intoxicated, lying as one dead. When aroused every muscle trembles; if the tongue is protruded it trembles, and there is inability to articulate. CROT-H may save her life. Would it be possible to think of graver states of sickness than such as are produced by the ophidia? When a physician sees these states coming on he immediately thinks of a class of remedies that can cover such a state, remedies like BAPT, ARS, SEC and the OPHIDIA, and sometimes ARN, PHOS and PYR. ***477***

PHOS AC — Chest complaints are acute; typhoid pneumonia; low forms of fever ending in chest troubles; not unlike PHOS. ***823***

PICRIC ACID

CALAD — He has the most tantalising craving for the opposite sex with no ability to perform coitus. Lascivious ideas. Such men stand on the street corner and feast on the forms of passing girls and their semen dribbles away; a state also found in PICRIC ACID and SELENIUM. ***308***

If a young man cannot keep away from women, he is not so bad off if he will only keep to one, but if he goes from one to many, until he stands upon the street corners and, in his lust, craves the innocent women that go along the street. FL-AC is suitable in that state, like PICRIC ACID and SEPIA, and these medicines are particularly suited to that condition of enfeeblement of the mind and that disorder of the economy that makes man so low, that we have the state described as "low mindedness". ***540***

MANG — No medicine will give you a sicklier face. When persons have bled out and have become waxy and pale the routinist thinks of CHINA, but when there has been no bleeding and this same state is present from breaking down of the blood corpuscles MANG is to be thought of. Chlorosis and pernicious anaemia would make one think of MANG, and also PIC AC and FERRUM. ***724***

PLATINA

CIC — He is suspicious and shuns people; despises others; overestimation of himself. In this it approximates PLAT, but there is no further resemblance between the two remedies. ***434***

When the desire is so violent that it drives her to secret vice the remedies are GELS, GRATIOLA, ORIGANUM, NUX VOMICA, PHOS, PLATINA and ZINC. ***561***

CALC PHOS — Intense sexual excitement (like PLATINA, GRATIOLA, ORIGANUM). ***337***

MANG — "Pain and contraction at the navel." something like PLUMB, although it is not said to draw like a string at the navel, like PLUMB and PLAT. ***725***

STAPH — Crawling etc. in the female

external genitals, COFF, PLAT, PETROL, APIS, TARENT HISP. *947*

Another feature of COFF is that the woman can scarcely wear the napkin during menstruation (PLAT). The parts are in a state of hyperaesthesia. The vagina is hot and sensitive, often preventing coition. *459*

ARG NIT — Here is a striking feature. "Patient cannot lie on the RIGHT side because it brings on so much palpitation." We have plenty of remedies with palpitation worse from lying on the left side, but remedies with palpitation worse lying on the right side are rare (ALUMN, BAD, KALM, KALI NIT, LIL TIG, PLAT, SPONG). This is uncommon, strange, rare and peculiar. *138*

LIL TIG — Pain in the back and down the spine; irritable and sensitive spine with trembling. It competes very closely with PLAT. *703*

PLUMBUM

NAT MUR — a waxy, greasy, shiny skin; other remedies with greasy, shiny skin are PLUMB, THUJA, SELEN. These remedies go deep into the life. Any remedy that can produce such wonderful changes is long acting. *772*

If you will compare LEAD in its poisonous effects on those who work in white lead you will see quite a counterpart of ALUMEN, and you will not be surprised to learn that PLUMBUM and this remedy antidote each other. They do so because they are so similar, they cannot live in the same house. ALUMEN is a great remedy to overcome lead colic in those who work in lead; it removes the susceptibility. *65*

CARBON SULPH — Retraction of navel (PLUMBUM). 392

CROTON TIG — It feels to her as if a string were attached behind the nipple pulling backward, a sharp, drawing, stinging pain that will in some instances keep her walking the floor night and day. Though it is but a little thing it is very important symptom to know with CROTON TIG. We see this drawing as with a string in the eye and in the breast, and also the symptom, very like the PLUMBUM symptom, drawing in the navel upon pressure, somewhat like a string. *481*

MANG — "Pain and contraction at the navel;" something like PLUMB, although it is not said to draw like a string at the navel, like PLUMB and PLAT. *725*

MOSCH — Drawing in at the umbilicus (PLB). *751*

PLAT — Violent cramping pains in the abdomen, drawing pains in the navel as if by a string which causes a sensation of retraction in the abdomen. Pressing bearing down pain in the abdomen. These pains are much like PLUMB, and PLAT has been used as an antidote to PLUMB. Pressing, drawing pains from incareerated flatus. The torpor of the intestinal canal is much like that which is found in PLUMB. *842*

PODOPHYLLUM

A certain class of physicians used to call PODO "vegetable MERCURY". PHYT ought to be called "vegetable MERCURY" because it is so full of symptoms analogous to MERC. *839*

In ARS the head symptoms alternate with physical symptoms. We find in PODO the peculiar feature that the headaches alternate with diarrhoea, and one or the other will be present. In ARN the mental symptoms alternate with uterine symptoms. The uterine symptoms, when observed, look like ARN, but these go away in the night and mental symptoms come on, the mind being heavy, gloomy and cloudy. ***156***

Very often the CINA child will flop over on its belly and get to sleep in that way. If it is turned on the side it wakes up again. While in the mother's arms it will go to sleep with the abdomen resting on the mother's shoulders, but when she puts it on the side in bed it wakes. If you had a child with copious gushing, violently foetid stool ameliorated by lying on the abdomen, and it would have another stool if it were lying any other way, PODO would be the remedy. ***438***

ALOE — "Feeling of weakness in abdomen as if diarrhoea would result." The weakness is sometimes very great, so much so that he has to go to bed with the diarrhoea, and you will often mistake it for PODO, so great is the exhaustion. PODO has great distension, tremendous gushing, much flatulence, great rumbling in the bowel and the trouble comes on at 4 o'clock in the morning. ***60***

Purging is sometimes present in ARS, but generally he does not have much purging such as we find in PODO, PHOS AC. . ***162***

The PHOS AC diarrhoea often ameliorates many of the symptoms and the patient feels better. If the diarrhoea slacks up the patient is worse and on come symptoms of tuberculosis, weakness, prostration, brain-fag. Some patients say they are never comfortable unless they have diarrhoea. PODO is the very opposite. Take the same child; the stool is very copious and runs all over the floor, the mother wonders where it all comes from, but the stool is so OFFENSIVE, a horrible stench, and the patient looks as if dying; mouth and nose drawn, countenance hippocratic, almost unconscious. There is painless stool in both, but PHOS AC has not the great prostration. In PHOS AC the stool is whitish-grey, like dirty white paint; in PODO it is yellow. ***822***

In proportion as there are coldness, blueness and scanty discharges (in cholera) CAMPH is indicated. In proportion as copiousness, blueness and coldness are present, VERAT is indicated. SEC has something of cholera in it. PODO has exhaustive stools; ARS anxious restlessness. ***1010***

In cholera-like states there are other remedies which relate to CUPR and which ought to be considered. PODO has cramps, mainly in the bowels. It has a painless, gushing diarrhoea with vomiting as well, and hence is useful in cholera morbus. The cramps in PODO are violent, they feel to him as if the intestines were being tied in knots. The watery stool is yellow, and if examined after a little while it looks as if corn meal had been stirred into it. The odour is dreadful, smelling like a PODO stool. If you say it smells like stinking meat that only partly describes it; it is not quite cadaveric but it is horribly offensive and penetrating. The stool is gushing, copious, and is accompanied by dreadful exhaustion. "It is a wonder where it all comes from!" says the mother, speaking of the exhaustive diarrhoea in an infant or in a child. The stool runs away gushingly, in prolonged squirts, with a sensation of emptiness, sinking, deathly goneness in the whole abdomen. ***491***

PSORINUM

In certain places it prevails and is taught that anything relating to syphilis must be treated with SYPH; that anything relating to gonorrhoea must be treated with MED, anything psoric must be treated with PSOR, and anything that relates to tuberculosis must be treated with TUB. That will go out of use some day; it is mere isopathy and it is an unsound doctrine. It is not the better idea of Homoeopathy. ***1001***

When well selected remedies act only for a short time, and the symptoms agree, CALC SULPH is one that should be thought of along with SULPH, PSORINUM and TUBERCULINUM. ***348***

TUB may well be considered a species of PSOR. ***1001***

GRAPH — From eruptions, catarrhal discharges, menstrual flow, ulcers, breath and perspiration there is marked offensiveness (like CARBO VEG, PSORINUM, KALI PHOS, KALI ARS). ***553***

ABROT — The emaciation begins IN THE LOWER LIMBS AND GRADUALLY SPREADS UPWARD so the face is last affected; that is the opposite of LYC, NAT MUR and PSOR. ***17***

MANG — Dreadful flushes of heat like PSOR, LACH, SULPH and GRAPH, coming on in women who have been anaemic for some time. ***725***

In old troublesome lingering haemorrhages starting up afresh on the slightest provocation SABINA will stop the gush, the acute stage, but it does not hold, the haemorrhage recurs and then an antipsoric is needed. SULPH is very commonly the remedy, but PSORINUM, though not laid down in the books for haemorrhages, after SULPHUR has exhausted itself, will often follow for this oozing and frequent recurrence. ***899***

CIMIC — There is a terrible mental state that alternates with physical states. It is an overwhelming sadness or gloominess, she is bowed down with sorrow. Sits and mopes in great sadness, like PSOR and PULS. ***31***

SULPH — Before the headache comes on there is a flickering before the eyes, a flickering of colour. Scintillations, stars, saw teeth zig-zags are forewarnings of a headache. These zig-zags come very often with that hungry all-gone feeling in the stomach. We have the same state of affairs, similar appearance of zig-zags and flickerings in both NAT MUR and PSOR before the headache. ***963***

SIL — Headache worse from cold air. PSOR wears a fur cap even in the summer. MAG MUR is better from wrapping up the head, but still wants to be in the air. ***927***

LYC and especially PHOS and PSOR have headaches with great hunger. At or about the beginning of the attack there is a faint all-gone hungry feeling which eating does not satisfy. Such is the nature of PHOS and PSOR when the appetite and the headache are associated. ***706***

PSORINUM leads all others in "hungry headaches", but PSOR wants to eat and cannot get enough. SANG has a hunger, but not for food; aversion at the thought and smell of food. PSOR can eat a wolf meal and so can PHOS. It is a false hunger with the headache in SANG. ***903***

NUX-M has prolonged and inveterate constipation; prolonged urging to stool followed by a soft stool (ALUM, CHINA, PSOR). The stool is difficult but soft. He wonders why he has to urge for a soft stool. ***803***

Nervous hunger in pregnant women, who cannot sleep unless they get up at night and eat crackers, calls for PSOR. ***765***

DULC — In dry, teasing coughs that are winter "colds" that go away in the summer and return in the winter. PSOR has a dry, teasing winter cough. ARS has a winter cough.. ***510***

There is another class of remedies having the stuffing up of the nose not relieved by the discharge. There is a constant desire to blow the nose, yet he gets no relief. This makes me think of LACH, KALI BI, PSOR, NAJA and STICTA. PSORINUM has the copious, watery, bland discharge from the nose, it may be excoriating, it has both. The stuffing up of the nose generally takes place in the open air; he is relieved in a warm, close room and by lying down; has some dyspnoea which is relieved by stretching the arms at right angles to the body. Hay fever is a psoric sickness. PSORINUM given in a single dose will so develop the symptoms that the case will be more clear. The attack is not the best thing to prescribe for. If it is too violent, a short acting remedy may be selected that will mitigate it. NUX VOMICA has a free, easy breathing in the open air, but when he goes into the warm room his nose stuffs up, which also occurs at night, though the water drips on the pillow yet he stuffs up like PULS, BRY and the IODINE preparations, IODIDE OF ARSENIC and CYCLAMEN. ***863***

PTELEA

MAG MUR — Right lobe of liver sore, painful while lying on it and when he turns over to the left he is uncomfortable, as it feels as if the liver dragged over to the left. NAT SULPH often cures that condition, and PTELEA has a somewhat similar condition. ***719***

CARD MAR — The most important of all the liver symptoms. Dragging pain in right hypochondrium when lying on left side; like ARN, MAG-M, NAT-S and PTEL........ ***397***

PULSATILLA

BELL is useful in simply the exaggeration of the whitish mucous flow. Where it has been thick and yellow and then stops suddenly from a cold and a coryza comes on, BELL is warthless. Always bear in mind that you select for suppressed catarrh a medicine that is within the sphere of the symptoms that have been suppressed. Hence the medicine for thick greenish-yellow discharges might be MERC, SULPH or PULS; then you are within the range of medicines capable of restoring the flow and at the same time beginning a curative effect on the state of the tissue, leaving the patient in a much better state. ***243***

When patients are under constitutional remedies, they need caution about certain kinds of food that are known to disagree with their constitutional remedy. A BRYONIA patient is often made sick from eating sauerkraut, from vegetable salads, chicken salad, etc. so that you need not be surprised, after administering a dose of BRY for a constitutional state, to have your patient come in and say that she has been made very ill from eating some one of these things. It is well to caution persons who are under the influence of PULS to avoid the use of fat foods, because very often they will upset the action of the remedy. It is well to say to patients who are under LYC, "See that you do not eat oysters while taking this medicine." These medicines are known to produce states in the stomach inimical to certain kinds of foods; certain remedies have violently inimical relations to acids, lemons etc. If you do not particularly mention the fact, and say, "You must not touch vinegar or lemons; nor take lemon juice while taking this medicine." you will have the remedy spoiled, and then wonder why it is. It is not an uncommon thing for a patient who has been under the influence of RHUS TOX, and has been doing well up to a certain time, after he has taken a bath, to have his symptoms return in the form of a RHUS state; the action of the remedy stops right there. He must of course take a bath, and yet it is true that some constitutional cases under RHUS must stop taking their ordinary bath in order to keep themselves under the influence of RHUS. It is the same with CALCAREA - a bath will often stop the action. *286*

STANNUM — The pain has been likened to the pulling of a string, gradually increasing and gradually letting up. The PULS pain is somewhat similar in its first half; it gradually becomes intense, but suddenly lets up with a snap; comes gradually and stops suddenly. Remember what is said about the BELL pain. It comes suddenly and reaches its intensity at once, where it may remain for hours, but ceases suddenly. *943*

Medicines having much trouble with the veins are often disturbed by hot bathing, weakness after a hot bath, weakness in warm weather, aversion to heat and desire for cold. It is the state of PULS. The PULS veins contract in cold weather and the shrivelling up makes the patient feel better, but the veins fill and become engorged in the warm air and after a hot bath. A tepid bath sometimes makes a PULS patient feel better, but a Turkish bath is generally distressing. Many of the complaints of AESC are of this sort; AESC often feels better in cold air. The symptoms of AESC are often brought out by temperature, especially the little stinging pains. It is characteristic of these superficial pains that they are nearly always ameliorated by heat, while the deeper affections are nearly always ameliorated by cold; Now in PULS, the stinging pains in the scalp and those over the body, here and there, are often ameliorated by the local application of heat, while the patient himself wants to be in the cold; in the same way AESC stinging pains are better from heat, while the patient himself is better from cold, although at times he is aggravated from cold, damp weather in rheumatic and venous conditions. *38*

FL-AC suffocates somewhat like PULS in a warm room. *537*

GRATIOLA — Complaints are better in the open air, but he is chilly in a warm room (like PULSATILLA). *560*

SABINA — The patient is disturbed by heat, is worse in a warm room or from too much clothing. Wants to be in the open air and wants the windows open (PULS). *896*

The mental state of BRY is usually relieved from cool air, he wants the windows open. Anxiety, confusion of mind, fear, etc. are ameliorated from being cool. Sometimes the delirium and the congestive fulness of the head affecting the mind will increase if the room becomes very warm, or from the heat of the stove, from becoming heated, or from warm covers. In children this will be noticed, whereas if the window is thrown up to relieve the stuffiness of the room the child will sleep quietly. Such remedies as BRY, APIS, PULS and many others come in here. *280*

The LIL TIG patient very commonly is a warm blooded patient. She is like the PULS patient; warm blooded, wants a cool room, likes to walk in the open air, except at times when the prolapsus is aggravated by walking. ***700***

The LIL TIG patient suffocates in a crowded room, in the theatre, in church, like APIS, IOD, KALI IOD, LYC and PULS. ***701***

It is in the nature of AESC to have FLYING PAINS all over the body, like PULS and KALI CARB; flitting, sharp, shooting, tearing pains, flying from one part to another; they seem at times to be scarcely more than skin deep. ***37***

CIMIC — You will find that when one set of symptoms becomes extremely severe others have temporarily subsided, and so they change about like PULS. But the symptoms have to be taken collectively to get the image of the patient. ***34***

You take a patient who is hot blooded, who is always suffering from the heat, from too much clothing and too warm a room, especially in the evenings, a patient that is tearful and sad, and may be a blonde. Why, you say, I am trying to describe a PULS patient. Well, yes, anyone can see that. PULS is a hot blooded patient, but after using that remedy for a while you will notice that the patient goes to the other extreme and becomes chilly and wants much clothing; the heat is taken out of the case. SIL is the natural follower of PULS and you would be astonished how often a patient leaving PULS runs toward SIL. SIL goes deeper into the case, it does more curing, and it is the natural chronic of PULS. Other remedies of course follow PULS, but SIL more frequently than any other medicine. Now that is the second step; the patient has gone from a warm into a cool state; the overheated state has been lost and he has gone into SIL, but when SIL has been administered for a while it cures the cold state and removes the chilliness of the patient (remember, however, that SIL at times has something of PULS in it; in some of its complaints it is aggravated from overheating) and the patient under SIL goes back to the warm state again, becomes warm blooded, wants the warm covers thrown off, wants to be lightly covered. Then it is that FL-AC comes in the series. FL-AC follows SIL as naturally as SIL follows PULS. They exist in threes, There are other remedies that exist in threes, but the most common ones you will think of will be SULPH, CALC and LYC; SULPH, SARS and SEP and COLOC, CAUST and STAPH, which often follow each other and rotate in this way. Do not let these facts make you give a routine remedy unless the symptoms agree, but it does help to remember that the remedies are somewhat similar. It is true that PULS, SIL and FL-AC are similar all along the line as to the nature of their symptoms. PULS corresponds to more acute disturbances, or to the earlier stages of chronic disease, the more active or violent operations of chronic disease. It will take off the wire edge of the disease, and it will be followed by some medicine that is complementary to it, always to be determined by the symptoms that arise. There are cases that would be greatly injured by so deeply acting a remedy as SIL if given in the beginning, that is, the suffering would be unnecessary; but if you commence with PULS you can mitigate the case and prepare it to receive SIL, providing the two would appear to be in a plane of agreement. A very serious case had better first receive PULS, and the way being paved by that remedy, follow it up with SIL.... .... ***539***

KALI SULPH — PULSATION ALL OVER THE BODY. Touch aggravates many symptoms. Many symptoms appear ON WAKING. Trembling and quivering. Walking ameliorates. Warm coverings aggravate, warm room aggravates, warm bed aggravates, warm wraps aggravate, bathing aggravates. Complaints dating back to suppressed eruptions. Post-scarlatinal nephritis. One does not need to reflect to perceive that this is PULS somewhat intensified. It takes up the work and finishes as a complement of PULS, unless, as in some instances, the patient becomes a cold and chilly subject and is better during rest, and then SIL will often be found to have what symptoms that remain. It is usual for a patient under a deep acting remedy to go to opposite modalities and hence PULS is so often followed by SIL; but this is not always true. When PULS has acted well for a time and because of opposite modalities SIL does good work for a while and then the patient swings back to the original state, symptoms and modalities, then it is that KALI SULPH is of great usefulness. What occurs is the same as when SULPH, CALC and LYC have rotated in a case too deep to be cured by a single remedy and a series of remedies has been what was required because the symptoms changed in such a manner that the series was homoeopathically suited. Quite unlike PULS, the KALI SULPH patient is easily angered and obstinate and VERY IRRITABLE. Seems to be thinking of something far away. ANXIETY in EVENING in bed, during the night and on waking. Aversion to work, to business and to company (like PULS). ***661***

SIL — In an old chronic case broken down with suffering the symptoms are worse after a bath, he wants warmth, dreads the cold, is always shivering. But when in the neck there is an acute inflammation, the very opposite is present; he suffers from flushes of heat, an irregular flushing fever, cold extremities while the upper part of the body is hot, sweat about the head and neck, sensation of heat and suffocation in a warm room. This will be present in quinsy and abscesses of the glands of the neck, if acute. SIL here shows its relation to PULS. The latter in its chronic manifestations is overburdened with heat, but in acute troubles is chilly. They are reversed as to their acute and chronic states. PULS in the beginning is chilly and sweating. ***930***

We often see one who is subject to quinsy progressing toward the IODINE state. He is always suffering from heat like a PULS patient; at times in the earlier stages, before any organic changes have taken place you may mistake IOD for PULS. But if you watch the patient you will observe the tendency toward emaciation and see that the two remedies soon part company. They are both hot, they are both irritable, they are both full of notions. The PULS patient is far more whimsical, more tearful, has greater sadness and has constant loss of appetite, while the IOD subject wants to eat much. The PULS patient often increases in flesh, although growing increasingly nervous. The IODINE patient becomes thin, has a ravenous hunger, cannot be satisfied, suffers from his hunger; he must eat every few hours and is better from eating. He also has great thirst. ***602***

When SULPH AC has cured the sensitiveness to cold the patient often becomes worse and requires PULS, which is the natural complement and antidote. ***976***

The first effect of OP is to constipate. Let several doses be given, and as the effects of the OP wear off he may have diarrhoea. OP eaters can seldom stop because a diarrhoea comes on. If you should ever have an OP case and diarrhoea comes on PULS will nearly always control it. But there are individuals who reverse that. ***458***

SIL — Begins to sweat as soon as he falls asleep (PULS, CON). ***934***

Compare CIMIC with PULS, SEP, NAT MUR, LIL TIG, CAUL and IGN. ***35***

CIMIC — Sits and mopes in great sadness, like PSOR and PULS. *31*

FL-AC — Reticence and silence; sitting and saying nothing. This reticence is like PULS and often belongs to the insane who will sit in the corner and say nothing all day, never uttering one single word, and hardly answering when spoken to. A patient sits in the corner and says nothing and does nothing, eats when food is offered, is led to her room when the time comes, resists nobody, answers nothing; such a state is found in PULS and is closely allied to FL-AC. *541*

IGN has another thing: "Thinks she has neglected some duty." That is very much like PULS, HELL and HYOS. Only AURUM believes that she has commited a great wrong. *596*

AGAR — Twitching and jerking of the eyes. You will observe this about the AGAR eyes; as the patient looks at you there is a pendulum-like action of the eyes; they go back and forth all the time; they oscillate, though he tries his best to fix his look on you. This stops only during sleep. A few other medicines have cured this symptom - CIC, ARS, SULPH, PULS, but AGAR also produces and cures it. *44*

AURUM MUR is one of the most useful remedies for catarrh of the nose in patients who are sensitive to the warm room. It classes with PULSATILLA and KALI SULPHURICUM, as both of these are better in the open air. *202*

CYCL — Stomach weak. Nausea after eating. Pork diragrees. The stomach symptoms are much like PULS. *496*

NUX-V — Stomach symptoms like PULS; worse in the morning; foul mouth in the morning also like PULS. *807*

NAT SULPH, SANG, PULS and LYC cure this alternation of diarrhoea and constipation. *903*

DULC is a medicine wonderfully useful in diarrhoea, at the close of summer, hot days and cold nights, with changeable stool; diarrhoea of infants. There seems to be no digestion; yellow, slimy stool; yellow-green stool, with undigested stool, frequent stool, blood in the stool and quite a mass of slime, showing a marked catarrhal state. This gets better and worse; this gets better under ordinary remedies; it will often get better from PULS, because PULS symptoms seem to predominate, and sometimes it is relieved by ARN. *504*

APIS — The anus protrudes with stool and seems to remain open, an open anus like PHOS and PULS. *121*

KALI SULPH — Orchitis after suppressed gonorrhoea (PULS). *665*

CLEM — Orchitis with much painful swelling and hardness. Now when the swelling has gone down - perhaps you gave PULS which was the remedy for the time, but it did not finish the case - there is induration of this portion. *447*

Inflammation of the parotid (mumps) changing to testes or mammae is generally cured by CARBO VEG or PULS, but ABROT has cured when these remedies have failed. *17*

ALUM is a suitable remedy again when the woman has a gonorrhoea which has been prolonged by palliation. She has been made comfortable by partly suitable remedies, but it seems that no remedy has been quite deep enough to root out the trouble, for it keeps coming back. In a discharge that keeps returning, better for a little while on PULS, and on this and that and the other thing and even on THUJA, given more especially because it is gonorrhoea than because she is a sick woman. 74

The routine prescriber always thinks of PULS, SEP etc. for bearing down pains in the female, but in a woman with spinal irritation etc. with the dragging down sensation as if the parts would drop into the world, AGAR is the best. *46*

LIL TIG — "Menses scanty, flow only when moving about." This will make you think of PULS, the menses being so scanty and becausse the PULS patient is of similar nervous temperament. PULS has scanty menstruation and relief in the open air. It also has much dragging down in the pelvis, though not so extreme as a rule as in LIL TIG. But there is much in LIL TIG quite different from PULS. *702*

KALI CARB — It is a severe labour, a prolonged labour; the uterus appears to be weak, and the pains are feeble; they are all in the back and do not go to the centre of operation as they should. Now this same kind of a pain may deceive you in taking another form. The pains begin in the back, appear to go to the uterus and then run up the back, which would turn you aside entirely from the KALI CARB pain into a pain that would indicate GELS. Sometimes these pains are so severe that they actually seem to prevent rather than encourage the contractions of the uterus; when the contractions of the uterus cease and the woman screams out and wants her hips rubbed, with pain in each side of the abdomen rather than in the centre, in the region where the broad ligament ought to be, CIMIC will make the pains regular. PULS is the medicine for the absence of marked contraction, in cases inclined to do nothing; in a case that is inactive when the os is sufficiently dilated and the parts relaxed, and the prediction is an easy and simple labour, but the patient does not do anything. It is a state of mildness or inactivity. PULS will very often in 5 minutes cause a very strong contraction of the uterus, sometimes in an almost painless way. *634*

When a mother has lost her infant and it is necessary to dry up the milk, LAC-C and PULS are the best remedies for this purpose, when no symptoms are present. They will do it speedily. The LAC-C patient is imaginative and sensitive to pain and her surroundings, hyperaesthesia and touchiness. PULS will be called for in the PULS constitution. *678*

SQUILLA — has a loose morning cough and a dry evening cough (ALUM, CARBO-VEG, PHOS-AC, SEP, STRAM, PULS). PULS and AQUILLA being strong here, but SQUILLA has a hard cough. The loose morning cough is worse than the dry evening cough. Patient chilly, cannot have the least draft, wants plenty of clothing and is very sensitive to cold; not so in PULS. *941*

MANG has not rapid inflammatory rheumatism, like PULS and BELL, but tenderness of the joints with not much swelling and aggravation from damp weather, like RHOD, RHUS and DULC. *726*

FERRUM — Rending pains in the limbs, dull aching in the limbs. These pass off when moving about quietly and gently, like PULS. *528*

GUAIACUM — Sore, swollen joints. The rheumatic joints are more painful from warmth (LAC-C, LED, PULS) and more comfortable when cool. *562*

PULS and LEDUM are the two principal remedies that want the feet in very cold water. *697*

MEASLES when they come out with that purplish colour very often require SULPH. SULPH is a great remedy in measles. A routinist can do pretty well in this disease with PULS and SULPH, occasionally requiring ACON and EUPH. *960*

The record of AIL in scarlet fever makes it worthy of further study; it ought to be reproved that we may have a fuller understanding of it. "Eruption plentiful, with a bluish tint. Typhoid scarlatina." "Eruption is slow to make its appearance, remains livid." "Body and limbs covered with an irregular patchy eruption of a very livid colour." Here you see but one type of scarlet fever. This low type of fever sometimes needs SULPH or PHOS or BELL or BAPT or LACH. When you see the rash perhaps you will say that looks like an ACON rash, but there is such scanty zymosis in the nature of ACON that it is no longer thought of. BELL is not suitable, for in that remedy the rash is shiny or smooth, the typical Sydenham rash. On the other hand you will say PULS has a measly rash, and often associated with a low form of fever, but not so low as the typhoid type, so PULS goes out of your mind. *52*

With RUMEX, PULSATILLA, SENEGA, ARS and NUX VOM you can patch up the last years of a phthisical patient. You will see ACETIC ACID recommended for the diarrhoea in phthisis. You patch him up year after year. Sometimes ARS is the remedy and it has to be more frequently repeated; sometimes it is LYC, PULS, PYR or ARN. *888*

If to the burning in the chest, the severe pains in the larynx and trachea while talking and cough ending in belching you add heat in the palms and soles, SANG will patch him up and mitigate the trouble. Many such cases get SULPH, but to their destruction. There is a class of remedies that suits these phthisical patients better than SULPH, SIL and GRAPH; such remedies as PULS, SANG, SENECIO GRACILIS and COCCUS CACTI, which will palliate, mitigate his sufferings and may even build him up so that he could take a medium potency of a deep remedy. ... *900*

If STANNUM brings back his old neuralgic pains and you know that he has not a long time to live, and seems to suffer much, PULS is the natural antidote. When a loose, easy cough is turned into one that is violent, dry and racking under STANN and seems to be prolonged, PULS will restore the loose cough. This is not a good action of the remedy; in incurable cases you can get the best results by not going too high..... *944*

When it is a case of septicaemia SULPH goes to the very root of it. When the feet burn, when there is a hungry feeling in the stomach, the night aggravation with sinking and exhaustion, and when throughout the body there is a sensation of steam rising or hot flushes one after another, you must give SULPH. Now, on the other hand, if in such a case, with the hot sweat and other general features, you have one rigor following another in rapid succession, and no end to them, you cannot get out of that case without LYC, which goes as deeply into the case as SULPH. When there is a continuous intermingling of little chillinesses and little quiverings throughout the body and the pulse has lost its proper relationship to the temperature, PYR must be administered. If there is a purplish appearance of the body, cold sweat all over, if there are remittent or intermittent chills, with thirst during the chill and at no other time and the face is red during the chill, you must give FERRUM, as no other remedy looks just like that. When one side of the body is hot and the other side is cold, and you find the woman in a tearful state, trembling with fear, nervous excitement and restlessness, give

PULS, which also has a septic state and is sufficient to overcome the septic condition. *972*

PYROGEN

The tendency to form abscesses is quite strong in CALC SULPH, and is quite similar to PYROGEN. *347*

The symptoms become most troublesome, the gagging and coughing and effort to expectorate because of the thick, ropy mucus are very distressing. He breaks out in a cold sweat, especially on the upper parts of the body. The chest is full of coarse rales from the tough mucus which he cannot expectorate. We think in such a case of remedies like ANT TART, PYR, KALI BICH etc. but SENEGA is just as suitable, especially when there is a great amount of dryness in the throat and larynx, dryness in the throat during sleep and observed on waking, and inability to expectorate the thick, ropy mucus. *915*

You will remove the sore bruised aching all over the body of a consumptive by ARN, and it will suit the cough and gagging and retching and make him sleep. Later PYR may be needed for the aching in the bones and distressing cough. You patch him up year after year. Sometimes ARS is the remedy and it has to be more frequently repeated; sometimes it is LYC, PULS, PYR or ARN. *889*

In PUERPERAL FEVER there is a continued oozing of black, offensive blood that will not coagulate; bleeding from every orifice of the body as well as from the uterus. Imagine a woman who is pregnant suffering from typhoid fever. She aborts and a low zymotic state comes on with the symptoms that I have described and with all the appearances as if she would bleed to death after the abortion. The blood will not coagulate and the flow continues. Or in a woman during a typhoid fever menstruation comes on. It is not a true menstrual flow, that is, it does not resemble the ordinary flow, because it is copious, dark and liquid, a continuous oozing with all the grave symptoms described, and especially the besotted countenance, the comatose state, the appearance as if she were intoxicated, lying as one dead. When aroused every muscle trembles; if the tongue is protruded it trembles, and there is inability to articulate. CROT-H may save her life. Would it be possible to think of graver states of sickness than such as are produced by the ophidia? When a physician sees these states coming on he immediately thinks of a class of remedies that can cover such a state, remedies like BAPT, ARS, SEC and the OPHIDIA, and sometimes ARN, PHOS and PYR. *477*

When it is a case of septicaemia SULPH goes to the very root of it. When the feet burn, when there is a hungry feeling in the stomach, the night aggravation with sinking and exhaustion, and when throughout the body there is a sensation of steam rising or hot flushes one after another, you must give SULPH. Now, on the other hand, if in such a case, with the hot sweat and other general features, you have one rigor following another in rapid succession, and no end to them, you cannot get out of that case without LYC, which goes as deeply into the case as SULPH. When there is a continuous intermingling of little chillinesses and little quiverings throughout the body and the pulse has lost its proper relationship to the temperature, PYR must be administered. 972

RANUNCULUS BULBOSUS

CROTON TIG, RHUS, RANUNCULUS, ANAC and CLEM at times look so alike that I am unable to tell them apart by their eruptions. They are all similar enough to each other to become universal antidotes. The others are all deeper acting than RHUS. The RANUNCULUS, the little buttercup, has cured epithelioma of the lids. It has cured cancerous affections, so we say it goes deep into the tissues. *446*

RHODODENDRON

PETR — Very sensitive to change of weather, like PHOS and RHOD; aggravated before a thunderstorm....................................... *819*

MANG has not rapid inflammatory rheumatism, like PULS and BELL, but tenderness of the joints with not much swelling and aggravation from damp weather, like RHOD, RHUS and DULC. *726*

SIL — Serous cysts in the vagina as large as a pea or an orange, projecting from the vagina or projecting upwards and flattened out in conformation with it. Many little cysts like hickory nuts grouped together. RHOD and SIL have cured these even when there was a paucity of other symptoms........ *933*

RHUS TOX

BELL and ACON have no manifestations of typhoid, even if the symptoms are present. Be sure that the remedy has not only the group of symptoms, but also the nature of the case. The typhoid case has a likeness in BRY or RHUS, but not in BELL. We owe no obedience to man, not even to our parents, after we are old enough to think for ourselves. We owe obedience to truth..... *769*

There are probably several varieties of urethral discharges, but there is one that is sycotic, and when that has been suppressed, it has produced a miasm with soreness in the bottom of the feet, in the knees and particularly through the back and loins and sciatic nerves, in the knees and ankle joints. Sometimes it affects the upper extremities, but particularly the lower. Most violent aggravation when keeping still, like RHUS, great aching that increases so long as he keeps still, he is very often compelled to keep the bed and then he constantly moves and turns. An antisycotic must be selected. While this group of symptoms would be cured by RHUS when the case is not sycotic, when the symptoms come from suppressed gonorrhoea MED or THUJA will cure *997*

It is not an uncommon thing for a patient who has been under the influence of RHUS TOX, and has been doing well up to a certain time, after he has taken a bath, to have his symptoms return in the form of a RHUS state; the action of the remedy stops right there. He must of course take a bath, and yet it is true that some constitutional cases under RHUS must stop taking their ordinary bath in order to keep themselves under the influence of RHUS. It is the same with CALCAREA - a bath will often stop the action. I only speak of these things to impress upon you the importance of feeding and treating your patient in accordance with the remedy; in accordance with principle and not by rule; do not have one list of foods for your patients; do not have a list of things for everybody. There is no such thing in Homoeopathy. *286*

Complaints of ACONITE and PULSATILLA come on from getting the feet wet, and these complaints rise upwards, come on through the feet and go upwards and affect the head. BELL complaints come on from exposure of the head and go downwards; sometimes affect the head, sometimes the chest, sometimes the stomach, sometimes centre in the abdomen, sometimes centre in the uterus and ovaries. RHUS has complaints from getting wet, but the complaints are in the parts that are wet. If he gets the legs wet he will have rheumatism in the legs. *241*

RUMEX is as sensitive to cold, to baths, and chilly surroundings as RHUS but it is aggravated by motion. *888*

KALI IOD — Old gouty subjects who must keep in motion, and must keep in the open air, who are always too warm and cannot endure any degree of warmth in the room, who suffer more from their gouty pains when keeping quiet, those who are fatigued when keeping quiet and can walk and move without fatigue in the open air, especially when it is cold, with enlarged joints, with restlessness, anxiety, nervousness, harshness of the temper and great irritability, alternating with weeping. This relief from motion will make the routinist give RHUS in many instances, but RHUS would have no relation to the case whatever. Remember, RHUS is a cold patient who is always shivering and wants to be by the fire, whose complaints are ameliorated by the heat, he is ameliorated in a warm room and becomes fatigued by continued motion, whereas KALI IOD does not become fatigued from continued motion. *639*

A strong feature of TUB is that its pains and aches are better by motion. I have seen this aching distress in the limbs many times where RHUS has acted temporarily or has failed; where RHUS seemed to be the remedy but was not deep enough to hold its action. Where RHUS was superficially indicated - or the deep action of the disturbance, the deep inheritance - the tired constitution, the chronic nature of the case prevents the action of RHUS, TUB cures these cases. Especially in girls that are book-keepers and shopkeepers, who have inherited phthisical constitutions, who have aches and pains during damp weather, in rainy weather, during a storm, when the weather changes, when the weather becomes cold; then it is that TUB cures when remedies such as RHUS have failed; these patients are better from motion, better by walking; worse during rest. 1006

BRY — Early in the case he was able to keep still, and found that he was better from keeping still, and that the mental state was better from keeping still, and that the anxious restlessness increased the more he moved, until finally a reaction comes and he is obliged to move. You would think, looking at the case superficially, that the patient is better from motion, as in RHUS, but in RHUS you will find that that the patient moves and in moving he gets feeble, and when he sits down the pains come on again. There is the distinction between the two, and yet they look alike if not examined carefully. *279*

The BRYONIA patient is ordinarily relieved from drinking, but if, when overheated, he drinks cold water, all of his rheumatic symptoms are worse, the cough is worse, and the headache is worse. He will have a violent headache after drinking cold water when heated. In RHUS patients complaints are worse from drinking cold water when heated. The headache increases into a throbbing and bursting pain tenfold greater than it was before drinking. *287*

ANAC — The eruptions are like RHUS in many respects; erysipelatous eruptions dark, dusky and of malignant types. It is an antidote to RHUS poisoning. Eruptions all over yellow vasicles are common. Intense itching of eruptios. Skin burns much. It seems closely related in its symptoms to all the RHUS family. *105*

RUTA — Compare RHUS, SEP, SIL and SULPH. RUTA is an antipsoric but not so deep as SIL and SULPH. *892*

You will see IPECAC patients tossing over the bed as much as they do when they need RHUS, turning and tossing and moving the hands and feet, with restlessness. *605*

RUTA — Extreme restlessness like RHUS. So restless he can't keep still; a nervous restlessness. *892*

RHUS sweats on the body; the head is dry. PULS sweats on one side of the head. *928*

TUB — Aching in the bones of the head, with soreness of the periosteum - and these are better for travelling about, like RHUS. Better by motion; worse keeping still. *1007*

SULPH is not so suitable in the cases (erysipelas) that come on with rapidity and great violence, with vesicles and enormous blebs, but it suits those cases in which there is first an appearance of a mottled dusky red spot on the face, and a little distance from it another spot and then another, and these, as it were, all run together, and after a week or so it develops into a sluggish erysipelatous state, and the veins seem to be distended, and he is passing into a state towards unconsciousness. You will be astonished to see what SULPH will do in such a case, which comes slowly as if there were a lack of vitality to develop it, a slow, sluggish erysipelatous inflammation. Whereas if it be ARS, APIS or RHUS-TOX it spreads with rapidity. ARS and APIS burn like fire, and RHUS has blisters upon the erysipelatous patches. *967*

CANTH — Erysipelas of the face, dorsum of the nose, involving the lids. RHUS is more commonly used in this condition, but when it is violent CANTH will often be indicated and preferable to RHUS. RHUS has the blisters and the burning, but in CANTH between your two visits the erysipelas has grown BLACK, it is dusky, a rapid change has taken place, and it looks as if gangrene would set in. Burning in the erysipelatous area and the skin around burns FROM THE TOUCH. In RHUS this is not so. *362*

You do not need to run for the surgeon in every case of appendicitis if you know BRY, RHUS TOX, BELL, ARN and similar remedies. The homoeopathic remedy will cure these cases, and if you know it you need never run after the surgeon except in recurrent attacks. *147*

A man past middle age flooded the bed at night as soon as he went to sleep. The medicines which have this are limited, and he had received them all. I found I must figure it out on another basis. I ascertained that when moving about at his work he had no difficulty in holding the urine, but when he sat down he had to make an effort to control it. At the time this condition developed he had been in Atlantic City and had bathed much in the ocean. Here were the aggravation and amelioration of RHUS, and RHUS cured him. Few would think of BRY in urinary trouble. When he moves the urine dribbles, when he walks it flows. He is relieved only by keeping quiet. BRY is aggravated by motion; RHUS is relieved by motion. *868*

CAUST — Retention of urine from straining of the muscles of the bladder. If the patient is chilled at the time the remedy may be RHUS. RHUS and CAUST are the two great remedies for paralytic weakness of muscles from being overstrained, or from being overstrained and chilled. *403*

HYOS; "Paralysis of the bladder after labour, so that the urine remains in the bladder, with no desire to urinate." The routine remedy for retention of urine after labour is CAUST. CAUST, like RHUS, is a great remedy for the effect of strain upon muscles and parts, and the violent effort that the woman passes through in expelling the child from the womb in many instances leaves all the pelvic muscles tired, relaxed, paralysed. *586*

PETR is of wonderful use and competes with RHUS in eczema of the genitals of either male or female. Eruptions on the scrotum, penis, vulva. RHUS produces violent inflammation of the skin of the genitals in male and female; erysipelatous inflammation; nodules, vesicles and LARGE blebs. PETR produces SMALL vesicles which itch, sting and burn. Herpetic eruptions which tend to become erysipelatous. PETR and RHUS are the most common remedies for eruptions on the scrotum and genitals. *819*

We would think of ALUM when singers break down in the voice from paralysis or from overwork of the voice. The voice lets down and becomes feeble and when taking cold there starts up a peculiar kind of tickling. ALUM is very useful in these cases. ARG MET was the remedy used by earlier homoeopaths for singers and talkers with much trembling and letting down of the voice before the value of ALUM was known in such conditions. Let me tell you something here about RHUS as I may not think of it again. Many old singers, after taking cold, have a weakness left in the voice, which they notice on beginning to sing. On beginning to sing the voice is weak and husky, but after using it a little while it improves. Give RHUS to all these patients, prima donnas, lawyers, preachers etc. They must warm up the voice and then they are alright, but they say "If I go back into the green room for a little while, when I commence to sing again I am worse than ever." The voice is better if they stay in a very hot room and keep it in use. This fits into the general state of RHUS. *76*

NIT-AC — Inflammation of throat, tonsils, uvula and soft palate. Uvula and tonsils oedematous (APIS, RHUS-T). Great swelling of the throat and tonsils. Ulceration of tonsils. *798*

ARUM — Hoarseness and rawness of the throat of public speakers when talking. Of course you would say any voice that is hoarse is aggravated when talking, but it is not always so. The RHUS hoarseness carries with it its characteristic relief from motion, and the use of the voice is motion of the larynx. When the RHUS PATIENT commences to use the voice he finds that he is hoarse, but after using the voice a little it loosens up, becomes freer, or in other words, it is better from motion. This may be so either in acute or chronic hoarseness. Now in ARUM as in PHOS the voice is ameliorated from clearing the vocal cords of a little mucus. It is not so in RHUS TOX, for it is a weakness, a paralysis from cold. It is well known under RHUS that the tendons and muscles that are rheumatic become weak, they are stiff on beginning to move and are ameliorated when they are warmed up; so it is with the voice.... *182*

KALMIA — "Wandering rheumatic pains in the region of the heart". "When articular rheumatism has been treated externally and cardiac symptoms ensue". Rheumatism that goes from the lower to the upper limbs. Not uncommonly you will meet such things. These "rubbers" that go around the streets with a strong liniment and considerable magnetism frequently cause a rheumatism to leave the knee joint and, when it does that, the heart is likely to be the organ that suffers. Then KALMIA, AURUM, BRYONIA, RHUS-TOX, LEDUM, CALC, ABROTANUM and sometimes CACTUS are remedies that prove suitable for such cardiac affections. *670*

It is not an uncommon thing for a man, while going down stairs, to fall backward, his feet slip from under him, and he strikes his back upon one of the steps and undergoes a sharp injury. Some will at once give RHUS TOX; I have known others to give ARN. HYPERICUM is to be given at once to prevent the kind of inflammation that may come from such an injury. Then there will be other tendencies such as drawings and rheumatic symptoms that will come on, calling for RHUS and finally CALC. Old weaknesses of the back with painfulness rising from a seat are often cured by RHUS followed by CALC, but HYPERICUM must first of all take care of the condition of the fibres of the cord and meninges. *591*

RUTA is sometimes overlooked and RHUS-T or ARG NIT given, or other remedies not fully related to the case are given because RUTA is not well known. It falls under a class of complaints that resemble RHUS, in that it is sensitive to cold, aggravated from cold, damp weather; and the complaints are often brought on from straining the part; overstraining and overexertion of parts, but principally confined to parts that are of a tendinous character; aponeurotic fibres; white fibrous tissue; the flexor tendons specially; flexor tendons that are overstrained by exertion. RHUS has something like this, but nothing like what is found in RUTA. *889*

Immediately after a sprain, for the inflammatory state you will most likely need to give ARN; and RHUS will probably follow. But when nodules form in the tendons as a result of the strain RUTA is called for. RUTA is a great remedy for a mere sprain; it has all the soreness and weakness of tendons. ARN, RHUS and CALC are often necessary in a routine way when there is absence of all symptoms except the strain alone. *891*

ALUM SIL — Straining of muscles from lifting, like RHUS TOX......................... *85*

ZINC — Aching in the dorsal, lumbar and sacral regions, better from walking and worse rising from a seat. (In RHUS the aching is in the sacral region and better when walking and coming on while sitting. CALC, RHUS, PHOS, SULPH and SEP have this in the highest degree. ZINC occupies a lower grade in the aggravation when rising from a seat, as do PETR and LEDUM.) *1014*

MED — The rheumatic inflammations are worse from motion, but where swelling is not present these patients act like RHUS patients; they are sensitive to cold, suffer from aching and torturesome pains, and find relief only from motion - like RHUS. *727*

MANG has not rapid inflammatory rheumatism, like PULS and BELL, but tenderness of the joints with not much swelling and aggravation from damp weather, like RHOD, RHUS and DULC. *726*

When the muscles become fatigued from playing fixed exercises, scales etc. for hours at a time, when the player has to do the same things over and over again, RHUS comes in, but it is an acute remedy and only holds for a short time. It is especially a RHUS condition when certain muscles become over-used and the patient takes cold and a weakness sets in; after a cold bath or plunge the muscles take on paresis; getting wet when tired brings on the RHUS state. For the chronic state which follows, PLUMB and sometimes CURARE will be indicated. *845*

Zona is a herpetic formation, great vesicular patches come out upon the body called "shingles", here we should compare THUJA, GRAPH, RHUS-T, KALI HYDR and MEZ. *997*

CLEM is rather singular about the eruptions. One would not think that from so harmless a little shrub so much trouble would come; but there are persons who are just as sensitive to this vine as to RHUS, and it resembles RHUS to a great extent in its manifestations. It produces just as poisonous a condition as RHUS. Here I might speak of several remedies which relate to the RHUS poison. There are many vesicular remedies that look like RHUS and all of them you will have to use more or less in their antidotal relations to each other, but it is well to be sure in a given case which one of them produced the poison. CROTON TIG, RHUS, RANUNCULUS, ANAC and CLEM at times look so alike that I am unable to tell them apart by their eruptions. They are all similar enough to each other to become universal antidotes. The others are all deeper acting than RHUS. The RANUNCULUS, the little buttercup, has cured epithelioma of the lids. It has cured cancerous affections, so we say it goes deep into the tissues. *446*

Another feature to be considered in CROTON TIG is its relation to RHUS. It is an antidote to RHUS. CROTON TIG is closely related in its vesicular eruption to the RHUS family (particularly RHUS TOX), ANAC, SEPIA and ANAGALLIS. The eruptions of CROT TIG very often select as a location the genital organs. RHUS does the same, and when the genital organs are the principal seat of the eruptions in RHUS poisoning CROT TIG will commonly be its antidote; also when the eruptions are most about the eyes and scalp CROT TIG will often furnish an antidote. When the symptoms however confine themselves to the palms of the hands CROT TIG is not the remedy, but it is ANAGALLIS. ANAGALLIS does upon the palms of the hands just what CROT TIG does upon the genitals. If you examine ANAGALLIS you will find that the eruptions will come out and desquamate, and no sooner does the surface look as if it would heal than a new crop comes out. RHUS is similar in that it locates upon the palms of the hands, but RHUS does not repeat itself upon inflamed surfaces. In the CROT TIG eruption there is some burning, but nothing like that of RHUS. The RHUS burning pain in eruptions that are marked is almost like fire. It is worse from the air, and it is better from dipping the part in water as hot as it is possible to endure it. *481*

ARUM — The sneezing is like an ordinary coryza, with repeated chills over the body and aching in the bones as if the bones would break, like NUX, EUPATOR, ARN, RHUS, BRY and ARS that have aching all over during "cold". *180*

RUMEX — In the most violent coryza there is a lack of the febrile symptoms of BRY, RHUS and ACON. It has not the constitutional symptoms, the aching of the limbs, the general soreness, the high fever and thirst. The condition seems to have localised itself.. ***888***

SENEGA. is a sort of cross between BRY and RHUS TOX. The violent symptoms are those of BRY, yet it is worse from rest, unlike BRY. The symptoms of SENEGA are not so much like RHUS TOX, but it has an amelioration like that of RHUS-T, better from motion, the pains being worse when at rest... ***914***

MERC has a well defined dysenteric condition. Slimy, bloody stools with much straining, he feels as if he could never finish, even when no more is passing, a "NEVER-GET-DONE" FEELING. This is the very opposite of NUX and RHUS in DYSENTERY. These are relieved if a little stool is passed, but MERC and SULPH will sit and strain, and all the salts of MERC have the same state.......................................738

MAG CARB — Dry cough before the evening chill, like RHUS TOX.......................... ***716***

TUB — Dry, hacking cough before the evening chill (RHUS-T)...................... ***1005***

ROBINIA

SULPH AC — The sour vomiting is most like ROBINIA... ***978***

RUMEX

PHOS, BELL and RUMEX have soreness of the larynx sore to touch, but the BROM soreness is commonly below the larynx and in the throat pit as well. ***275***

SENEGA — "Dry cough with aphonia; worse in cold air and from walking", is like PHOS and RUMEX. These two remedies cause a cough which commences when he goes out into the air.. ***915***

SQUIL — Dry cough at 11pm.,worse from cold water and cold air (RUMEX). BELL has cough at 11pm.,worse from uncovering, red face, congestion in head. LACH has cough soon after going to sleep, which may be 11pm.. ***942***

RUTA GRAVEOLENS

CINA is useful in sensitive women, sensitive nervous women, who are always worse from using the eyes and get pain in the head from sewing. It is like RUTA in that respect, symptoms of eyestrain......................... ***437***

SPIG has from a mere neuralgic state what RUTA has from eyestrain. Latent errors of vision.. ***937***

MANG — Aching of the eyes on looking at near objects, especially a near light. I have used this medicine often with that symptom and cured when there was pain in the eyes from sewing, reading fine print and doing anything that would concentrate vision. RUTA in nervous, gouty constitutions, when there is pain in the eyes and complaints from sewing and reading fine print for a long time. RUTA is especially a remedy for artists who work with a magnifying glass............ ***723***

SIL — Rheumatism of the soles of the feet. Cannot walk (ANT-CRUD, MED, RUTA). ***934***

SABINA

CYCL; Desires lemonade (NIT AC, BELL, SAB). 496

SABADILLA

The remedies having the dyspnoea are ARSENIC, IODIDE OF ARSENIC, IODINE, KALI HYDR and SABADILLA; these are the ones I have found most frequently indicated in the asthmatic forms of hay fever.. ***864***

SAMBUCUS

SPONG — Wakens at night in great fear, and it is some time before he can rationalise his surroundings (AESC, LYC, SAMB, LACH, PHOS, CARBO VEG). ***938***

SANGUINARIA

STANNUM — The pain sometimes begins with sunrise, increases until noon and gradually diminishes, and ceases with sunset. On the other hand, it may begin at any time, as often at 10am. and increasing for 10 or 20 minutes, then gradually decrease until gone. A few other remedies have these sun headaches. KALM has a similar headache, not so regularly increasing and diminishing, but especially worse at noon. CACT has a sun headache. NAT MUR has never been known to cause it, but has cured it, especially when beginning at 10am., and worse from 2 to 3pm. SANG has headache coming and going with the sun. ***942***

SIL — Headache once a week (GELS, LYC, SANG, SULPH). Headache up through the back of the neck and especially to the right side of the head. Resembles SANG. ***927***

SEPIA is suited to old fashioned bilious headaches. It is better from vomiting; the pain gradually increases, loathing of food; then nausea, vomiting and the patient falls asleep and wakens without the headache. SANG resembles it, is better vomiting, better in a dark room; the direction is different, however. ***920***

The author has cured many violent sick headaches ending in vomiting bile, and cases in the habit of taking calomel with CARD MAR (SANG). ***396***

INFLAMMATION OF THE STOMACH so that he vomits everything he eats. The gout goes to different parts and in this instance it goes to the stomach and then BENZ-AC, ANT-C or SANGUINARIA is likely to be useful. ***258***

SANICULA

AGN — There is a growing weakness of the rectum and constipation, and he presses hard at stool, which often fails and slips back, like SIL, SANIC and THUJA. ***49***

SARSPARILLA

FL-AC follows SIL as naturally as SIL follows PULS. They exist in threes. There are other remedies that exist in threes, but the most common ones you will think of will be SULPH, CALC, LYC; SULPH, SARS, SEP; COLOC, CAUST, STAPH, which often follow each other and rotate in this way. ***539***

LAC-C — Escape of gas from the vagina. The fermentation of mucus and other substances in the bladder causing the escape of gas when urinating is found only under SARS; the urine flows with a loud noise. It is not uncommon for a child to break wind when urinating and the urine passes with a gurgling noise; this is cured by SARS. *677*

SECALE

SARS — Eruptions appear in the spring. All the venous remedies are braced up by winter and go down in the spring, as LACH, SEC and HAMAM. *905*

Now in PULS, the stinging pains of the scalp and those over the body, here and there, are often ameliorated by the local application of heat, while the patient himself wants to be in the cold; in the same way AESC stinging pains are better from heat, while the patient himself is better from cold, although at times he is aggravated from cold, damp weather in rheumatic and venous conditions. Again, in SECALE we see that the little sharp pains that follow the course of the nerves are better from heat, but the patient himself wants to be in the cold air, or to be uncovered, except the spot of pain, which he wants kept warm. We notice the same thing running through CAMPH; during the twinges of pain he wants the windows closed and wants hot applications; but as soon as the pain is over he wants the windows up and desires to be uncovered so that he can breathe. *38*

SARS — Weakness over the whole body; a paralytic feeling. Weakness of the mind and the tissues. All the organs are slowed down weak, sluggish, become congested. Weakness and dilatation of the veins, tendency to form varices in the limbs, varicose ulcers, haemorrhoids, varicose veins of the face and body. SECALE also produces great weakness of tissue, with venous stasis, ulceration and gangrene. But the two remedies, though similar in appearance, differ in regard to heat and cold. *905*

CAMPH — The more violently the patient suffers the sooner he is cold, and when he is cold he must uncover, even in a cold room. This is somewhat like SECALE. In SEC the patient when cold wants to uncover, to be in a cold room, and it also has frenzy, and so there is nothing in what we have yet seen to distinguish SEC and CAMPH. But there is another thing that runs through CAMPH by which a distinction can be made. The coldness, frenzy and heat very often intermingle. When the CAMPH patient is becoming cold, he has spells of heat which come over him. *355*

Prematurely old, a man of 40 looks to be 80, feet swollen, totters about on a staff. NUX will palliate in the early periods of breakdown, but the time comes when he is weak in body and mind and must have such remedies as SARS, LACH, SEC etc. ... *905*

LAUR — When convalescence is attended by weak heart, if there is cold skin and external heat is objectionable, it should be compared with CAMPH, AMM-C and SECALE.. *694*

CANTH — Restlessness causing him to move constantly, a rage and delirium intermingled with amorous frenzy. This kind of mental conduct in CANTH is similar to what will take place in HYOS, PHOS and SEC, a violent delirious state intermingled with sexual ideas and talk. *362*

The convulsions of CUPR spread from the extremities to the centre; ie. the little convulsions, merely cramps, are first felt in the fingers, and then in the hands and later in the chest and whole body. In CIC the little convulsions of the head, eyes and throat spread down the back to the extremities with violent contortions. The convulsions of SEC sometimes begin in the face. ***433***

When a CHINA patient bleeds a little, for instance, in confinement, right in the midst of the bleeding convulsions come on. You would scarcely need to think of any other remedy. SEC is the one other medicine that has this, but the two do not look alike. SEC wants the covers all off and the windows open even in very cold weather. If a draft of air blows on a CHINA patient while in labour, she may go into convulsions. .. ***439***

When the uterus is continually oozing, but every little while the flow increases to a gush, and with every little gush of bright red blood the woman thinks she is going to faint, or if there is gasping, and the quantity of the flow is not sufficient to account for such prostration, nausea, syncope, pallor, IPECAC is the remedy. When with the gushing of bright red blood there is an overwhelming fear of death, ACONITE. If your patient, while going through the confinement, has had a hot head, an uncontrollable thirst for ice cold water, and after the confinement everything has gone on in an orderly way, and the placenta has been delivered, and although you have no reason to expect such haemorrhage, it comes on, PHOS will nearly always be the remedy. In those withered women, lean and slender, who are always suffering from the heat, who want the covers off and want to be cool, who have had a tendency to ooze blood from the uterus, and now have a haemorrhage which is alarming, either with clots or only an oozing of dark liquid blood, you can hardly do without SECALE. ***607***

In the uterine haemorrhage compare SABINA with IPECAC, which has a gush of bright red blood fully as copious as SABINA, but at the beginning of that gush, before it has kept on long enough to produce exhaustion, the face becomes pale, there is nausea and a feeling of faintness, syncope, all out of proportion to the amount of blood lost. MILLEFOLIUM produces a gushing flow, but it has a continuous dribbling day after day, a continuous flow of bright red blood. SECALE looks like SABINA and when it is indicated it should never be given in large quantities. It has the expulsive bearing down, labour-like pains with the expulsion of large clots and copious flow but the flow is dark and offensive and after a short time it becomes thin and watery, leaving a brown stain difficult to wash out; at times tarry, copious and continuous, as if the uterus had no ability to contract. If you observe the cases in which during labour or abortion curde ERGOT had been used, you will notice that the patient has feeble uterine contractions as a resultant condition, and this will be seen during the menses or in the next labor. The symptompsof ERGOT last for years; it is another psora. Large doses may kill the foetus and cause abortion, but she will continue to bleed; the uterus will not contract when she most needs contractions. It produces a paralytic condition, and this is the state we prescribe SECALE for. We seldom prescribe it for its primary effect, but rather for the state of subinvolution, when the uterus retains the secundines. There is a continuous oozing of dark and offensive flow. The picture is more complete if we find that no matter how cool the room is she does not want heat, but wants to be uncovered and she is a lean, shrivelled, scrawny, hungry patient with dusky skin; she never takes on fat; is not robust. It produces varicose of the skin and the skin about the toes becomes dusky, and over the shine bones are dark spots, and she wants to lie with the extremities uncovered. Such patients lose flesh and become shrivelled. ***898***

APOC — "Shreds of pieces of membrane with the fluid blood. Menorrhagia continuing or paroxysmal", that is, a continuous flow until the patient is exhausted. That is like PHOS and IPECAC and SECALE. 128

PULS — Most troublesome cases of prolapsus. It competes with SEP, BELL, NAT MUR, NUX-V and SEC; all of these are remedies with great relaxation, bearing down; some have even cured procidentia. ***870***

Carbuncles that come upon the neck and upon the back begin with a pustule, and then several come, and they are surrounded by little pustules and papules and there is pitting upon pressure. For these carbuncles you will need to study particularly ARS, ANTHR, LACH, SEC and CROT-H. They are the medicines that have in their nature malignancy and manifestation. ***477***

MERC — Paralysis of the lower limbs, and twitching, jerking and quivering of the paralysed parts. ARG NIT, PHOS, SEC, STRAM and MERC have twitching of the muscles of the paralysed limb. ***741***

In cholera characterised by superabundance of cramps, CUPRUM is the simillimum. For those with coldness, blueness and scanty sweat, vomiting and purging, CAMPH is the remedy. These are called "dry cholera", they sink down and die without exhaustive discharges. In proportion as there are coldness blueness and scanty discharges, CAMPH is indicated. In proportion as copiousness, blueness and coldness are present VERAT is indicated. SEC has something of cholera in it. PODO has exhaustive stools; ARS anxious restlessness. ***1010***

CROT-H — In PUERPERAL FEVER there is a continued oozing of black, offensive blood that will not coagulate; bleeding from every orifice of the body as well as from the uterus. Imagine a woman who is pregnant suffering from typhoid fever. She aborts and a low zymotic state comes on with the symptoms that I have described and with all the appearances as if she would bleed to death after the abortion. The blood will not coagulate and the flow continues. Or in a woman during a typhoid fever menstruation comes on. It is not a true menstrual flow, that is, it does not resemble the ordinary flow, because it is copious, dark and liquid, a continuous oozing with all the grave symptoms described, and especially the besotted countenance, the comatose state, the appearance as if she were intoxicated, lying as one dead. When aroused every muscle trembles; if the tongue is protruded it trembles, and there is inability to articulate. CROT-H may save her life. Would it be possible to think of graver states of sickness than such as are produced by the ophidia? When a physician sees these states coming on he immediately thinks of a class of remedies that can cover such a state, remedies like BAPT, ARS, SEC and the OPHIDIA, and sometimes ARN, PHOS and PYR. ***477***

SELENIUM

NAT MUR — In old lingering cases where the skin looks transparent as if the patient would become dropsical, a waxy, greasy, shiny skin; other remedies with greasy, shiny skin are PLUMB, THUJA, SELEN. These remedies go deep into the life. Any remedy that can produce such wonderful changes is long acting. ***772***

CALAD has the most tantalising craving for the opposite sex with no ability to perform coitus. Lascivious ideas. Such men stand on the street corner and feast upon the forms of passing girls and their semen dribbles away; a state also found in PICRIC ACID and SELENIUM. ***308***

SENECIO GRACILIS

A patient much debilitated with bronchial catarrh; susceptible to cold, to every change in weather, from change to damp weather, to every draft, to change of clothing; always taking new "cold". There is burning in the chest behind the sternum; thick, tough, ropy expectoration; spasmodic cough, and every cough ends in belching; eructations of gas, empty eructations. If to the burning in the chest, the severe pains in the larynx and trachea while talking and cough ending in belching you add heat in the palms and soles, SANG will patch him up and mitigate the troubles. Many such cases get SULPH, but to their destruction. There is a class of remedies that suits these phthisical patients better than SULPH, SIL and GRAPH; such remedies as PULS, SANG, SENECIO GRACILIS and COCCUS CACTI, which will palliate, mitigate his sufferings and may even build him up so that he could take a medium potency of a deep remedy. But the deeper remedies ought to be avoided if the vital force is low, if the body is too much damaged to be repaired. Hahnemann warned against the use of PHOS in such cases of deficient vitality. SANG is a surface remedy; it does excellent palliation. *900*

SENEGA

There are a few remedies that have, in such high degree, this coarse rattling in the chest of old people, that it is well to emphasise it. BAR-C is one of them. SENEGA, AMMONIACUM and BARYTA MURIATICA should be compared. When there is coarse rattling in the chest all the time in an old person, an octogenarian, who is pretty comfortable in summer, but miserable all winter from the coarse rattling in the chest, and there are no other symptoms, AMMONIACUM will keep him comfortable. *226*

With RUMEX, PULSATILLA, SENEGA, ARS and NUX VOM you can patch up the last years of a phthisical patient. *888*

SEPIA

ARG NIT, NIT AC and HEPAR will cure the inflammatory stricture before it becomes a complete and permanent fibrinous stricture. It is only very rarely that you will be able with your medicines to cure a stricture after it has taken on permanency, after it is many years old, but as long as the inflammation keeps up there is hope. I remember one very old one that was cured by SEP. I did not at first know of its presence, but prescribed SEP on the symptoms of the case, and the patient came back with great suffering in the urethra and confessed to me that he had had gonorrhoea and had been troubled for years with a stricture. That inflammation was aroused anew and after it ran its course it really left the passage clear and there was never any more trouble with the stricture. That was a very unusual result. I have many times prescribed for patients with the utmost endeavours to do the same thing, and have cured the patient in other respects but the stricture would remain. *576*

FL-AC follows SIL as naturally as SIL follows PULS. They exist in threes. There are other remedies that exist in threes, but the most common ones you will think of will be SULPH, CALC, LYC; SULPH, SARS, SEP; and COLOC, CAUST, STAPH, which often follow each other and rotate in this way. Do not let these facts make you give a routine remedy unless symptoms agree, but it helps to remember that remedies are somewhat similar. ***539***

Compare CIMIC with PULS, SEP, NAT MUR, LIL TIG, CAUL and IGN. ***35***

CROTON TIG is closely related in its vesicular eruption to the RHUS family (particularly RHUS TOX), ANAC, SEPIA and ANAGALLIS. ***481***

RUTA — Compare RHUS, SEP, SIL and SULPH. RUTA is an antipsoric, but not so deep as SIL and SULPH. ***892***

PODO —The body is offensive; offensive sweat; compare SEP, MERC, ALOE, SULPH, MUREX, NUX-V. ***851***

Women needing SULPH are full of HOT FLASHES, such as they are likely to have at the climacteric period, and here it competes with LACH and SEP. SULPH and SEP are suitable in the most violent cases of dysmenorrhoea in girls and even in those of advanced age. ***972***

When a man arrives at the state where he wants to go somewhere else, that he wants to go away from home, that he is disturbed at home, that everything annoys him at home, that he no longer loves his children as he once did, he needs FL-AC. "Feeling of indifference to those he loves best." The SEPIA state is like this, but SEP is more frequently indicated in women. The woman will say, "Doctor, there is one thing I regret very much, and that is, I do not seem to enjoy my children, my home, my companions, my husband and my friends. There is a sort of alienation." Such is the way it is told when it is SEPIA. In the man it is more commonly FL-AC, in the woman more commonly SEPIA, but this need not necessarily be so. SEPIA corresponds more closely to the condition of the uterus and ovaries, and such conditions as the woman alone can have. (Compare CALC.) ***540***

If a young man cannot keep away from women, he is not so bad off if he will only keep to one, but if he goes from one to many, until he stands upon the street corners and, in his lust, craves the innocent women that go along the street. FL-AC is suitable in that state, like PICRIC ACID and SEPIA, and these medicines are particularly suited to that condition of enfeeblement of the mind and that disorder of the economy that makes man so low, that we have the state described as "low mindedness". ***540***

NAT-C — Headache, chilliness and palpitation, better from eating (IGN, SEP, SULPH). ***765***

CARBO VEG — Awful occipital headache, or headache over the eyes, or headache involving the whole head, with pounding like hammers. These states are like KALI BICH, KALI IOD and SEPIA. Many of these headaches are due to stopped catarrhal conditions. ***373***

SIL — Weight in the occiput as if it would be drawn back, with a rush of blood to the head, like CARBO VEG and SEPIA. .. ***927***

SIL — Flushes in the face during the day (SULPH, SEP, LACH). ***934***

Abdomen sunken in NUX, while in CALC and SEP it is engorged. ***808***

ALOE — There is much pain in the hepatic region, burning and heat etc. Mostly in the right hypochondrium you will find distension and fullness. It is pre-eminently a liver medicine. It is not as deep in its action as SULPH. You will often find that ALOE will serve as a palliative, when it will have to be followed by SULPH, SULPH AC, KALI BICH or SEPIA, the medicines that follow

ALOE and are complementary to it, finishing its work. *59*

PULS — Little, mild, gentle, florid, plethoric, warm-blooded girls, who kick the covers off at night and have nocturnal enuresis. Yellow, sallow, sickly girls who lose their urine in their first sleep call for SEP. Losing the urine in the first sleep is looked upon as a strong symptom, but you can figure it out, and hence it is NOT SO. All those cases that have to make an effort to hold the urine during the day lose it in their first sleep; for then the mind is taken off it, and as soon as the mind is taken off it the urine dribbles. CAUST and SEP are remedies looked upon as curing involuntary urination during the first sleep, but I have cured it with many other remedies. *868*

PSOR — Old gleet, painless discharge; the "last drop"; relaxed and cold genitals; a drop of white or yellow pus after a well selected remedy (SEP, SULPH, ALUM). *856*

CARBO AN — There are many uterine troubles, with burning, stinging, smarting, a yellow-brown saddle over the bridge of the nose, something like the mottled yellow saddle of SEP. *370*

CANN SAT — Leucorrhoea in little girls (SEP). *361*

The routine prescriber always thinks of PULS, SEP etc. for bearing-down pains in the female, but in a woman with spinal irritation etc. with the dragging down sensation as if the parts would drop into the world, AGAR is the best. Those slender, nervous, restless women with tingling and creeping must have AGAR. *46*

PULS — Most troublesome cases of prolapsus. It competes with SEP, BELL, NAT MUR, NUX-V and SEC; all of these are remedies with great relaxation, bearing down; some have even cured procidentia. *870*

PODO — Prolapsus of the uterus; prominent are MUREX, SEP, NAT MUR. SEP is better sitting or lying; worse walking. Aversion to coition; hot flushes; constipation with sense of lump in the rectum, or better by stool. MUREX has the following: The only relief is to press on the vulva; not better lying down; she then has pains in the back and hips compelling her to walk; yet this aggravates. *851*

Vomiting of pregnancy really depends upon the constitutional state and the remedy that is to cure must be a constitutional remedy. SULPH, SEP and KALI CARB are among the remedies commonly indicated. Sometimes ARS is needed. Of course, if a pregnant woman has simply disordered her stomach and has vomited bile a few times the remedy might be IPECAC. When a pregnant woman has no constitutional symptoms at all, and upon examining the case you find nothing but the nausea, overwhelming deathly nausea, with continuous vomiting day and night, a single dose of SYMPHORICARPUS RACEMOSA will help. *633*

SPONG — at times, after great dyspnoea, white tough mucus forms in the air passages, difficult to expectorate; it comes up and often has to be swallowed (ARN, CAUST, LACH, KALI-C, KALI-S, NUX-MOSCH, SEP, STAPH). *939*

SQUILLA — has a loose morning cough and a dry evening cough (ALUM, CARBO-VEG, PHOS-AC, SEP, STRAM, PULS). *941*

GELS — There is a sense of weakness and goneness in the region of the heart, and this weakness and goneness often extend into the stomach, involving the whole lower part of the left side of the chest and across the stomach, creating a sensation of hunger, like IGN and SEPIA. *545*

GELS — There are cardiac nervous affections like DIGITALIS, CACTUS and SEPIA. SEPIA is not known to be as great a heart remedy as CACTUS, but it has cured many cases of heart troubles. SEPIA has cured endocarditis, and a remedy that will take hold in endocarditis and root it out must be a deep acting remedy. *545*

In acute endocarditis the principal remedies are SPONG, ABROT, SEP, and KALM. NAJA in valvular diseases................. *941*

SPONGIA — Hypertrophy of the heart (KALM, NAJA, SEP). *939*

DULC — Eruptions upon the scalp that look so much like crusta lactea that DULC has been found a very useful medicine. Extreme soreness, itching, and the itching is not relieved by scratching, and the scratching goes on until bleeding and rawness take place. Eruptions that come out upon the face, upon the forehead, all over the nose, but especially on the cheeks, which become completely covered with these crusts; eczema of infants. Children only a few weeks old break out with these scalp eruptions, and DULC is one of the medicines that you will need to know. It is about as frequently indicated as any of the medicines. SEPIA, ARS, GRAPH, PETR, SULPH and CALC are about equally indicated, but of these, in this climate at least, I think SEP is probably more frequently indicated. 507

CROTON TIG — The eruptions are often about the eyes, on the temples, over the face and on top of the head. The appearance is so nearly like SEPIA that the two very often cannot be distinguished. SEP has the same vesiculation intermingled with pustules, the bleeding and rawness of the surface and the eruption of new crops. SEP is more frequently indicated in this raw, bleeding state of the scalp, in crusta lactea, or the eruption of children than CROTON TIG. *480*

BORAX, SEP, ARS and NAT-C are the remedies most inclined to produce ulceration of the tips and knuckles of the fingers, and also the toes. *763*

ZINC — Aching in the dorsal, lumbar and sacral regions, better from walking and worse rising from a seat. (In RHUS the aching is in the sacral region and better when walking and coming on while sitting. CALC, RHUS, PHOS, SULPH and SEP have this in the highest degree. ZINC occupies a lower grade in the aggravation when rising from a seat, as do PETR and LEDUM.) *1014*

When EUP PER has been apparently indicated by intermittents, and it has not proved of sufficient depth to root out the intermittent, there are two remedies, either of which is likely to follow it, and these are NAT MUR and SEP. These two remedies are very closely related to EUP PER, and take up the work where it leaves off, when the symptoms agree. *513*

SILICA

HEPAR has served a valuable purpose in its ability to establish suppuraiton around foreign bodies if INDICATED BY THE GENERAL SYMPTOMS OF THE PATIENT SIL is another remedy capable of establishing inflammation and suppuration and removes little foreign bodies that cannot be located. A little abscess will form, and the little mite will be discharged. It is well to be reminded that if a bullet were encysted in the lungs it would be well, if the symptoms called for HEPAR or SIL, to consider whether it might not be injurious to give a remedy that would establish suppuration. It might be that the bullet is resting in a vital place, in a network of arteries, and it would be well not to establish suppuration in this vital region. Deposits of a tubercular character are often located in a place that they can be easily suppurated out, and the action of the remedy on them would be the same as a foreign body. Hence it is that HEPAR, after its administration, will very often establish a crop of boils all over the economy because in the skin there are small accumulations of sebaceous matter and these will be suppurated out. SULPHUR also does this, so that it may be well to be careful and not to give SIL or SULPH or HEPAR too often or too high in patients that have encysted tubercle in the lungs. *576*

Another thing running through CALC is a PYAEMIC state, in which there are abscesses in deep muscles. Abscesses deep in the neck, deep in the thigh, in the abdomen. I have seen not only the abscesses go away, but also the pyaemic state which was prior to it. We have but a few medicines that will do it. There is something singular about this. Why does CALC favour the resorption of that fluid and encourage the part to become calcareous? It is more than I am able to explain, but it does it - when the symptoms agree. But SULPH and SIL, when their symptoms agree, hasten suppuration. But CALC has that peculiar action of concentrating and contracting. One may be indicated in one case, the other in the other case. There are times when SIL is indicated and the abscess is in such a dangerous place that if SIL is given the result that naturally belongs to the spreading of that abscess is dangerous; in such an instance the surgeon must be called in to drain the abscess in a safe manner, even when we know that if the abscess were located in a safe place, it would be better for the patient to have the remedy he needs. *314*

STRAM — Pus forms abscesses with excruciating pain (HEPAR, MERC, SIL, SULPH). *950*

CALC FLUOR is similar to SILICA in suppuration. *331*

Persons who are always grinding kaolin and the various products that are used in the manufacture of china and the workers in stone especially require CALC and SIL, but those who work in the coal mines often require SULPH. *960*

PULS is a hot blooded patient but after using that remedy for a while you notice that the patient goes to the other extreme and becomes chilly and wants much clothing; the heat is taken out of the case. SIL is the natural follower of PULS and you would be astonished how often a patient leaving PULS runs toward SIL. SIL goes deeper into the case, it does more curing, and it is the natural chronic of PULS. Other remedies of course follow PULS, but SIL more frequently than any other medicine. When SIL has been administered for a while it cures the cold state and removes the chilliness of the patient (remember, however, that SIL at times has something of PULS in it; in some of its complaints it is aggravated from overheating) and the patient under SIL goes back to the warm state again, becomes warm blooded, wants the warm covers thrown off, wants to be lightly covered. Then it is that FL-AC comes in the series. FL-AC follows SIL as naturally as SIL follows PULS. They exist in threes. It is true that PULS, SIL and FL-AC are similar all along the line as to the nature of their symptoms. There are cases that would be greatly injured by so deeply acting a remedy as SIL if given in the beginning, that is, the suffering would be unnecessary; but if you commence with PULS you can mitigate the case and prepare it to receive SIL, providing the two would appear to be in a plane of agreement. A very serious case had better first receive PULS, and the way paved by that remedy follow it up with SIL. ***539***

KALI SULPH — Walking ameliorates. Warm coverings aggravate, warm room aggravates, warm bed aggravates, warm wraps aggravate, bathing aggravates. Complaints dating back to suppressed eruptions. Post-scarlatinal nephritis. One does not need to reflect to perceive that this is PULS somewhat intensified. It takes up the work and finishes as a complement of PULS, unless, as in some instances, the patient becomes a cold and chilly subject and is better during rest, and then SIL will often be found to have what symptoms that remain. It is usual for a patient under a deep acting remedy to go to opposite modalities and hence PULS is so often followed by SIL; but this is not always true. When PULS has acted well for a time and because of opposite modalities SIL does good work for a while, and then the patient swings back to the original state, symptoms and modalities, then it is that KALI SULPH is of great usefulness. ***661***

It is well known that MERC is not followed well by SIL. SIL does not do useful work when MERC is still acting or has been acting. This is the time that HEPAR becomes an intercurrent remedy. SIL follows well after HEPAR and HEPAR follows well after MERC and thus HEPAR becomes an intercurrent in that series. ***574***

In this relationship to syphilis and mercury HEPAR is closely allied to STAPH, ASAF, NIT-AC, SIL etc. ***575***

STAPH — Nightly bone pains. ASAF, MERC, SIL. ***948***

The relationship between TUB and CALC is very close. They are interchangeable; that is, the one may be indicated for a while, and then the other. They are both deep acting remedies - also SIL is closely related to TUB, on the same plane of action, going deep into the life in a similar way; CALC, TUB, SIL and the SILICATES. ***1003***

TUB is a deep acting constitutional remedy because it is a product of disease from a very deep seated constitutional condition, like SIL and SULPH. ***1001***

Sometimes it is true it will appear to you that ACON is capable of coping with all there is in the disease. But there seems to be a lingering something that holds on, and such medicines as ARN and BELL and IP and BRY do have to come in to finish up the attack - or sometimes SULPH. Very commonly SIL. So we have to study the relations of medicines. ***30***

RUTA — Compare RHUS, SEP, SIL and SULPH. RUTA is an antipsoric, but not so deep as SIL and SULPH. ***892***

CHIN-ARS — Overconscientious about trifles (SIL, THUJA). ***428***

CALC — "Imagines someone is walking beside her." In the proving of SIL that was observed very strongly. It has been observed in PETR. ***317***

SULPH, SIL and SANG have periodic weekly headaches. ARS has a headache every two weeks. Not that these remedies will not cure other headaches, for SANG has also a headache every 3 days. *901*

MAG MUR — The head symptoms are troublesome. SIL will be given in cases where MAG MUR should be given, because the SIL headache is ameliorated from wrapping up the head. MAG MUR has it also. *718*

SIL and KALI CARB are the two principal remedies for the paroxysmal cough that comes on from scratching the auditory canal. I have seen them choke and gag and vomit when they needed KALI CARB after scratching the auditory canal. Spasmodic cough from scratching the auditory canal belongs principally to SIL and KALI CARB, but MANG has cured it. *724*

PSOR — Horribly offensive discharge from the nose; gluey discharge from the nose; offensive like MERC, SIL, CALC-P, HEPAR. *853*

MERC — Purulent formation in the Antrum of Highmore and fistulae from the mouth to the antrum. FL-AC and SIL are more frequently indicated in these fistulae, especially if the bone is involved. *737*

AGN — There is a growing weakness of the rectum and constipation, and he presses hard at stool, which often fails and slips back, like SIL, SANIC and THUJA. *49*

The symptoms usually found in an inflamed breast after confinement are: aching in the back and bone pains; fever and shivering. PHYT has these and falls into the very nature of the case. GRAPH has it only in a limited way. If there is high fever; congestion to the head; throbbing carotids; much redness, and the redness radiates from the nipple, BELL is the remedy. When the entire gland is as heavy as a stone, and hard, and the patient is sensitive to motion and touch, BRY. MERC when the general symptoms agree. HEP and SIL after suppuration is inevitable, especially when the only comfort is obtained from heat. *837*

Constant accumulation of mucus, more forms as soon as he clears it. Hemming all the time and annoying everybody. ARG MET, SIL, SULPH, PHOS and MANG all do that. Each hem brings up a mouthful of mucus. . *726*

HYPERICUM — Slight or irritation inflammation of the lower part of the [spinal] cord; it feels lacerated and sore, and aches and never passes over until the results of the injury right in the spot have been removed. These injuries have been cured after years by CARBO AN, SIL and THUJA, and other remedies as indicated. *591*

PETR — Hands and feet burn, wants the palms and soles out of bed. Do not be too sure of SULPH because the soles burn, or too sure of SIL because the feet sweat. Sweating of single parts. *819*

MAG MUR — Foot sweat is another symptom like SIL. *719*

The remedies having the dyspnoea are ARSENIC, IODIDE OF ARSENIC, IODINE, KALI HYDR and SABADILLA; these are the ones I have found most frequently indicated in the asthmatic forms of hay fever. If the complaint has been developed after being overheated at about that time, you will find that SILICA, PULSATILLA and CARBO VEG must be carefully compared....... *864*

If to the burning in the chest, the severe pains in the larynx and trachea while talking and cough ending in belching, you add heat in the palms and soles, SANG will patch him up and mitigate the troubles. Many such cases get SULPH, but to their destruction. There is a class of remedies that suits these phthisical patients better than SULPH, SIL and GRAPH; such remedies as PULS, SANG, SENECIO GRACILIS and COCCUS CACTI, which will palliate, mitigate his sufferings and may even build him up so that he could take a medium potency of a deep remedy. *900*

Some of our most stubborn cases of intermittent fever will relapse and continue relapsing, even when such remedies as SIL and CALC and the deeper acting remedies have been indicated, have acted well, have broken the fever, and in a few weeks, from exposure to cold, from sitting in a draft, from being fatigued, from mental exertion, from overeating and disordering the stomach this ague has returned. Any of these circumstances will bring back these stubborn cases of intermittent fever when TUB is needed. *1001*

There is that peculiarity that runs through sycosis which gives you a hereditary disease, and asthma corresponds to that disease. Hence it is that SIL is one of the greatest cures for asthma; it does not cure every case, but when SIL corresponds to the symptoms, you will be surprised how quickly it will eradicate it. While IPECAC SPONG and ARS will correspond just as clearly to the supervening symptoms and to everything that you can find about the case, yet what do they do? They palliate; they repress the symptoms, but your asthma is not better off, your patient is not cured *793*

SPONGIA TOSTA

There is that peculiarity that runs through sycosis which gives you a hereditary disease, and asthma corresponds to that disease. Hence it is that SIL is one of the greatest cures for asthma; it does not cure every case, but when SIL corresponds to the symptoms you will be surprised how quickly it will eradicate it. While IPECAC, SPONG and ARS will correspond just as clearly to the supervening symptoms and to everything that you can find about the case, yet what will they do? They palliate; they repress the symptoms; but your asthma is no better off, your patient is not cured. ARS is one of the frequently indicated remedies for the relief of asthma; so also are BRY, IPECAC, SPONG and CARBO-VEG, but they do not cure; although surprisingly at times where a patient is sitting up, covered with a cold sweat, wants to be fanned by somebody on either side of the bed, dyspnoea is so distressing that it seems almost impossible for the patient to live longer, to get another breath, then CARBO VEG comes in and gives immediate relief and the patient will lie down and get a very good night's rest. But what is the result? On comes the asthma again the very next cold. NAT-S goes to the bottom of this kind of a case.............. *793*

ARG NIT — Here is a striking feature. "Patient cannot lie on the RIGHT side because it brings on so much palpitation." We have plenty of remedies with palpitation worse from lying on the left side, but remedies with palpitation worse lying on the right side are rare (ALUMN, BAD, KALM, KALI NIT, LIL TIG, PLAT, SPONG). This is uncommon, strange, rare and peculiar. *138*

STANNUM

CALC — The expectoration is sweetish very often, like PHOS and STANNUM....... *328*

There are two remedies having this weakness of the chest and you cannot easily tell them apart. Weak voice, weak chest; a feeling that it is so difficult to breathe, and so difficult to talk, and so difficult to cough because the muscles of the chest feel so weak. These two medicines are ARG-M and STANNUM. ***135***

AMM-C is a good palliative in the last stages of consumption. A dose of AMM-C when there is great coldness, prostration and weakness in the chest. It is not unlike that sensation of weakness in the chest which is like STANNUM. He can hardly cough out loud, and because of the weakness he cannot expel the mucus, like ANT-T. ***100***

STAPHISAGRIA

You with have a class of cases where the warts have been caused to disappear by calomel, which makes them shrivel up and fall off, such is the old school treatment. Sometimes a patient comes to you with erratic symptoms and you may study for hours over these symptoms and see very little order in them, you will realise that the leading features have been left out and that something is lacking. Someone has applied nitric acid or calomel or something else and driven these figwarts away. These condylomata should not come without having some constitutional basis, these warts have a cause, and that cause seems to be less able to make the patient sick if he has the warts, he feels better when he has the warts. Strange to say, when these warts have been suppressed we get symptoms of NIT AC, THUJA, MERC and STAPH. ***997***

HYPERICUM'S action is upon the nerve sheaths and meninges, with stitching, tearing, rending pains along the nerves, wherever there are injuries. Now, there is another remedy that we want to know.If you have a clear cut or incised wound made with a sharp instrument, or if you have made such an opening with your knife while practising surgery, if you have opened the abdominal cavity and the walls of the abdomen take on an unhealthy look and there are stinging, burning pains STAPHISAGRIA is the remedy that will make granulation come immediately. STAPH is also a wonderfully useful remedy where the sphincter stretchers have been. STAPH is the natural antidote to stretching. When the urethra of a woman has been stretched for stone in the bladder, STAPH is useful. I remember a case of stretching of the urethra; after the operation the patient was in great distress, screaming and crying, bathed in a cold sweat, head hot and body in cold sweat., STAPH was given to her, and in a few minutes she went to sleep. Where coldness, congestion to the head, and rending, tearing pains occur from stretching sphincters, or from tearing, parts for the purpose of operation, death is likely to occur, and STAPH is closely related to that tearing lacerating and stretching of fibres which causes such suffering. ***591***

Syphilitic complaints are commonly worse at night and such anti-syphilitic remedies as ASAFOETIDA, MERCURIUS, STAPHISAGRIA, HEPAR, NIT-AC etc. are all worse at night. ***186***

In this relationship to syphilis and mercury HEPAR is closely allied to STAPH, ASAF, NIT-AC, SIL etc. ***575***

Violent congestive headaches that come on a few hours after an altercation or controversy, or little misunderstandings with somebody that he cannot talk back to will be covered by STAPH, but BRY also has that. STAPH is suited to irritable, violent, nervous, excitable people that get into violent altercations or disputes. If a headache comes on such a patient may need BRY. If in a chronic state a patient says "Doctor, if ever I have a dispute with a man over anything I come down with nervous excitement, sleeplessness, headaches." You do not have to work long on that case, because more than likely STAPH will be suitable. *280*

I have seen syphilitic iritis of the most severe character cured with STAPH, HEPAR, NIT AC, MERC, KALI IOD and many other remedies. The inflammatory process stops at once, there are no adhesions, no deformity and no troubles remaining behind. *638*

CAUST — Dryness of the mouth and throat; rawness of the throat; must swallow constantly on account of a sensation of fullness in the throat, a nervous feeling in the throat. This is often a forerunner of Paralysis. The STAPH patient when excited will keep up a constant swallowing and this goes on until it becomes a source of great annoyance. *401*

MERC — Black teeth and early decay of the teeth in syphilitic children, like STAPH. *737*

When piles are so painful that she breaks out in sweat, becomes anxious, and pulsates all over, on the slightest touch or at stool, NIT AC has been useful. (Compare PAEONIA and STAPH.) *799*

SPONG — at times, after great dyspnoea, white tough mucus forms in the air passages, difficult to expectorate; it comes up and often has to be swallowed (ARN, CAUST, LACH, KALI-C, KALI-S, NUX-MOSCH, SEP, STAPH). *939*

PSOR — Hot flatus, burning the anus; smells of boiled eggs, ARN and STAPH. *855*

STICTA

There is another class of remedies having the stuffing up of the nose not relieved by the discharge. There is a constant desire to blow the nose, yet he gets no relief. This makes me think of LACH, KALI BI, PSOR, NAJA and STICTA. PSORINUM has the copious, watery, bland discharge from the nose, it may be excoriating, it has both. The stuffing up of the nose generally takes place in the open air; he is relieved in a warm, close room and by lying down; has some dyspnoea which is relieved by stretching the arms at right angles to the body. NUX VOMICA has a free, easy breathing in the open air, but when he goes into the warm room his nose stuffs up, which also occurs at night, though the water drips on the pillow yet he stuffs up like PULS, BRY and the IODINE preparations, IODIDE OF ARSENIC and CYCLAMEN. *864*

STRAMONIUM

HYOS — Now to give you some idea as to the grading of this general type of insanity it should be compared with STRAM and BELL. You heard in the lecture on BELL that it is violent, its fever most intense. There is much excitement. In STRAM, when we reach that, you will see that his delirium, his insanity, is expressed in terms of extreme violence. These three run so close together that something can be brought out by associating them together. When considering HYOS in its mental state it is well to realise that it seldom has much fever in its insanity. It has a fever sometimes in the low form, but when HYOS is thought of in relation to the febrile state the intensity of the heat would be in this order: BELL, STRAM, HYOS. Now, BELL is very hot in its mental states, STRAM is most violent and active, murderously violent, is moderately hot in its fever, as a rule. HYOS has a low fever, sometimes none at all with its insanity. When one comes to take into consideration the violence of its delirium, or the maniacal actions, then it changes the order. The order as to violence of conduct would be: STRAM, BELL, HYOS. *582*

"Anxiety on hearing running water. A fear of water." That runs through BELL, HYOS, CANTH and, of course, the nosode HYDROPHOBINUM (LYSSIN). STRAM has the fear of water. STRAM has the fear of anything that might look like water, shining objects, fire, looking glass. Fear of things that have in any manner whatsoever the resemblance to fluids, and hence the sound of fluids. HYDRO-PHOBINUM (LYSSIN) has cured "involuntary urination on hearing running water." It has cured a chronic diarrhoea when that symptom was present. *583*

Our lamented Hering, one of the ablest teachers the world ever had, classes BELL for typhoid fever when the delirium and the heat are somewhat like BELL, but let me tell you just what will take place. When you give BELL for the delirium in typhoid fever - for such a delirium as looks like BELL - you may subdue the delirium, but other manifestations will rise in that fever. You will not subdue the fever, but you will subdue the patient. The patient will be sick longer, will go into a greater state of prostration than if you had let that delirium alone. But STRAMONIUM fits perfectly Hering's description of a case in which he says BELL should be given. **234**

HELLEBORUS — Complete unconsciousness in connection with cerebral congestion, or inflammation which has gone on to hydrosephalus, cerebro-spinal meningitis, or inflammation of the brain, with stupefaction. Even early in the disease HELLEBORE lacks the wildness and acute delirium found in STRAMONIUM and BELLADONNA. It is passive. *566*

In the brain complaints of STRAM the forehead wrinkles and in the chest complaints of LYC the forehead wrinkles, and their wrinkles are somewhat alike. You go to a semiconscious patient suffering from cerebral congestion and watch him; he is wild, the eyes are glassy, the forehead wrinkled and the tendency is to activity of the mind. That is not LYC, but STRAM. By close observation these practical things will lead you to distinguish almost instantaneously between STRAM in its head troubles and LYC in the advanced stage of pneumonia. *709*

SQUILLA has a loose morning cough and a dry evening cough (ALUM, CARBO-VEG, PHOS-AC, SEP, STRAM, PULS). *941*

ARG NIT, PHOS, SEC, STRAM and MERC have twitching of the muscles of the paralysed limbs. *941*

STRONTIUM CARBONICUM

After a surgical operation, where there has been much cutting, a great state of prostration, coldness, oozing of blood, almost cold breath, of course the Materia Medica man, if there is one around, will say, "Why, give him CARBO VEG, of course." Yes, you will, but it will not help him. It may disappoint you. But if you are a surgeon, know your surgical therapeutics better than a Materia Medica man, you will say, "No, STRONTIUM CARB is what I want!" It relieves that congestion all over the body; he gets warm and has a comfortable night. STRONTIUM CARB is the CARBO VEG of the surgeon. **592**

STRYCHNINE

CIC — Great agitation; child grasps at one's clothing in a frightened manner. This is likely to occur before the convulsion, great horror in the countenance, yet he has no recollection of the horror when he comes out of the convulsion. That state of anxiety and fear comes after the attack has begun, though the convulsions have not yet come on. Between the convulsions the patient is mild, gentle, placid and yielding, which distinguishes it from NUX VOM and STRYCHNINE convulsions. The NUX convulsions are all over the body and are worse from touch and draft, blueness and purple colour of the body, but between the convulsions the patient is very irritable. **434**

SULPHURIC ACID

"Aphthae in mouth and on tongue." "Aphthae on tongue and inside of cheek." This alone is not an indication for BORAX, although BORAX is one of the medicines when the mouth is so sore that the child lets loose its hold of the nipple or bottle. Many prescribers give BORAX on that indication alone but the constitutional state ought to be hunted up, so that there may be constitutional foundation for the remedy. SULPH AC is more frequently indicated. **268**

A marked feature of the KALI BICH throat is its oedematous uvula. This symptom is also found in APIS, KALI-I, LACH, MUR-AC, NIT-AC, PHOS, SULPH-AC and TAB. **620**

SULPH — Often with the coryza the discharge excoriates the lips and the nose. At times the fluid that remains in the nose smarts like fire, and when it comes in contact with the child's lip it burns, so acrid is it; almost like the condition under SULPH AC, so red will be the parts that are touched by it. **953**

SULPHUR

When well selected remedies act only a short time, and the symptoms agree, CALC SULPH is one that should be thought of along with SULPH, PSORINUM and TUBERCULINUM. **348**

At the present day it is fashionable to use the cautery, to make local applications to stop leucorrhoea and other discharges and to heal up ulcers. Now when these external conditions go there is an anaemic state established in the economy, the patient becomes waxy and pallid, sickly looking, and these catarrhal discharges come on as a relief because of the suppression of some other condition. For instance, since the suppression of a leucorrhoea the woman has had a thick bloody or watery discharge from the nose. ARS is frequently suitable to the constitution when an ulcer has been dried up by salves, or an old ear discharge has been stopped by the outward application of powders. The doctor thinks he has done a clever thing in stopping such discharges, but he has only succeeded in damming up the secretions which are really a relief to the patient. Such medicines as SULPH, CALC and ARS are suitable for the catarrhal discharges that come from these suppressions in broken down constitutions.... **159**

The catarrhal state wherein BELL is useful is simply the exaggeration of the whitish mucous flow. Where has been thick and yellow and then stops suddenly from a cold and a coryza comes on, BELL is worthless. Always bear in mind that you select for suppressed catarrh a medicine that is within the sphere of the symptoms that have been suppressed. Hence the medicine for thick greenish-yellow discharges might be MERC, SULPH or PULS; then you are within the range of medicines capable of restoring the flow and at the same time beginning a curative effect on the state of the tissue, leaving the patient in a much better state. ***243***

Patients who have a tendency to phthisis are subject to abscesses about the region of the rectum that break inside or out and form complete or incomplete openings. These seem to take the place of what would otherwise come, and if healed by operation or other external means, the tendency is to end in chest trouble, either in the form of a fixed catarrh or tubercular infiltrations. SIL is one of the remedies that turns the constitution into order and in one to five years the opening ceases to be necessary and it will heal. Surgeons heal it up at once and for a time the patient is comfortable, but in a few years he breaks down. CAUST, BERB, CALC, CALC PHOS, GRAPH, SULPH etc. are suitable in such cases. SIL here follows THUJ well. ***932***

OP — The sluggishness and painlessness are most striking. The inaction is shown in the lack of reaction to the properly selected homoeopathic remedy. It competes here with SULPH. On studying the case you may find many OP symptoms, and when given thus indicated, it rouses the system out of its sluggishness and causes reaction. ***810***

In old cases of suppressed malaria, SEPIA brings back the chill, but its most useful sphere is after a bad selection of the remedy and the case becomes confused. In a case confused by remedies think of CALC, ARS, SULPH, SEP and IPECAC. Never give CHINA or NAT MUR for irregular symptoms and stages. ***925***

The author has many times observed that gummata in throat and anus will take on destructive ulceration in old broken down cases after SULPH has been given and that SYPH will restrain it and establish repair. SULPH often produces prolonged aggravation when there are many tissue changes in advanced stages of syphilis. Such changes are most likely gummata. The effort of SULPH is to remove the results of disease, which the patient cannot stand. It often causes suspicion of latent syphilis when such aggravations are very severe after SULPH high. SULPH low will not be followed by such results. After such prolonged aggravation SYPH should be considered. Latent syphilis often exists where it is least expected. ***987***

Much vertigo Aphasia. In some of these cases of brain syphilis SULPH and CAUST have caused prolonged suffering and weakness. SYPH will act favourably. ***987***

GUAIACUM — In psoric cases complicated with syphilis and mercury and other violent drugs we find use for this a most neglected remedy. It is closely related to CAUSTICUM, SULPHUR and TUBERCULINUM. ***562***

GRAPH is as broad and deep as SULPH, showing the great similarity to this great remedy in chronic cases. ***554***

TUB is a deep acting constitutional remedy because it is a product of disease from a very deep seated constitutional condition, like SIL and SULPH. ***1001***

MANG — Irritability and low-spirited, like SULPH and GRAPH. It is similar to ARG MET, PHOS, GRAPH and SULPH in its underlying tendency to tuberculosis. .. ***723***

ALOE is more nearly related to SULPH in its venous condition than to any other remedy. If you study together, side by side, ALOE, KALI BICH and SULPH you will be astonished at their wonderful relation to the stomach and bowels. ***58***

CALC has burning in the vertex, and this is often present with coldness of the forehead, or the whole head may feel cold except for a burning spot on the vertex. CALC will again have cold head and icy cold feet when walking in cold air, or in very cold weather; but as soon as the feet get warm, they go to the other extreme and burn so that he puts them out of bed. This has often led inexperienced practitioners to prescribe SULPH because that is a keynote of SULPH. All keynote prescribers give SULPH whenever the patient puts the feet out of bed, but a number of remedies have burning feet, hot feet, so we are not limited to SULPH. ***321***

NUX is closely related to SULPH and often antidotes the overaction of SULPH. It seldom goes to the bottom and antidotes the constitutional action of SULPH, but it will remove its exaggerated action, its superficial action. ***808***

To appreciate that late development, and to see it in BARYTA CARB from all of its symptoms and peculiar features, leads to such remedies as GRAPH, SULPH and CALC, but nothing compared to this remedy. . ***221***

STRAM — High grade inflammation which it carries to the finish. Pus forms abscesses with excruciating pain (HEPAR, MERC, SIL, SULPH). ***950***

Another thing running through CALC is a PYAEMIC state, in which there are abscesses in deep muscles. Abscesses deep in the neck, deep in the thigh, deep in the abdomen. You will be astonished to learn that CALC will take care of the abscess (when symptoms agree) and it will not break. I have many times seen an abscess disappear when fluctuation was most positive. I have seen those abscesses disappear when pus was shown to be present by the needle; I have seen not only the abscesses go away, but also the pyaemic state which was prior to it. We have but a few medicines that will do it. There is something singular about this. Why does CALC favour the resorption of that fluid and encourage the part to become calcareous? It is more than I am able to explain, but it does it - when the symptoms agree. But SULPH and SIL, when their symptoms agree, hasten suppuration. But CALC has that peculiar action of concentrating and contracting. One may be indicated in one case, the other in the other case. There are times when SIL is indicated and the abscess is in such a dangerous place that if SIL is given the result that naturally belongs to the spreading of that abscess is dangerous; in such an instance the surgeon must be called in to drain the abscess in a safe manner, even when we know that if that abscess were located in a safe place, it would be better for the patient to have the remedy he needs. ***314***

TUB — Complaints worse standing; must move. This is as marked in this remedy as in SULPH. ***1007***

BARYTA MUR — Dread of bathing, like SULPH. ***229***

PSOR is closely allied to SULPH. The patient dreads to be washed. The skin over the body, especially the face, looks filthy, though it has been well washed. ***851***

PULS — Much clothing and covering aggravate. Often he cannot wear flannels or woollen clothing because they irritate the skin, causing itching and eruptions like SULPH, and this is not surprising, since SULPH and PULS are antidotes. There is no remedy like PULS to antidote SULPH when it has been used every spring to "cleanse the blood". Some people use SULPH until the skin becomes red, hot, easily irritated and aggravated by clothing. PULS is the antidote. Old cases of psoriasis; little flat, brownish patches about the size of the thumbnail, which itch tremendously, in old SULPH patients are covered by PULS. ***858***

NAT-P — The body smells sour (like HEPAR, SULPH, LYC)...................................... ***773***

PODO — The body is offensive; offensive sweat; compare SEP, MERC, ALOE, SULPH, MUREX, NUX-V. ***851***

MANG — Dreadful flushes of heat like PSOR, LACH, SULPH and GRAPH, coming on in women who have been anaemic for some time. ***725***

NAT-C — Headache, chilliness and palpitation, better from eating (IGN, SEP, SULPH). ***765***

You will see one suffering from the AESC backache, on attempting to rise from sitting, make many painful efforts before he finally succeeds. This is found in SULPH, PETR and is also cured by AGAR. ***39***

SIL — Headache once a week (GELS, LYC, SANG, SULPH).................................. ***927***

PSOR — Increased growth of hair on the face; a fuzz (NAT-M, SULPH, CALC). ***856***

PULS — Eyes are ameliorated by washing in warm water, or tepid water; even cold water feels good to the eyes. The SULPH patient is made worse by bathing; the eyes smart, burn and become increasingly red after washing in water. ***860***

AGAR — Twitching and jerking of the eyes. You will observe this about the AGAR eyes; as the patient looks at you there is a pendulum-like action of the eyes; they go back and forth all the time; they oscillate, though he tries his best to fix his look on you. This stops only during sleep. A few other medicines have cured this eye symptom - CIC, ARS, SULPH, PULS, but AGAR also produces and cures it. ***44***

SIL — The parotids enlarge from every cold and get hard (BAR-C, CALC, SULPH).... .... ***928***

ALUM is not a medicine that would be selected for a cold settling in the throat, not a remedy for acute sore throat, but it is a deep acting anti-psoric and acts for months. Its greatest use is as a remedy for taking cold. In this respect it is like SIL, GRAPH and SULPH. ***72***

CARBO AN — The glands of the throat and axillae grow purple and indurated with no tendency to soften. Some of these medicines, after infiltrating a gland, will hurry up the inflammatory action, produce sloughing, rapid breaking down, with pus - like HEPAR, MERC and SULPH. ***368***

MANG — Constant accumulation of mucus (in larynx), more forms as soon as he clears it. Hemming all the time and annoying everybody. ARG MET, SIL, SULPH, PHOS all do that. Each hem brings up a mouthful of mucus. ***726***

DIG — "Loss of appetite and violent thirst." Most doctors give SULPH when the patient drinks much and eats little. ***501***

PHOS — Awful sinking, gone feeling in the stomach. This sometimes comes at 11 o'clock, like SULPH. ***830***

ALOE is not as deep in its action as SULPH. You will often find that ALOE will serve as a palliative, when it will have to be followed by SULPH, SULPH AC, KALI BICH or SEPIA, the medicines that follow ALOE and are complementary to it, finishing its work. *59*

In PSOR we find the haste of SULPH, the flatulence of OLEAN and ALOE, and difficulty of expelling a soft stool like ALUM, CHINA and NUX-M. *855*

SIL was one of the greatest remedies for the chronic diarrhoea in the soldiers of our Civil War. It cured a fair percentage of those sick from sleeping on damp ground, eating all sorts of food until the stomach and bowels were prostrated, from long marches, from going into the South from the cold North, from becoming overheated. It is like SULPH in these symptoms. *932*

AGAR — Sensation as if the rectum would burst, even after stool (MERC, SULPH). *45*

ALOE is like SULPH again, in that it drives him out of bed in the early morning with diarrhoea and there are times when he puts the feet out from underneath the covers to cool them off; the soles of the feet burn and he uncovers them. *60*

Like SULPH, CALC SULPH has cured morning diarrhoea. *352*

GUAIACUM — Morning diarrhoea (SULPH). *563*

KALI BICH also has a morning diarrhoea like SULPH. *621*

LIL TIG has a very urgent diarrhoea driving out of bed in the morning; he must make great haste. You may get this confused with SULPH, because LIL TIG has great heat in the head, emptiness in the stomach and great burning of the palms and soles. *701*

KALI-BICH — Diarrhoea after beer, like ALOE, CHINA, GAMBOGIA, LYC, MUR-AC and SULPH. *621*

CUPR is especially suitable to young men who have become PREMATURELY OLD FROM VICES, from strong drink, from late nights and various abuses, and these cramps are not unlikely to occur in such subjects. CUPR and GRAPH are the two remedies for cramps coming under these circumstances, but whereas CUPR is said to produce cramps that prevent the act (of coition), GRAPH is said to bring on the cramps during the act. These two remedies however, compete closely with each other, and hence if GRAPH corresponds to the constitution of the patient, it should be given, and the same in regard to CUPR. SULPH also has cured this state. *489*

PSOR — Old gleet, painless discharge; the "last drop"; relaxed and cold genitals; a drop of white or yellow pus after a well selected remedy (SEP, SULPH, ALUM). *856*

Now, in these thick passive discharges (of gonorrhoea) that are long-standing, old cases, we are very much troubled to find remedies. These old stubborn cases that still remain yellow and still remain thick. They will not yield to ordinary remedies and they come under a peculiar class of remedies, ARG-M, ALUM, ALUMN, SULPH. Ones not usually thought of in the early period, but the general constitutional state of the patient forms his symptoms. *133*

The condition (vomiting of pregnancy) really depends upon the constitutional state and the remedy that is to cure must be a constitutional remedy. SULPH, SEP and KALI CARB are among the remedies commonly indicated. Sometimes ARS is needed. Of course, if a pregnant woman has simply disordered her stomach and has vomited bile a few times the remedy might be IPECAC. When a pregnant woman has no constitutional symptoms at all, and upon examining the case you find nothing but the nausea, overwhelming deathly nausea, with continuous vomiting day and night, a single dose of SYMPHORICARPUS RACEMOSA will help. *633*

ALUM — Induration here and there so that it favours lupus and epithelioma in one who is subject to these swellings and eruptions. ALUMINA and ALUMEN, like ARS, LACH, SULPH and CON are medicines that relate to these troubles. Some of these have made brilliant cures where there is infiltration. *71*

KALI SIL has cured most stubborn cases of eczema where SULPH and GRAPH seemed indicated and failed. *660*

TARENT-H has cured a dry, itching eczema of the extremities and other parts of the skin after ARS and SULPH have failed. *994*

DULC — Eruptions upon the scalp that look so much like crusta lactea that DULC has been found a very useful medicine. Extreme soreness, itching, and the itching is not relieved by scratching, and the scratching goes on until bleeding and rawness take place. Eruptions that come out upon the face, upon the forehead, all over the nose, but especially on the cheeks, which become completely covered with these crusts; eczema of infants. Children only a few weeks old break out with these scalp eruptions, and DULC is one of the medicines that you will need to know. It is about as frequently indicated as any of the medicines SEPIA, ARS, GRAPH, DULC, PETR, SULPH and CALC. *507*

CHAM — "Burning of the soles at night; puts the feet out of bed." All the routine prescribers, whenever the patient is known to put the feet out of bed, give SULPH, yet there is a large list of remedies with hot feet, burning soles and all of them will put the feet out of bed, of course, to cool them off. There is no reason why they should all get SULPH. *423*

Like SULPH, NAT-S has burning of the soles of the feet at night, and the burning extends to the knees; burning from the knees down. It has also, like SULPH, great burning in the top of the head. *793*

PETR — Eruptions disappear of themselves or are suppressed. Hands and feet burn, wants the palms and soles out of bed. Do not be too sure of SULPH because the soles burn, or too sure of SIL because the feet sweat. Study closely the skin symptoms and compare with GRAPH and SULPH. *819*

ZINC — Aching in the dorsal, lumbar and sacral regions, better from walking and worse rising from a seat. (In RHUS the aching is in the sacral region and better when walking and coming on while sitting. CALC, RHUS, PHOS, SULPH and SEP have this in the highest degree. ZINC occupies a lower grade in the aggravation when rising from a seat, as do PETR and LEDUM.) *1014*

BERB — Finally the gouty deposits become prominent in the fingers, and after the gout has determined itself then we have sore fingers; but these correspond more particularly to LEDUM, SULPH, AESC and LYC where the disease has become marked and located in the joints. *261*

KALI CARB, SULPH, CARBO VEG and DROSERA are perhaps more frequently indicated than other medicines in such coughs as follow pneumonia or measles. *635*

SIL — Slow recovery after pneumonia (LYC, SULPH, PHOS, CALC). Flushes, rattling in the chest. Flushes in the face during the day (SULPH, SEP, LACH), rattling in the chest like ANT TART, flushes like SULPH and LYC. *934*

"Doctor, I have never been quite well since I had pneumonia." The catarrhal state has settled in his chest and there is a chronic tendency to take cold. These cases are threatening to go into phthisis and will hardly be likely to recover without KALI CARB. In this tendency for catarrhal states to locate in the chest KALI CARB should be thought of as well as PHOS, LYC and SULPH. *627*

Deposits of a tubercular character are often located in a place that they can be easily suppurated out, and the action of the remedy on them would be the same as a foreign body. Hence it is that HEPAR, after its administration, will frequently establish a crop of boils all over the economy because in the skin there are small accumulations of sebaceous matter and these will be suppurated out. SULPHUR also does this, so that it may be well to be careful and not to give SIL or SULPH or HEPAR too often or too high in patients that have encysted tubercle in the lung. *577*

Many excellent homoeopathic physicians have said to me, "I do not agree with you as to the danger of SULPH in phthisical cases. I have cured cases of phthisis with SULPH." So have I, many of them. But I did not refer to curable cases, but to those cases that are well developed and have grave symptoms. It is well to know all the elements in the case; then if you have administered a remedy and killed your patient, you know at least what you have done. It is better to know what you have done if you have killed your patient than to be ignorant of it and go on and kill some more in the same way. *577*

Do not be afraid to give the anti-psoric remedies when there is a history of tuberculosis in the family, but be careful when the patient is so far advanced with tuberculosis that there are cavities in the lung, or latent tubercles, or encysted caseous tubercles. Your anti-psorics might rouse him into a dangerous condition. Do not suppose however that it is dangerous to give SULPHUR because one's father and mother have died of tuberculosis. SULPHUR may be just the remedy to prevent the child from following the father and mother. *635*

RUMEX — In the morning hurried to stool like SULPH. It is common for phthisical cases to have a morning diarrhoea, and many of them look like SULPH. When the morning diarrhoea is gushing, RUMEX will palliate; it will allay the extreme sensibility fo the lungs, will ward of the sensitiveness of cold and will patch him up. RUMEX is not so deep as SULPH, but it is an anti-psoric. It is limited however to the early stages, will carry a chronic case so far, but it will require to be followed by another anti-psoric. CALC follows it well. "Serious attack of diarrhoea in an old man of 70, after failure of SULPH." The SULPH patient with a cough, especially in phthisis, commonly wants cool air, cooling things; though the stomach symptoms are sometimes ameliorated from hot drinks, yet he wants cool, refreshing air. *887*

If to the burning in the chest, the severe pains in the larynx and trachea while talking and cough ending in belching you add heat in the palms and soles, SANG will patch him up and mitigate the troubles. Many such cases get SULPH, but to their destruction. There is a class of remedies that suits these phthisical patients better than SULPH, SIL and GRAPH; such remedies as PULS, SANG, SENECIO GRACILIS and COCCUS CACTI, which will palliate, mitigate his sufferings and may even build him up so that he could take a medium potency of a deep remedy. ... *900*

NUX and RHUS in DYSENTERY are relieved if a little stool is passed, but MERC and SULPH will sit and strain, and all the salts of MERC have the same state.... ***738***

AIL — "Eruption plentiful, of a bluish tint. Typhoid scarlatina." "Eruption is slow to make its appearance, remains livid." "Body and limbs covered with an irregular patchy eruption of a very livid colour." Here you see but one type of scarlet fever. This low type of fever sometimes needs SULPH or PHOS or BELL or BAPT or LACH. ***52***

SYMPHORICARPUS RACEMOSA

Vomiting of pregnancy really depends upon the constitutional state and the remedy that is to cure must be a constitutional remedy. SULPH, SEP and KALI CARB are among the remedies commonly indicated. Sometimes ARS is needed. Of course, if a pregnant woman has simply disordered her stomach and has vomited bile a few times the remedy might be IPECAC. When a pregnant woman has no constitutional symptoms at all, and upon examining the case you find nothing but the nausea, overwhelming deathly nausea, with continuous vomiting day and night, a single dose of SYMPHORICARPUS RACEMOSA will help. ***633***

SYPHILINUM

In certain places it prevails and is taught that anything relating to syphilis must be treated with SYPH; that anything relating to gonorrhoea must be treated with MED, anything psoric must be treated with PSOR, and anything that relates to tuberculosis must be treated with TUB. That will go out of use some day; it is mere isopathy and it is an unsound doctrine. It is not the better idea of Homoeopathy. ***1001***

TABACUM

The most common form of sea-sickness I have found to be the following: awful deathly nausea, great pallor, cold body, profuse sweat and exhaustion, ameliorated by fanning, by the open air, by closing the eyes, by quiet and darkness, and aggravated by warmth. TAB is generally the remedy for such cases. ***818***

CUPR — Convulsions where a limb will first flex and then extend - an alternation of flexion and extension. In a child you will see the leg all at once shoot out with great violence, then up against the abdomen again with great violence, and then again shoot out. It is hard to find another remedy that has that. TAB has it, but not many others. ***493***

A marked feature of the KALI BICH throat is its oedematous uvula. This symptom is also found in APIS, KALI-I, LACH, MUR-AC, NIT-AC, PHOS, SULPH-AC and TAB. ***620***

TARENTULA CUBENSIS

PYR — VIOLENT BURNING IN AN ABSCESS (ARS, ANTHR, TARENT-C).... ***872***

You will remove the sore bruised aching all over the body of a consumptive by ARN, and it will suit the cough and gagging and retching and make him sleep. Later PYR may be needed for the aching in the bones and distressing cough. You patch him up year after year. Sometimes ARS is the remedy and it has to be more frequently repeated; sometimes it is LYC, PULS, PYR or ARN. These medicines help him along, and they have often to be changed, but finally the breakdown occurs, and these medicines are no longer suitable. An awful dyspnoea gradually creeps on the patient; there is craving for air; the breathing space is becoming diminished. Dropsy comes on in the extremities. The heart gives out; there is emaciation; the hippocratic countenance is seen; there is cold sweat, blue face, sinking. Even now we can palliate with TARENT-C. Sometimes it has to be repeated. It will relieve for days and give a euthanasia, not a stupefaction as produced by morphine, benumbing the senses, but an actual comforting. ***889***

TARENTULA HISPANICA

STAPH — Crawling etc. in the female external genitals, COFF, PLAT, PETROL, APIS, TARENT HISP, the latter has: While outer parts feel as if insects were biting and crawling, better from heat or cold. ***947***

THUJA

SIL has also cured fistulous openings. Patients who have a tendency to phthisis are subject to abscesses about the region of the rectum that break inside or out and form complete or incomplete openings. These seem to take the place of what would otherwise come, and if healed by operation or other external means, the tendency is to end in chest trouble, either in the form of a fixed catarrh or tubercular infiltrations. SIL is one of the remedies that turns the constitution into order and in one to five years the opening ceases to be necessary and it will heal. Surgeons heal it up at once and for a time the patient is comfortable, but in a few years he breaks down. CAUST, BERB, CALC, CALC PHOS, GRAPH, SULPH etc. are suitable in such cases. SIL here follows THUJ well. ***932***

SIL — Complementary to CALC, PULS, THUJA. ***935***

SQUIL in its internal nature is quite like THUJA in regard to its spurting urine and its spasmodic cough. ***941***

CINNB is closely related to THUJA.. ***745***

NAT-S— In chronic gonorrhoea, with greenish or yellowish-green discharge. Instead of gonorrhoea running off into a white, gleety discharge, it keeps up a yellowish, thick, greenish discharge. It competes here with THUJA and MERC, both of which are antisycotics. ***793***

The dreadful EFFECTS OF VACCINATION are often cured by SULPH. In this it competes with THUJA and MALANDRINUM. ***960***

Oysters seem to poison the LYC patient, just as onions are a poison to the THUJA patient. The OXALIC ACID patient cannot eat strawberries. ***704***

CHIN-ARS — Overconscientious about trifles (SIL, THUJA). ***428***

AGN — There is a growing weakness of the rectum and constipation, and he presses hard at stool, which often fails and slips back, like SIL, SANIC and THUJA. *49*

ALUM is a suitable remedy again when the woman has a gonorrhoea which has been prolonged by palliation. She has been made comfortable by partly suitable remedies, but it seems that no remedy has been quite deep enough to root out the trouble, for it keeps coming back. In a discharge that keeps returning, better for a little while on PULS and on this and that and the other thing and even on THUJA, given more especially because it is gonorrhoea than because she is a sick woman. The patient is tired and worn out, and when you come to look at the whole patient and you see the paretic condition, the continued return of the discharge that has been palliated by remedies, think of ALUM both in the male and in the female. *75*

PSOR is indicated (in old gleet) above all others if there is an unusually offensive state of the genitals. THUJ if the odor is of a nauseating, sweet character; warts exposed by rolling back the foreskin; sweet odor in spite of washing. *856*

STAPH — Dry, sensitive warts about the genitals from sycosis or from the abuse of mercury, which causes a tendency to warty growths. Moist, red, offensive warts belong to THUJA. *947*

When the case is of sycotic origin, small or large gelatinous polypi form in the larynx and they are sore, causing loss of voice or cracked voice, when they cause choking or uneasiness, HEPAR is one of the remedies. HEPAR, CALC, ARG NIT and NIT AC and sometimes THUJA are the remedies related to such conditions.. .... *575*

NAT MUR — In old lingering cases where the skin looks transparent as if the patient would become dropsical, a waxy, greasy, shiny skin; other remedies with greasy, shiny skin are PLUMB, THUJA, SELEN. These remedies go deep into the life. Any remedy that can produce such wonderful changes is long acting. *772*

CINNB — Fig warts (THUJA). *744*

SABINA has all the wart-like excrescences found in THUJA and found in sycosis. The THUJA wart is a little sensitive wart, appears to be covered with a thin film and bleeds from the slightest touch. SABINA cures warty excrescences about the anus, cauliflower excrescences, gonorrhoeal warts about the vulva and about the male genitals. *898*

STAPH — Meibomian tumours (CON, THUJA), in irritable children (KREOS). *946*

Slight of inflammation or irritation of the lower part of the [spinal] cord; it feels lacerated and sore, and aches and never passes over until the results of the injury right in the spot have been removed. Such injuries, if taken early, can be cured by HYPERICUM. It is in the remedy. These injuries have been cured in after years by CARBO AN, SIL and THUJA, and other remedies as indicated. *591*

TUBERCULINUM

When well selected remedies act only a short time, and the symptoms agree, CALC SULPH is one that should be thought of along with SULPH, PSORINUM and TUBERCULINUM. *348*

GUAIACUM, is closely related to CAUSTICUM, SULPHUR and TUBERCULINUM. *562*

I remember starting out to prove TUB on an

individual I suspected would be sensitive to it from his history and symptoms. The first dose almost killed him, and, considering the use that that substance is put to in diagnosing the disease in cattle, it seemed to stir him up. He became emaciated and looked as if he would die. I let it alone and watched and waited patiently and the symptoms of AGAR came up and established the relationship between these two remedies, and confirmed Hering's observation of the relationship of AGAR to the tubercular diathesis. AGAR cured him and fattened him up. *47*

KALI SULPH — PREDISPOSITION TO PHTHISIS. It is frequently indicated after TUB. *661*

Losing flesh and craving for meat in those who are tubercular, or in those that are from tubercular parents. Patients suffering from dry cough. There are persons who have simply this tendency who go along year after year in this withered state, with the little hacking cough, not rousing up into much. Finally some favourable circumstance arises and the tuberculosis comes on rapidly after it has remained in a sluggish state for a long time. There are a few remedies more likely to be associated with that condition than any others - ARS, CALC, LYC, MAG CARB and TUB. They fit into this lingering state, this prelude to active phthisis. They sometimes set a patient thriving, but mind you, these cases are hard cases to manage. They are difficult to find remedies for. Their trouble is so latent, the symptoms do not come out and sometimes you will have to read between the lines. They are the one-sided cases spoken of by Hahnemann. 716

BAR-C — Knots of lymphatic glands down the neck under the ear (BAR-M, TUB). 225

APOC — "Hydrocephalus, with great stupor." That is the last stage of it where there is great prostration, loss of flesh, stiffness of all the limbs, with dropsical swellings. Many times in hydrocephalus pains shoot along the nerves and attack the joints. Then it is that such remedies as APIS and CALC and APOC take hold with wonderful depth. The first permanent and substantial indication that the remedy is working in a hydrocephaloid case is that it increases the flow of urine, which has been scanty all the time. For hydrocephalus study TUB. *125*

VALERIAN

MOSCH cures many hysterical girls who have come to adult age without ever learning what obedience means. They are self-willed, obstinate and selfish. When they have been encouraged to resort to crafty cunning, to have every whim gratified from infancy to eighteen years of age they become fit subjects for MOSCH, ASAF, IGN and VALER. *750*

VERATRUM ALBUM

CAMPH — The air as it leaves the chest feels like that from a cellar, like CARBO VEG and VERAT. *356*

SPONG — Dry, spasmodic cough, troublesome cough; cold things taken into the stomach aggravate. (VERAT is better from cold water, but the cough is aggravated.) *940*

SABAD — Head covered with cold sweat. Many of the symptoms are closely related to VERAT, especially in the cold sweat on the forehead with complaints. *894*

ARN follows well after ACON and is complementary to ACON, IPECAC and VERATRUM. *148*

AMM-C — Sometimes it is an exhaustion with vomiting, exhaustion as in VERAT, with coldness, blueness, sinking, dyspnoea. *98*

Those cases going on for a while as melancholic, low spirited; she believes she has sinned away her day of grace, yet she has lived an upright life; sad; imagines strange things, does strange things, until finally violent delirium comes on; she screams aloud; exhorts people to repent; face red and eyes flashing; exhorts and prays in incoherent speech. In such cases STRAM should be compared with VERAT. *950*

VERATRUM VIRIDE

AIL — The congested condition of the skin is present even when there is no rash, a passive congestion of the veins. Quite a number of medicines have that, but VERAT V produces such a vasomotor paralysis that a line upon the skin made by pressure will remain a long time. *51*

VESPA VULGARIS

PODO — Great soreness of the abdomen before and during the menstrual period (APIS, CIMIC, VESPA, LACH, but these are not so likely to have diarrhoea and, if so, it is not as copious). 849

WYETHIA

A peculiar kind of itching coming on in some hay fevers is an itching in the roof of the mouth, on the soft palate, and for relief the patient must draw the tongue back and forth over the soft palate with this coryza, sneezing etc. WYETHIA will cut this attack short. When the itching extends to the larynx and trachea with great irritability and sensitive to cold NUX VOM. *894*

ZINC

In many medicines reaction (to medicine) is slowed down, but in BELL it is intensified. So it is in NUX VOMICA and ZINCUM. *239*

Running through CADMIUM SULPH we find it is spasmodic and nervous - it affects muscles like ZINC. It is found in its crude state associated with ZINC. *304*

ABROT — The diarrhoea is his great relief like NAT-S and ZINC. *18*

LAC-C — Severe pain in the region of the right ovary ameliorated by the flow of bright red blood is again somewhat like LACH. These pains take alternate sides. ZINC also has pain in the ovaries ameliorated by the flow; she never feels well except when menstruating, hysterical at all other times but well at the menstrual period is ZINC. *677*

When the desire is so violent that it drives her to secret vice the remedies are GELS, GRATIOLA, ORIGANUM, NUX VOMICA, PHOS, PLATINA and ZINC. *561*

In AGAR and ZINC the spine is affected and both of these have aggravation from stimulants. *45*

ALUM is a spinal remedy and aggravation from spirituous drinks is in keeping with some other spinal remedies. You can find it in ZINC. The ZINC patient cannot drink wine, for all of his complaints are aggravated by it. *73*

Sometimes the scarlet fever patient will go into convulsions because the rash fails to come out. APIS is sometimes a suitable remedy and must be compared with BRY, CUPRUM and ZINC. *120*